Pharmacognosy and Phytochemistry

(Vol. I)

Pharmacognosy and Phytochemistry
(Vol. I)

Dr Hemalatha K
Assistant Professor
Acharya & BM Reddy College of Pharmacy
Soladevanahalli
Bengaluru, Karnataka
India

Dr Pulak Majumder
Associate Professor
Sri Adichunchanagiri College of Pharmacy
BG Nagar, Karnataka
India

TECHSAR™
NEW DELHI

Published and Printed by
Techsar Pvt. Ltd.
4435-36/7, Ansari Road, Daryaganj
New Delhi-110 002 (India)
E-mail: tech_info@techsarworld.com
Website: www.techsarworld.com

ISBN: 978-81-95966-27-1

Reprint 2025

Preface

Pharmacognosy is the scientific study of substances derived from terrestrial, marine, and microbial sources, and has just lately expanded to include phytotherapy and nutraceuticals. As a result, public interest in pharmacognosy is anticipated to grow in the future as the biochemical function of phytomedicines, nutraceuticals, and natural pharmaceuticals in general becomes more thoroughly understood.

Pharmacognosy and Phytochemistry (Vol-I) is the outcome of the authors' tireless efforts to incorporate the extensive collection of traditional and current informations, which has long been a prerequisite of the curriculum in Pharmacy. The field of pharmacognosy has consistently benefited from the wealth of knowledge available on a variety of natural drug-related topics, such as their history, alternative medical systems, categorization, identification, cultivation, collection, manufacture and adulteration of medicines of natural origin, etc. This book is intended to provide a significant contribution to the field of pharmacognosy in the light of all this thorough information on the subject. The inclusion of commercial versions of the pharmaceuticals is one of the book's unique features.

The book is formatted with five units separated into 12 sections. Every chapter provides academics with a reasonable grounding on the subject. Unit one deals with the introduction of pharmacognosy with its history, scope, source and qualitative analysis. Unit two describes the cultivation, collection, processing and storage of drugs of natural origin along with plant genetics. In unit three, information focused on plant tissue culture and edible vaccines. Unit four, describes pharmacognosy in various systems of medicine traditional medicine and secondary metabolites. Plant products, marine medicinal plants, natural allergens, hallucinogenic and teratogens are included in unit five.

By carefully assembling the well-written chapters with tidy, well-labelled illustrations, the writers are able to completely apprehend their goal. Graduate students in pharmaceutical sciences, as well as undergraduate and professional doctoral pharmacy students, may confidently recommend this book. Furthermore, anyone with a scientific interest in herbal medicine and complementary and alternative medicine will find the information beneficial. The educators of aspiring pharmacists and other healthcare professionals will especially warmly embrace this volume.

The authors express their sincere obligation to Almighty, parents and spouses for inspiring them to write a book that is urgently needed by various arena of students all in one location. The authors will constantly look for comments and suggestions to raise the book's overall quality.

Authors

Contents

UNIT I

Introduction to Pharmacognosy

Objectives

- To understand the basic concept of Pharmacognosy, and its origin, history and scope.
- Explains the botanical knowledge to classify drugs of various sources.
- To know the methods of crude drug evaluation and adulteration.
- Describes the quantitative microscopy of crude drugs.

1.1 INTRODUCTION

The resilient relationship between plants and humans was genuinely established over the time. Humans relied on Mother Nature for every aspect of life especially food and medicine. Exploration of herbs for medication in human ailments began since time immemorial. Plants are used as remedy to maintain health–physically, mentally, spiritually and also in specific clinical conditions. There is no clear time indication which can provide lime light on the beginning of utilization of plants by humans for medicinal purposes but archaeological evidence suggests that it might be during the Paleolithic age, with the first written evidence dating back to the Sumerians.

The botanicals or natural drugs are plant derived products, consumed by humans since centuries. They are composed of naturally occurring substances which have constituents with health enhancing or medicinal activities.

Worldwide various ethnic populations developed their own tactics for plant utilization throughout their cultures, customs, religious rites, food habits and medicinal practices. As an example, the countries like Africa, Asia and Latin Americans utilize traditional medicine to encounter their primary healthcare needs because of the remote access to conventional clinical treatment. They use herbals or botanicals at home as first line treatment in high fever which may result from malaria in children population. The complete relationship between man and vegetation is called 'Ethnobotany'.

The growing popularity of herbal medicines since last few decades led this market in greater heights. Currently, the global market for herbal medicines stands at over US $80 billion annually and is growing steadily upwards.

The humans received an immense contribution from plant kingdom towards health when there was no other source of medicine like synthetic medicine or any such concept like surgery. Various plant species contain numerous bioactive components like alkaloids, phenols, tannins, cryogenics, glycocides, terpeniods, etc., which all possess various effective roles in human body like anti-infections, anti-bacterial, etc. For instance, alkaloids and antihistamine derived from the bark of *Alstonia boonei* are useful in the treatment of human ailments such as fever, dizziness and high blood pressure. Even the most renowned herbals, such as ginger (*Allium sativum*) and garlic (*Zingiber officinale*) are spicy additions in regular food provisions that also have long been used to maintain human health since long. Some of the plants are described below for their investigations in older times.

Table 1.1 Examples of plants for investigation in olden times

Herb	Drug / chemical	Basic investigation
Digitals (*Digitalis* sp.)	Digoxin	Europeans started to utilize the leaves of this plant in heart therapy during the eighteenth century.
Ipecac (*Cephaelis* sp.)	Emetine	Brazilian Indians and others South American tribes used roots and rhizomes of this plant to cure dysentery and induce vomiting to the patients.
Opium (*Papaver somniferum*)	Codeine, morphine	Ancient Sumerians, Egyptians and Greeks used opium latex for the treatment of headaches, arthritis and inducing sedation.
Ephedra (*Ephedra* sp.)	Ephedrine	Crude drug has been used by Chinese for respiratory ailments since 2700 BC.
Cinchona (*Cinchona* sp.)	Quinine	Peruvian Indians used *Cinchona* for the treatment of fevers.
Colchicum (*Colchicum* sp.)	Colchicine	The use of Colchicum has been used in Europe since 78 AD for the treatment of gout.

World Health Organisation (WHO) has constituted 252 essential drugs list as basic and essential medication therapy where 11% of drugs out of the list are exclusively of plant origin and a significant number are synthetic drugs obtained from natural precursors. Some remarkable drugs in this area obtained from plants include digoxin from *Digitalis* spp., quinine and quinidine from *Cinchona* spp., vincristrine and vinblastine from *Catharanthus roseus*, atropine from *Atropa belladonna* and morphine and codeine from *Papaver somniferum,* etc. Even more, about 60% of anti-tumour and anti-infectious drugs from natural origin are already on the market or under clinical trials. In management of type-2 diabetes across the world, more than 400 traditional plants or plant derived products are on action yet more. Galegine, a phyto-bioactive substance produced by the herb *Galega officinalis*, provided the pharmacological and chemical basis for the discovery of metformin which is the foundation therapy for type-2 diabetes. Several anticancer agents including vincristine, taxol, vinblastine, derivatives, irinotecan and topotecan and etoposide derived from epipodophyllotoxin are in clinical use worldwide.

There is an appropriate coexistence of medicinal system and social development in ancient times. The development of allopathic system of medicine, which is also known as modern system of medicine also gradually developed over time on the basis of efforts made by people over the method of scientific and observational even though, the base is still laid on depth of traditional medicinal knowledge and its therapeutic applications. This continuous interest towards exploration of medicinal plants by human beings has brought about today's modern and sophisticated stage of herbalism. The multidimensional tactic uniting of botanical, phytochemical, biological and molecular techniques are the modern keys for discovery of new drugs by exploiting natural sources. In last few decades, a clear shift has been observed in world population from herbal to modern synthetic medicine due to its comparably prompt action in human body and easy accessibility. As a result, people become more vulnerable to various clinical ailments, deterioration and degenerations.

The revitalization of herbal components and their use has been evolving throughout the world. Medicinal plants are now in a 'come-back' phase with the last two decades where people slowly shifted their focus back to the natural remedies. Technological and methodological advances have made the discovery, validation and manufacture of high-value phytochemicals a reality and botanical therapeutics have come of age.

1.2 BACKGROUND

Origin of Pharmacognosy

The word **'pharmacognosy'** derives from the Greek word **Pharmakon**, 'a drug' and **gignosco**, 'to acquire knowledge' is probably the oldest modern science, and generally the study of crude drugs of plant and animal origin (in the form of tinctures, teas, poultices, powders, and other herbal formulations), and it incorporates authentication and quality control of such drugs, based on macroscopic and microscopic examinations of crude drugs.

The term pharmacognosy was first introduced by the Austrian physician Schmidt in 1811 and then in 1815 by Seydler in a work titled *Analecta Pharmacognostica*. Like any other scientific area, since the introduction of Pharmacognosy some 200 years ago, it has evolved over the years.

'Pharmacognosy' represents the oldest branch of the pharmacy profession and one among the five major divisions in pharmaceutical curriculum. The ancients gathered herbs, animals, plants, and minerals and concocted them into ill-flavoured pungent mixtures. Such substances extend beyond the category of crude drugs and their derivatives include a variety of commercial products: allergens, allergenic extracts, antibiotics, immunizing biological, flavouring agents, condiments, beverages, insecticides, rodenticides, and herbicides. In a restricted sense, Pharmacognosy implies a particular knowledge of methods of identification and evaluation of drugs.

Definitions

The discipline of Pharmacognosy has evolved in definition over the years. While the fundamental connectedness among all definitions includes an understanding of drug entities, the combined descriptive variations from subtle to distinctive need highlighting. In the 1800s, Pharmacognosy was defined as "the simultaneous application of various scientific disciplines with the object of acquiring knowledge of drugs from every point of view". By timely modifications over the time the modern pharmacognosy definition has been evolved.

Pharmacognosy is defined as the *science of biogenic or naturally derived drugs, pharmaceuticals, and poisons, and it incorporates various modern analytical techniques to authenticate and quality control of crude drugs as well as purified active extracts, fractions, and components, and even medicinal foods.*

Pharmacognosy is linked with many other areas of science and a complete understanding of this field has to be taken into account, but not be limited to botany, chemistry, enzymology, genetics, pharmacology, toxicology, horticulture, quality control, and biotechnology. The areas of science which embrace Pharmacognosy, as well as ancillary fields, are pharmaceutics, pharmcoeconomics, pharmacovigilance, regulatory law, and conservation.

1.3 ADVANCES IN PHARMACOGNOSY

Drug use from medicinal plants has advanced from the formulation of crude drugs to the isolation, identification, and assessment of bioactivity of active compounds in drug discovery. Modern Pharmacognosy involves the broad study of natural products from various sources including plants, bacteria, fungi, and marine organisms.

Pharmacognosy has always been a translational or multidisciplinary science, and during the evolution of the scope of this subject area, phytochemistry and phytochemical analysis have become integral parts of Pharmacognosy. Molecular biology has become essential to medicinal plant drug discovery through the determination and implementation of appropriate screening assays directed towards physiologically relevant molecular targets, and modern Pharmacognosy also encapsulates all these relevant new areas into a distinct interdisciplinary science.

The emphasis and focus of research in Pharmacognosy have changed significantly, from focusing on identification of drugs, including the isolation of active principles, and more recently, the investigation of biological activity. Research in ethnobotany, ethnomedicine, and ethnopharmacology has also become an important element in Pharmacognosy.

Pharmacognosy has played a pivotal role in the discovery and development of new drugs and therapies, and has been continuing to do so even today. It also formed the basis of the development of the subject "Pharmacy". However, it is rather unfortunate that Pharmacognosy is somewhat neglected nowadays as a major subject area within the modern Pharmacy curricula, especially in the West.

For the sake of new hypes of modern medicine, one should not forget the usefulness traditional medicines based on plants. It has never been more important for any modern pharmacist to have proper knowledge about traditional medicines. One of the best examples of the usefulness of not neglecting indigenous herbal remedies is *Artemisia annua* (common name: qinghaosu), which has long been used in China for the treatment of intermittent fever or malaria. Extracts from this plant were studied in the West from the 1980s onward, resulting in the development of a new class of effective anti-malarials, the artemisinins.

1.4 DEVELOPMENT OF THE SCIENCE OF PHARMACOGNOSY

General History

The history of Pharmacognosy is as old as human existence. Therefore, it is very hard for any Pharmacognosist to identify the tangible origin of this science. The word 'drug' derives from

Latin term *'Droog' which* means 'dried', when dried plants were commonly used as medicine. Broadly, history of pharmacognosy can be classified into three major stages.

First stage before eighteenth century, very few documents and recorded evidences are available showing use of natural products by humans.

Second stage involves nineteenth century, which is the time when basic subject evolved. In this century, the name pharmacognosy came into practice. Initially, the subject was more likely descriptive botany of medicinal plants. But as the time progressed, it changed the course and encompassed extraction, isolation and other advanced techniques.

In twentieth century, which may be regarded as the third stage of development, series of discoveries resulted in complete metamorphosis of the subject.

From last few decades, Pharmacognosy is studied in more systematic manner. As herbal wave continues to sweep the world, importance of natural products is at the pinnacle. People are expecting natural products to fit in modern framework. As a result of this there is a series of new herbal formulations in the market.

Pharmacognosy in Ancient Times (Before the Nineteenth Century)

The ancient Egyptians documented their knowledge about medicine on paper made from *Cyperus aquaticus* commonly called acquatic sage or papyrus. *Papyrus Ebers* (around 1500 BC), *Berlin Papyrus, Edwin Smith Paprus, Kahun Medicak Papyrus* are some of the oldest handbooks which contain information of illness and treatments. In ancient Egypt and Mesopotamia clay tablets were used to document knowledge of drugs which date back to 3000 BC. Chinese pharmacopoeia, the Pen Tsao, attributed to the legendary Emperor Shen Nung (written between 3000 and 2730 BC), appears to be the oldest pharmacopoeia on the earth. This treatise includes recipes and therapeutic uses of many Chinese traditional medicines. Ancient India, information about drugs was documented in several Ayurvedic texts which still exists. Apart from *Atharvaveda* there are several books like *Charak Samhita, Sushrut Samhita, Astang Hridaya, Madhav Nidan* and *Bhava Prakash* were written on plants for their use in various clinical conditions.

In *papyrus*, crocus, dried ox-bile juice, castor oil, and so on were well mentioned for their utilization. In about 77 AD, Dioscorides, a Greek doctor, kept a record of about 600 kinds of crude drugs in his, *De Materia Medica*, a book that had played an important role in pharmacology and botany by the fifteenth century.

The *Historia*, written by Pliny (23-79 AD), gave a brief account of nearly 1000 species of plants, most of which could be used as medicines. Wild herbs were used to treat illnesses in the Soviet Union before the eleventh century.

Galen (131-200 BC) a Greek pharmacist worked on extraction of chemical constituent from the plants. He developed various methods of extraction therefore the branch of pharmacy which deals with extraction of chemical constituents from plants and animals is called galenical pharmacy.

Hippocrates (460-360 BC) a Greek scientist worked on human anatomy and physiology, particularly on circulatory system and nervous system. He prepared the famous oath for physicians, which is still taken by the physicians. He is known as father of medicine.

In eighteenth century, Pharmacognosy was much closely related to botany. In old days, drugs from natural origin were used in crude form as powder or decoction.

Pharmacognosy in Early Modern Times (1815-1930)

It was at the beginning of the nineteenth century that pharmacognosy came into its real being. In 1815, C.A. Seydler, a German who used the word "pharmakognosie" in his book, *Analecta Pharmacognostica*, was referred to as the father of pharmacognosy. 'Pharmakognosie' etymologically means knowledge about crude drugs. In 1825, Martius, a German scholar, set up "pharmakognosie" as a subject to study in college, and then a new discipline named 'Pharmakognosie' emerged. According to Martius, Pharmacognosy, as a part of merchandizing, was a study to research drug base taken from nature to test its purity and to check impurities or adulterants. From then on, German scholars published works, named pharmakognosie, on plant and animal drugs successively. In 1880, Gendō Oi, a Japanese scholar, translated 'Pharmakognosie' as 'Pharmacognosy'. Japanese early study of pharmacy was based on quoting and researching Chinese herbs.

In 1806, Serturner, a German, clarified the cell to be the basic unit of plant structure, and then microscopes were used to research the internal structure of crude drugs. In 1857, Schleiden published a book,*Grundriss der Pharmakognosie des Pflanzenreiches* (foundation of pharmacognosy of plants), in which he gave a detailed description of microstructure of a great many plant crude drugs. Later, Berg in 1865 and Vogl in 1887 published anatomical atlas of crude drugs successively, which furthered the development of identifying crude drugs by the use of microscopes, and then this method became the most important one to identify crude drugs.

Meanwhile, the qualitative and quantitative methods of chemistry were used in crude drug identification. Fluorescence analysis and chromatography were used in sequence in the later half of the nineteenth century and in the beginning of the twentieth century, both of which enriched the research field of pharmacognosy and promoted a greater development than the early methods of identifying crude drugs by shape and smell.

Pharmacognosy in Modern Times (1930 to the Late 1990s)

Since the 1930s, development of biology and chemistry enriched methods and ways of studying pharmacognosy. The development of the bioassay of intensity of drug action (biological potency) advanced the study of active ingredients of crude drugs and strengthened their quality evaluation. Chemical and physical methods, such as colorimetry, spectrophotometry, and fluorescence analysis, were applied to identify crude drugs . When Pharmacognosy developed on lines of morphology and chemistry, many new disciplines emerged.

For example, with accumulation of chemical composition of plants in type and number, a new sub-discipline, plant chemotaxonomy, came into being through exploration of chemical composition of plants and their genetic relationship. The new discipline not only had taxonomical significance but also pushed for new sources of crude medicines.

Later in the nineteenth century, development in science expanded the arena of pharmacognosy. Modern pharmacognosy has become a kind of multidisciplinary subject which embraces phytochemistry, analytical pharmacognosy, pharmacotherapy, medicinal plant biotechnology, herbal formulations and nutraceuticals. Zoopharmacognosy is branch of pharmacognosy which involves observation of animal behaviour for discovery and development of new drugs. Nowadays drugs from natural origin are studied, formulated and regulated in the framework of modern medicine.

From ancient times to the middle of the nineteenth century, pharmacology had been in its traditional stage for all countries in the world. At that time, knowledge about medicines came mainly from senses and practical experience, and the major contents for any medicinal book were mostly about medical effectiveness and partly about its name, origin, morphology, and identifying sensory characteristics. Due to underdeveloped science, people could hardly know all the details about medicines.

Therefore, the problem of identifying the authenticity and quality of crude drugs arose. With advancement in bioscience and widespread application of microscope, pharmacognosy made great progress in the middle of the nineteenth century and finally became an independent subject. The early work of pharmacognosy was establishing quality standards for crude drugs in business.

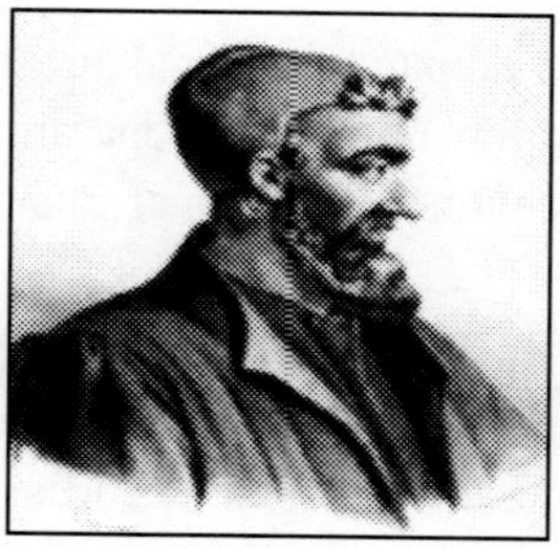

Fig. 1.1 Galen

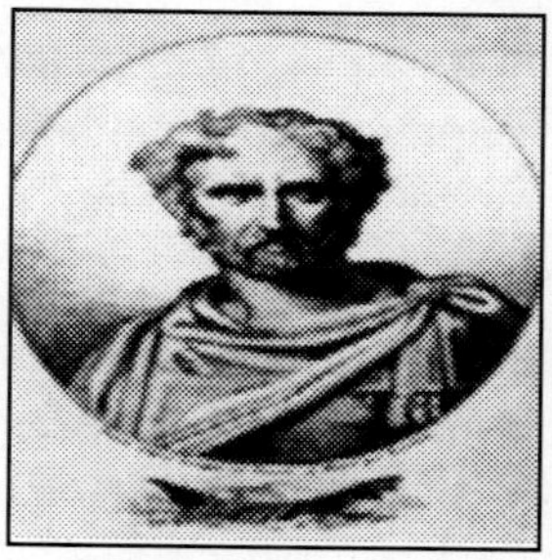

Fig. 1.2 Pliny

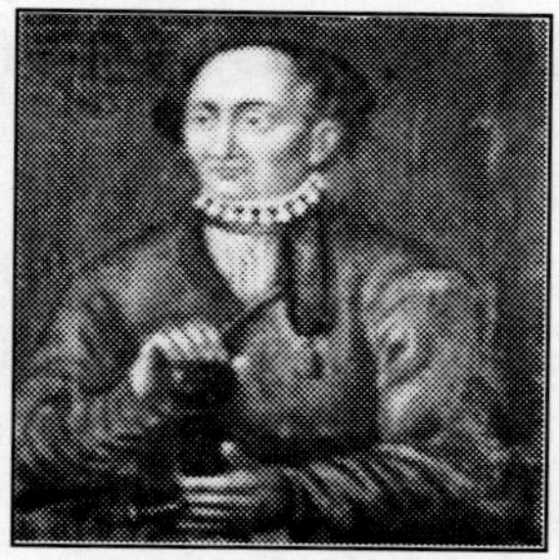

Fig. 1.3 Theophrastus

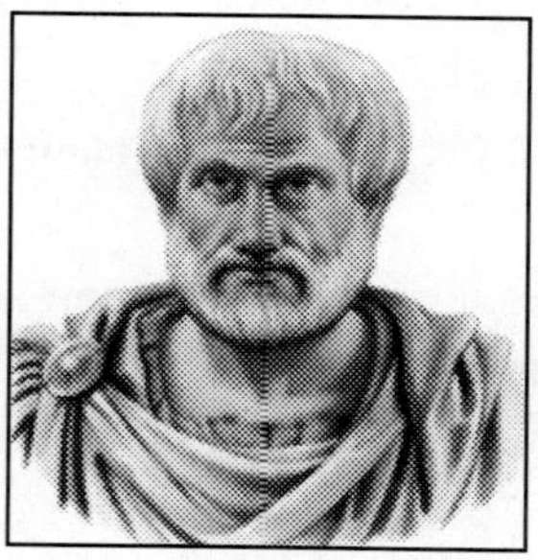

Fig. 1.4 Aristotle

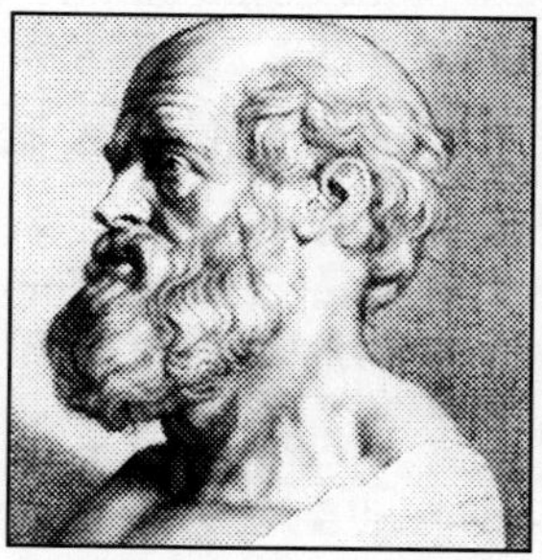

Fig. 1.5 Hippocrates

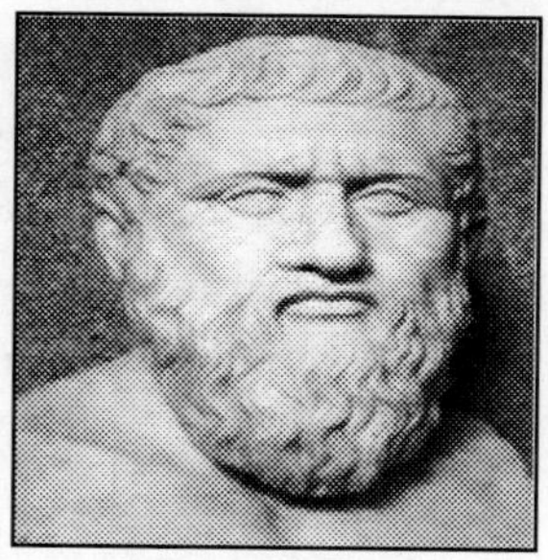

Fig. 1.6 Plato

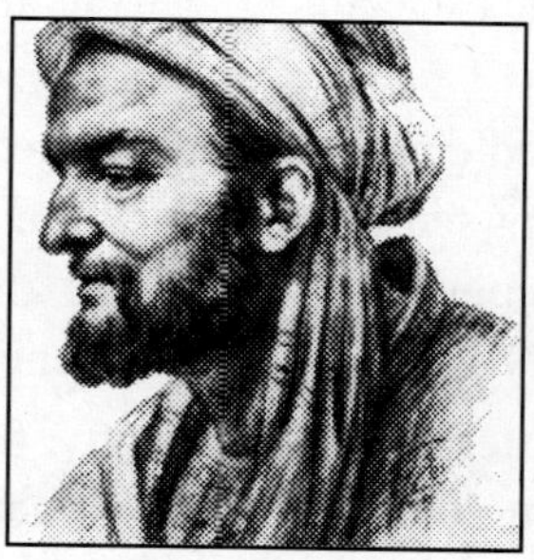

Fig. 1.7 Ibn Sina

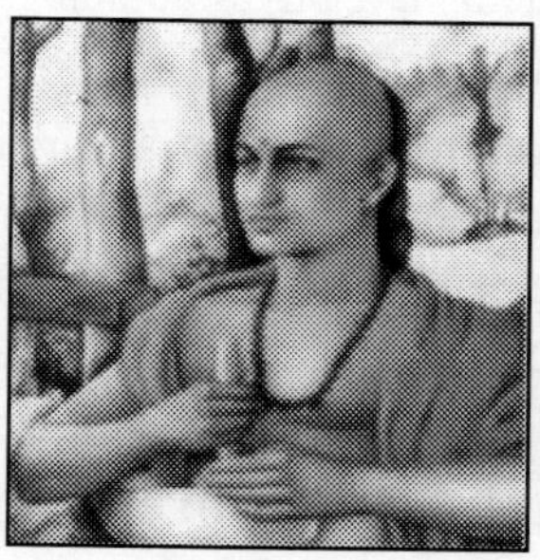

Fig. 1.8 Charaka

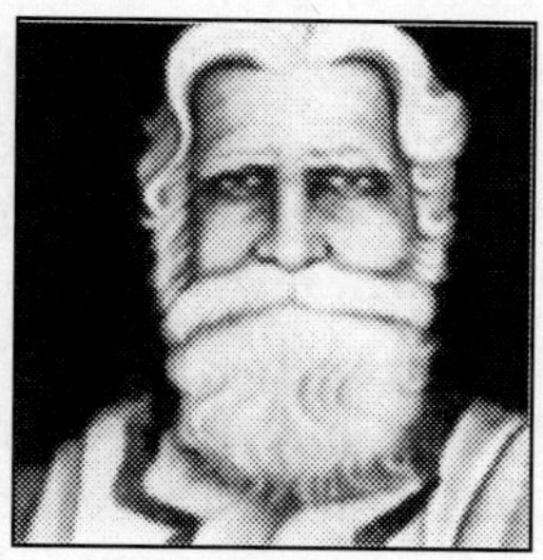

Fig. 1.9 Sushruta

The development of modern pharmacognosy took place by simultaneous advancements in the areas of organic chemistry, biochemistry, biosynthesis and modern methods and techniques of analysis like paper chromatography, thin layer chromatography, gas chromatography, and high performance liquid chromatography.

Through high performance thin layer chromatography (HPTLC), column chromatography and other techniques, namely, UV spectroscopy, NMR spectroscopy, IR spectroscopy a large number of active constituents isolated from different plants were found to possess various pharmacological activities.

1.5 SCOPE OF PHARMACOGNOSY

It generally indicates the area of activity, predetermined and limitations, but somewhat flexible range of understanding, thought or action.

- Pharmacognosy has broad scope in the field of Pharmacy such as preparation of galenicals, analysis of phytoconstituents, herbal preparation, synthesis of steroidal hormone, preparation of antibiotics, perfumes, flavouring agents, cultivation and collection of medicinal plants, tissue culture and isolation of phytoconstituents.
- Phytochemistry has undergone significant development in recent years. The technology involving extraction, purification and characterization of pharmaceuticals from natural sources is a significant contribution to the advancement of natural and physical sciences.
- The knowledge of chemotaxonomy, biogenetic pathways for formation of medicinally active primary and secondary metabolites, plant tissue culture and other related fields is essential part of implementation from pharmacognosy.
- Drug discovery from natural products/medicinal plants, herbal therapy, phytotherapy, natural medicines, and phytopharmaceuticals.
- Current research in drug discovery from medicinal plants involves a multifaceted approach combining botanical, computational, phytochemical, biological, and molecular techniques. It is evident that drug discovery from medicinal plants continues to provide new and important leads against various pharmacological targets.
- Pharmacognosy has always been a field of multidisciplinary science, and during the expansion of the orbit of this area, phytochemistry, phytomedicine, and phytochemical analysis have become important parts of this field.
- Molecular biology has become an extremely important area for medicinal plant drug discovery analysis through the determination and application of convenient screening assays directed physiologically related molecular targets, and modern pharmacognosy encapsulates all of these relevant new research areas into a distinct interdisciplinary natural product science.
- The insistence and focus of research in pharmacognosy have alternated significantly, from focusing on isolation and structure elucidation of drugs, including the information of active constituents, along with their biological activity as well as structure activity relationship (SAR) studies.

- Advanced researches in the field of ethnobiomedicine, ethnobotany, and ethnopharma-cology has also become an essential element in the orbit of pharmacognosy.
- Pharmacognosy deals has important association with medicinal chemistry, pharmacological studies and formulations (pharmaceutics).
- Fast development of advanced phytochemistry and pharmacological testing ways and methods, new plant derived drugs are finding their way into medicine as single phytochemical, rather than in the mixture form of traditional herbal preparations.
- Different sub-branches of pharmacognosy, such as analytical, industrial, and clinical, have been established as a modern and professional offshoots of specialized pharmacognosy to meet the most productive advancements and collaborations in this field.
- Furthermore, molecular, metabolomic, and genomic pharmacognosy have been introduced as the new and promising targets of research for accommodating future supply and demands in biomedicine, molecular biology, biotechnology, and analytical chemistry of traditional natural medicines and folk medicinal plants.

1.6 FUTURE OF PHARMACOGNOSY

Medicinal plants are of great value in the field of treatment and cure of diseases. Over the years, scientific research has expanded our knowledge of the chemical effects and composition of the active constituents, which determine the medicinal properties of the plants. It has now been universally accepted that the plant drugs and remedies are far safer than that of synthetic medicines for curing the complex diseases like cancer and AIDS. Enormous number of alkaloids, glycosides and antibiotics have been isolated, identified and used as curative agents. The modern developments in the instrumental techniques of analysis and chromatographical methodologies have added numerous complex and rare natural products to the armoury of phytomedicine. To mention a few, artemissinin as antimalarial, taxol as anticancer, forskolin as antihypertensive, rutin as vitamin, P and capillary permeability factor and piperine as bioavailability enhancer are the recent developments. Natural products have also been used as drug substitutes for the semisynthesis of many potent drugs. Ergotamine for dihydroergotamine in the treatment of migraine, podophyllotoxin for etoposide, a potent antineoplastic drug or solasodine and diosgenin that serve for the synthetic steroidal hormones are the first-line examples of the recent days.

Little more needs to be said about the present-day importance of medicinal plants, for it will be apparent from the foregoing that the plant themselves either in the form of crude drugs or even more important, for the medicinally active materials isolated from them, have been, are and always will be an important aid to the physicians in the treatment of disease.

1.7 DEFINITION OF TERMS

The following are some essential terms belonging to the discipline of pharmacognosy which are widely used.

Chromatography

This is a laboratory method used for separating mixtures of chemical compounds based on the principle of adsorption. Different bonding properties of the molecules to be separated are very important for achieving good separation which is usually achieved when the relative amounts of each solute are distributed between a moving stream known as the mobile phase and a contiguous stationary phase. The mobile phase can be a liquid or a gas, while the stationary phase is either a solid or a liquid. Chromatography is used in quantitative and qualitative analysis of biological and chemical substances and is particularly useful in the separation of isomers and natural materials.

Although chromatography is mainly associated with purification, it also has wider applications for the identification of compounds based on their chromatographic behaviour.

Crude Drugs

Any product that has not been advanced in value or improved in condition by grinding, chipping, crushing, distilling, evaporating, extracting, artificial mixing with other process or treatment beyond what is essential to its proper packing and the prevention of decay or deterioration pending manufacture.

Crude drugs can be classified into two groups: organized and unorganized (details given in the last part of this topic).

Ethnobotany

This is the study of the relationships between plants and the people in the field. It includes the use of plants for furniture, shelter, transportation, as well studying the use of plants in medicine, alternative methods of healing, wild food, agricultural crops, and in religious ceremonies.

Ethnopharmacology

This is the scientific study correlating ethnic groups with their health and how it relates to their physical habitats, and their methodologies in creating and using plant based medicines.

Extraction

This is a way of separating the desired substance(s) from a mixture using a suitable solvent in which the desired substance is soluble. In other words, extraction techniques are used to separate compounds based upon their different solubility in two immiscible solvents. This is a laboratory procedure commonly used when isolating or purifying natural products.

Herbs

This term is more appropriately applied when referring to culinary plants and refers to crude materials, which may be obtained from lichens, algae, fungi, or higher plants such as leaves, flowers, fruits, seeds, stem, back, roots, rhizomes, or other parts which may be entire, fragmented, or powdered.

Medicinal Plants

These are either wild or cultivated plants used for the management and treatment of ailments, example: *Mentha piperita.*

Metabolomics

This is the systematic study of chemical processes that involve metabolites that represent unique fingerprints left behind producing somewhat of a metabolite profile.

Natural Products

A generic term which can be an entire organism (plant, animal, microorganism, etc.), part of an organism (leaf, flower, isolated glands, etc.), an extract, an exudate, a partially fractionated preparation, or isolated pure compounds.

Phytotherapy

It is a part of pharmacognosy that is concerned with the clinical use of crude drug extracts or partially purified mixtures from plants. It can also be referred to as the area dealing with the scientific studies of the bioactivities of plant based medicines, as well as their clinical uses.

Spectroscopy

This is the study of the interaction of atoms and molecules with light also referred to as electromagnetic radiation. Such information provides insight into the measurement of the radiation intensity as a function of wavelength.

1.8 SOURCES AND COMPOSITION OF DRUGS

A large number of drugs are used in the clinics for the cure of various ailments. These drugs are diverse in chemical structure and are obtained from a wide variety of sources. In earlier days, simple chemical substances and different parts of plants were employed as medicinal agents, but most drugs currently used in therapeutics are synthetic in nature. However, natural sources are still used for obtaining some drugs mainly because their synthesis is difficult and uneconomical. Drugs are mainly obtained from the following sources.

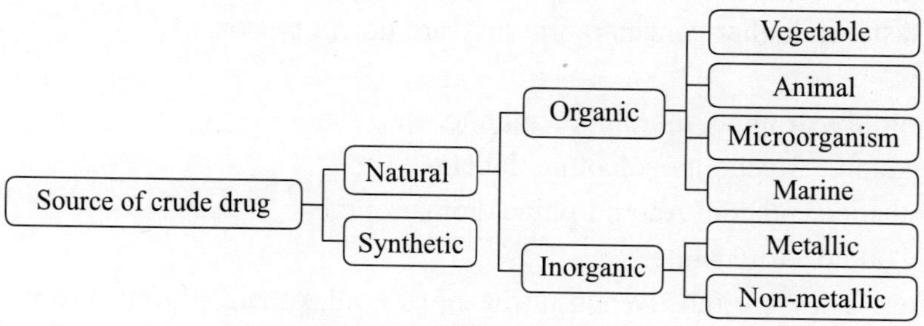

Fig. 1.10 Source of drugs.

(i) Natural Sources of Drugs

Active principles of drugs are mainly present in crude form in minute amounts. These active principles are separated by various techniques or may be used as such in some cases.

(A) Organic Drugs

Main natural sources of organic drugs are vegetable, animal, microorganisms and marine.

1. Vegetative source

The drugs obtained from vegetative origin. It is a very old and important source of drugs; various parts of the plants are still used for drugs.

Table 1.2 The following are the active constituents of crude drugs act as potent source of therapeutic agents

Part of the plant	Name of the plant	Active Principle	Use
Root	Rauwolfia Ipecacuanha	Reserpine Emetin	Antihypertensive, emetic
Flower	Clove Pyrethrium	Eugenol Pyrethrin	Local anaesthetic insecticide, rubefacient
Bulbs	Urginea	Squill	Emetic, rodenticide
Rhizome	Ginger	Gingerol	Carminative
Bark	Cinchona	Quinine	Antimalarial
Leave	Belladona Digitalis	Atropine Digitoxin	Anti-muscarinic Cardiac stimulant
Seed	Nux-vomica Physostigma	Strychnine Physostigmine	Rodenticide Anti-glaucoma
Wood	Sandal wood Quassia	Sandal wood oil Quassin	Urinary antiseptic Stomachic

(a) **Alkaloid:** These are complex, alkaline, nitrogenous compounds mostly obtained from plants and also animals. They are alkaline nitrogenous organic compounds which combine with acids to form crystalline salts without production of water. They are readily soluble in alcohol but sparingly soluble in water but their salts are soluble in water.

A few of them are liquid, which nearly contain C, H and N only. The solid alkaloids contain oxygen in addition and are colourless crystalline. Most of the alkaloids are closely related to pyridine and some may be prepared synthetically from pyridine bases. They are mostly bitter in taste. In higher concentration they are potent poisons.

Examples:

Solid alkaloid: Atropine, morphine, quinine, etc.

Liquid alkaloid: Arecholine, nicotine, lobeline.

Semi-synthetic/synthetic: Apomorphine, homatropine.

Animal alkaloid: Adrenaline.

(b) **Glycosides:** They are mostly non-nitrogenous bodies mainly occurring in plants. They are non-nitrogenous compounds having sugar attached to non-sugar part by ether linkage, mainly contain C, H and O. Some may have in addition N and a few S. They do not combine with acids to form salts. They are mostly soluble in alcohol, less soluble in water and insoluble in ether. Some are highly active, while others are practically inert. These are hydrolysed by acids and liberate aglycone (non-sugar part).

Examples: Digitoxin, scillarin, digoxin, etc.

(c) **Saponins:** These are plant glycosides which have distinctive property of frothing. They are a group of non-nitrogenous substances usually glycosides, soluble in water and form froth when shaken. It can split up on hydrolysis into sugar and aglycone (sapogenin). Toxic saponins are called sapotoxins.

Examples: Digitonin, senegin, glycyrrhizin, etc.

(d) **Resins:** These are resin-like substances which are oxidative products of volatile oils. They are produced by some plants. They are invariably composed of a large number of substances which may be acid, alcohol or ester in chemical composition, basically secretions of plant tissues. They are bitter, amorphous solids and insoluble in water, but soluble in alcohol, ether, etc. They are soluble in alkalis forming non-detergent resin soaps.

Examples: Resin of Jalap, podophyllin.

Types of resin combinations

Oleo-resins: They are natural plant exudates which are semisolid mixtures of resins and volatile oils, e.g., crude turpentine.

Gum-resins: They are mixture of resins and gums, e.g., asafoetida.

Balsams: They are oleoresins containing benzoic acid or cinnamic acid, e.g., benzoin, balsam of Peru, etc.

(e) **Tannins:** Tannins are non-nitrogenous phenol derivatives characterised by their astringent action on the mucous membrane. They mainly occur in leaves and barks of the plants having irritant or astringent action. They react with iron to form blue colouration. They precipitate metallic salts, alkaloids and proteins. Some are glycosides, i.e., occur in combination with sugar.

Example: Tannic acid obtained from nut galls.

(f) **Gums and Mucilage**

Gums: Gums are secretory products of plants which are used as emulsifying agents for oils and, suspending agents for insoluble substances. They are amorphous, colloidal, complex polysaccharides. They dissolve in water forming viscid adhesive fluid known as mucilage.

Examples: Acacia, Tragacanth.

Mucilage: They are thick, gluey substance produced by most plants and some microorganisms. It is a polar glycoprotein. It occurs in various parts of nearly all classes of plant, usually in relatively small percentages, and is frequently associated with other substances, such as tannins and alkaloids. Mucilage in plants is thought to aid in water storage and seed germination, and to act as a membrane thickener and food reserve.

Table 1.3 Difference between gums and mucilage

Gums	Mucilage
1. Gums are produced by plant when it is injured or diseased by a process "gummosis"	1. Mucilage is a normal product of plant growth.
2. Gum is produced outside the plant cell.	2. Mucilage is produced inside the cell.
3. Gums are soluble in water to form adhesive solution.	3. Mucilage is not soluble in water, and form slimy solution with water.
4. Gums are made up of sugar, salts of uronic acid, e.g., gum acacia, tragacanth gum.	4. Mucilage is made up of ester and sulphuric acid, e.g., mucilage is present in agar, senna, isapgol.

(g) Oils: Oils are obtained from vegetable, animal and mineral sources. Oils are of 3 types: Volatile, fixed and mineral.

mm

(i) Volatile oils: These are also called essential, ethereal, aromatic or flavouring oils as they are responsible for the aroma and odour of plants and flowers. They are composed of diverse chemical compounds such as alcohols, aldehydes, ketones, esters, sulphur compounds, etc. They are mainly present in the flowering parts of plant, leaves and fruits and give characteristic smell to plants. They are mainly obtained by a process of distillation without being decomposed. They do not form soap with alkalis. They are less soluble in water but more soluble in organic solvents. Alcoholic solutions of these oils are known as essences and are used in perfumery. They do not leave a grease spot on paper. On exposure to air and light, they tend to oxidise and turn rancid.

Examples:

Liquid volatile oil: Eucalyptus oil, clove oil.

Solid volatile oil: Camphor, menthol, thymol.

(ii) Fixed oils: They are esters of higher fatty acids (oleic, palmitic, stearic acids) and glycerines, obtained from fruits, seeds and some other parts of the plants. They are non-volatile and as such cannot be distilled without decomposition, so obtained by process of expression. They are insoluble (immiscible) in water, sparingly soluble in alcohol and freely soluble in ether. They are liquid at ordinary temperature. They leave a permanent grease spot on paper. They turn rancid on heating. They form soap with alkalis.

Examples:

Vegetable oils: Olive oil, castor oil, mustard oil.

Animal oils: Cod liver oil, shark liver oil.

(iii) Mineral oils: These are obtained by boring the earth and do not belong to organic class. Some are used in medicinal preparations and contain only C and H.

Example: Liquid paraffin.

(h) Waxes: They are esters of higher fatty acids and higher monohydric alcohols. They are firmer in consistency and have higher melting, points.

Example: Yellow and white bees wax.

2. Animal sources

From animal source relatively few but important drugs are obtained. It includes:

(i) Hormones: Insulin, thyroxin, gonadotropins, etc.

(ii) Vitamins: Cod liver oil (vit. A).

(iii) Vaccines/sera: Anti-rabies vaccine (ARV), anti-tetanic serum (ATS), anti-diphtheric serum, etc.

(iv) Replacement therapy: Liver extract.

3. Microbial source

Microorganisms are also an important source of drugs. Certain bacteria, fungi and actinomycetes produce antibiotics which form a major group of therapeutically useful drugs.

Example: Penicillin G from *Penicillium notatum* (fungi), Streptomycin from *Streptomyces griseus* (bacteria), Bacitracin from *Bacillus subtilus* (bacteria).

4. Marine source

The drugs are obtained from sea. The major sources of such drugs are sponge, cone snail, bryozoa, coral, sea algae, etc. Some examples are given below.

Table 1.4 Drugs from marine source

Compound ame	Marine Organism	Chemical Class	Use
Cytarabine (Ara-C)	Sponge	Nucleoside	Cancer
Eribulin Mesylate (E7389)	Sponge	Macrolide	Cancer
Vidarabine (Ara-A)	Sponge	Nucleoside	Antiviral
Ziconotide	Cone snail	Peptide	Analgesic
Bryostatin 1	Bryozoa	Polyketide	Cancer, Alzheimers
Pseudopterosins	Soft coral	Diterpene glycoside	Wound healing
PM00104	Nudibranch	Alkaloid	Cancer

5. Tissue culture

Tissue culture is gaining increasing popularity across many different industries, including pharmaceuticals. The following compounds are harvested from plants by tissue culture for pharmaceutical medicines. Alkaloids like, tropaine, cocaine, atropine, scopolamine, hyoscyamine, etc. berberine (high blood pressure, diabetes), valepotriates (antitumor and cytotoxicity activities), taxol (ovarian cancer), etc.

(B) Inorganic Sources

Drugs obtained from inorganic sources have been simply classified into metals and non-metals. Metalloids which show intermediate properties. The elements either occur in native state or combined state.

1. **Metals:** Minerals are the main source of metals.

Table 1.5 Various sources of metals

Agent	Use
Magnesium sulphate	Purgative
Calcium carbonate	Astringent
Copper sulphate	Emetic
Ferrous sulphate	Haematinic
Zinc sulphate	Astringent
Bismuth subnitrate	Antiseptic
Lead acetate	Local sedative, antiseptic

2. **Non-metals**: These are also used for various purposes.

Table 1.6 Various sources of non-metals

Agent	Use
Iodine (Pot. iodide)	Expectorant
Bromine (Pot. bromide)	Sedative
Hydrogen peroxide	Antiseptic
Sulphur	Insecticide, disinfectant
Carbon (charcoal)	Adsorbant

(ii) Synthetic Sources of Drugs

Synthetic drugs are prepared in the laboratory with the help of inorganic and organic substances. Majority of drugs are obtained synthetically or semi-synthetically. Numerous drugs which were originally obtained from plants are now prepared synthetically.

For example, ether and chloroform (volatile anaesthetics), sulfonamides and quinolones (antimicrobial drugs), paracetamol (analgesic), pentobarbital and thiopental (hypnotic and parenteral anaesthetics), etc.

1.9 ORGANIZED DRUGS, UNORGANIZED DRUGS

Table 1.7 Difference between organized drug unorganized crude drugs

Organized (cellular) drug	Unorganized (acellular) drug
1. Cellular structure present.	1. Cellular structure is absent.
2. Organized drugs are part of plant, animal like, fruits, seeds, and roots.	2. Unorganized drugs are obtained from parts of plant and animal by extraction, distillation incision, expression.
3. To study organized drug properly, there T S or L C is taken and studied under microscope.	3. For study of unorganized drug physical constituent like density, viscosity, refractive index, optical rotation and chemical test are important criteria.
4. They are solid in nature.	4. They are solid, semi-solid, or liquid.
5. Ex. clove, fennel, dill, digitalis.	5. Lemon oil, starch, catechu.

Some unorganised drugs are described below.

They are classified into several groups:

1. Gums and mucilage and resins and resin combinations (described early in vegetative source of drugs).
2. **Dried juices:** The juices obtained from fleshy leaves (aloes) or from the stems of the trees (kino).
3. **Dried latex:** Latex is a product present in special tissue of plant. It is a white, aqueous, suspension, the suspended particles are protein, sugar, minerals, alkaloid, resin, or starch. Under microscope, small particles of oil globules are easily detectable, e.g., opium, papain, gutta percha.

4. **Extracts:** Pharmaceutical origin drugs are obtained by alcoholic or hydro-alcoholic solutions and adjusting the product to a standard strength, e.g., agar, black, catechu, gelatin.

1.10 CLASSIFICATION OF CRUDE DRUGS

Mother earth nurtures a vast diversity of flora and fauna. Nearly about 2.5 lakh plant species exist on the earth among them about 10,500 genres and 300 families are identified. The use of medicinal plants in human ailments has been present since time immortal and even today many of such natural drugs are important as commercial products. Around 200 plant families are currently cultivated as medicinal crop where among 35-40 species are cultivated as large-scale field corps.

The various medicinal plants are known for their therapeutic or curative actions and till date the natural drugs have been the key choice as a source of drug discoveries and inventions. But human inquisitiveness and exploring tendency not only restricted them in research on terrestrial plants or animals, it has gone beyond the boundaries even in mysterious world of marine organelles where nearly five lakh species have their habitats. This exploration leads a new source of potential therapeutic agents from natural source of unending search.

Crude drug is defined as an unprocessed natural substance used as drug either directly or indirectly without changing or modifying its chemical composition.

Crude drugs are classified into two distinct categories for better grouping. They are:

(a) Organized drugs

(b) Unorganized drugs

(a) Organized Drugs

- Organized crude drugs consist of organs or parts of the plants.
- They mostly originate from plant sources.
- They possess cellular organization in the form of anatomical features.
- Morphological parts or the entire plant can be considered for organized drugs.
- In organized drugs the microscopical and anatomical studies are preeminent.
- They can be used as medicine either directly, by modifying or by extracting the active ingredient.
- The medicines prepared from organized crude drugs include herbal teas, herbal extracts, tinctures, etc.
- Organized crude drugs are extensively used for the isolation and purification of active constituent of therapeutic significance.
- *Examples:* Cinchona bark, sandalwood, quassia wood, senna, digitalis leaves, nux vomica seeds, rauwolfia roots, etc.

(b) Unorganized Drugs

- The unorganized drugs consist of plant, animal or mineral originated prepared or exudate liquid or semisolid products, which are no longer any parts or organ of plant.
- Unorganized drugs may be solid, semisolid or liquid.

- Physical, chemical and analytical standards are applied for testing their quality and purity.
- It does not have the morphological or anatomical organization. Hence, microscopical studies are not required.
- Unorganized drugs such as essential oils, fixed oils, fats and waxes obtained from vegetable or animal sources, extracted from plant, become the direct commodity for use.
- Unorganized crude drugs may be miscellaneous mineral products (example, *shilajit).*
- *Example:* Plant exudates (gums, oleogums, oleogum resins), plant lattices (opium), aloetic juices (aloes), dried extracts (black and pale catechu), agar, alginic acid, etc.

In order to study and arrangement of the crude drugs we should adopt some particular sequence of system referred as classification of drugs. Such system should have certain advantages, i.e., simple and easy method along with it must overcome confusions and ambiguities about drug selection and process.

Each system of classification has own merits and demerits due to its wide distribution. In the purpose of study the drugs are classified in seven different ways. It includes:

1. Alphabetical classification
2. Taxonomical classification
3. Morphological classification
4. Pharmacological classification
5. Chemical classification
6. Chemotaxonomical classification
7. Sero-taxonomical classification

1. Alphabetical Classification

It is an old, primitive and simplest method of classification of crude drugs. Such type of classification is based on the first alphabet of the name of crude drugs. The names might be in Latin, English (common names) or sometimes local language (vernacular names). This system of classification has been adopted in various standard books or dictionaries such as:

1. Indian Pharmacopoeia (IP)
2. British Pharmacopoeia (BP)
3. British Herbal Pharmacopoeia (BHP)
4. United States Pharmacopoeia (USP) and National Formulary (NF)
5. British Pharmaceutical Codex (BPC)
6. European Pharmacopoeia (EP), etc.

According to the Latin names, European Pharmacopoeia arranged the crude drugs. Whereas United States Pharmacopoeia (USP) and British Pharmaceutical Codex (BPC), have arranged crude drugs in English.

Merits:

- This method is very easy and quick to use.
- No chance of repetition of entries and is devoid of confusion.
- Easy to find the location, tracing and addition of drug entries.

Demerits:

- No relationship between previous and successive drug entries.
- No idea about their chemical or physical properties.

Examples:

A-Acacia, B-Benzoin, C-Cinchona, D-Dill, E-Ergot, F-Fennel, G-Gentian, H-Hyoscyamus, I-Ipecacuanha, J-Jalap, K-Kurchi, L-Liquorice, M-Mints, N-Nux vomica, O-Opium, P-Podophyllum, Q-Quassia, R-Rauwolfia, S-Senna, V-Vasaka, W-Wool fat, Y-Yellow bees wax, Z- Zeodary.

2. *Taxonomical Classification*

In this classification the crude drugs are classified according to kingdom, subkingdom, division, class, order, family, genus and species as follows.

- **Kingdom**: Planate represents the entire plant groups exist in the earth.
- **Class:** Angiospermae (angiosperms) represents the group of plants that produce flowers and Gymnospermae (gymnosperms) which don't produce flowers.
- **Subclass:** The plant class which produces two seed leaves known as Dicotyledonae (dicotyledons, dicots), similarly Monocotyledonae (monocotyledons, monocots) are the plants with one seed leaf.
- **Superorder:** It represents a group of correlated plant families, which areclassified in the order in the way thought to have developed their differences from a common ancestor.
  Dicotyledonae have six superorders: i) *Magnoliidae, ii) Hamamelidae, iii) Caryophyllidae, iv) Dilleniidae, v) Rosidae, vi) Asteridae,* etc., and in the Monocotyledonae it have four superorders, i.e., *Alismatidae, Commelinidae, Arecidae*, and *Liliidae.*
- **Order:** Each superorder is further divided into several orders.
- **Family:** Each order is divided into families. These are plants with many botanical features in common, and are the highest classification normally used.
- **Subfamily:** The family may be further divided into a number of subfamilies, which group together plants within the family that have some significant botanical differences.
- **Tribe:** A further division of plants within a family, based on smaller botanical differences known as tribe.
- **Subtribe:** A further division based on even smaller botanical differences is called subtribe.
- **Genus:** This is the part of the plant name that is most familiar. The normal name that you give a plant—like withania (Ashwagandha).
- **Species:** This is the level that defines an individual plant. Together, the genus and species name refer to only one plant, and they are used to identify that particular plant.
  The species is further often divided into subspecies that contain plants not quite so distinct that they are classified as varieties.

Merits:

- It is helpful for studying evolutionary developments.

Demerits:

- This system also does not correlate in between the chemical constituents and biological activity of the drugs.

3. Morphological Classification

In this system, the drugs are arranged according to the morphological or external characters of the plant parts or animal parts, i.e., which part of the plant are used as a drug, e.g., *organized* drugs and *unorganized* drugs.

Table 1.8 Examples of organized drugs

Parts of plant	Examples
Woods	Quassia, Sandalwood and Red Sandalwood
Leaves	Digitalis, Eucalyptus, Gymnema, Mint, Senna, Spearmint, Squill, Tulsi, Vasaka, Coca, Buchu, Hamamelis, Hyoscyamus, Belladonna, Tea
Barks	Arjuna, Ashoka, Cascara, Cassia, Cinchona, Cinnamon, Kurchi, Wild cherry.
Flowering parts	Clove, Pyrethrum, Saffron, Santonica, Chamomile

Table 1.9 Examples of unorganized drugs

Source	Examples
Dried latex	Opium, Papain
Dried Juice	Aloe, Kino
Dried extracts	Agar, Alginate, Black catechu, Pale catechu, Pectin
Waxes	Beeswax, Spermaceti, Carnauba wax

Merits:

- Morphological classification is more helpful to identify and detect adulteration. This system of classification is more convenient for practical study especially when the chemical nature of the drug is not clearly understood.

Demerits:

- The main drawback of morphological classification is that there is no correlation of chemical constituents with the therapeutic actions.
- Repetition of drugs or plants occurs.

4. Pharmacological Classification

Grouping of drugs according to their pharmacological action or of most important constituent or their therapeutic use is termed pharmacological or therapeutic classification of drugs. This classification is more relevant and is mostly followed. Drugs like digitalis, squill and strophanthus having cardiotonic action are grouped irrespective of their parts used or phylogenetic relationship or the nature of phytoconstituents they contains.

Table 1.10 Examples of crude drugs for their pharmacological action

Pharmacological category	Example
Laxatives	Senna, Isabgol
Carminatives	Fennel, Coriander, Cardamom
Emetics	Ipecac
Biter	Quassia, Cinhona
Cardio tonics	Digitalis, Strophanthus
Antihypertensive	Rauwolfia
Expectorants	Vasaka, liquorice
Anticancer	Vinca, Taxus, Podophyllum
Antimalarial	Artemesia, Cinchona
CNS stimulant	Tea, Coffee
CNS depressant	Belladonna, Opium

Merits:

- This system of classification can be used for suggesting substitutes of drugs, if they are not available at a particular place or point of time.

Demerits:

- Drugs having different action on the body get classified separately in more than one group that causes ambiguity and confusion. Cinchona is antimalarial drug because of presence of quinine but can be put under the group of drug affecting heart because of antiarrhythmic action of quinidine.

5. *Chemical Classification*

In this classification system the active constituents are classifying factor. Depending upon the presence of phytochemicals the crude drugs are classified. The plants contain various constituents in them like alkaloids, glycosides, tannins, carbohydrates, saponins, etc. The drugs with similar chemical constituents are grouped into the same group irrespective of their morphological or taxonomical characters. The examples are shown below.

Table 1.11 Examples of crude drugs for their phytoconstituents

Active chemical constituents	Example
Alkaloids	Cinchona, Datura, Nux vomica, Ipecac
Glycosides	Senna, Aloe, Ginseng, Digitalis
Volatile oils	Clove, Coriander, Fennel, Cinnamon
Tannins	Catechu, Tea

Contd.

Resin	Benzoin, Tolu Balsam
Enzymes	Papain, Caesin
Lipids	Bees wax, Lanolin

Merits:

- It is a popular approach for phytochemical studies.

Demerits:

- Ambiguities arise when particular drugs possess a number of compounds belonging to different groups of compounds.

6. Chemotaxonomical Classification

It is a combine approach between taxonomical and chemical identity of drug. This system of classification relies on the chemical similarity of a taxon, i.e., based on the existence of relationship between constituents in various plants. There are certain types of chemical constituents that characterize certain classes of plants. This gives birth to entirely a new concept of chemotaxonomy that utilizes chemical facts/characters for understanding the taxonomical status, relationships and the evolution of the plants.

For example, tropane alkaloids generally occur among the members of Solanaceae family, thereby, serving as a chemotaxonomic marker. Similarly, other secondary plant metabolites can also serve as the basis of classification of crude drugs. The berberine alkaloid in Berberis and Argemone, Rutin in Rutaceae members, Ranunculaceae alkaloids among its members, etc., are other examples. Even though identification of multiple species like eucalyptus can also be possible by applying the taxonomical and chemicals inputs.

Merits:

- It is the latest system of classification that gives more scope for understanding the relationship between chemical constituents, their biosynthesis and their possible action.

Demerits:

- No correlation upon therapeutic actions of the drug.

7. Serotaxonomical Classification

This method of classification is comparatively new and more advance. It can be explained as the study about the application or the utility of serology in solving the taxonomical problems. Serology can be defined as the study of the antigen-antibody reaction. Antigens are those substances which can stimulate the formation of the antibody. Antibodies are highly specific protein molecules produced by plasma cells in the immune system. Proteins are carriers of the taxonomical information and commonly used as antigen in serotaxonomy.

It expresses the similarities and the dissimilarities among different taxa, and these data are helpful in taxonomy. It determines the degree of similarity between species, genera, family, etc., by comparing the reaction with antigens from various plant taxa with antibodies present against a given taxon.

Merits:

- It helps in comparing non-morphological characteristics, which helps in the taxonomical data. This technique also helps in the comparison of single proteins from different plant taxa.

Demerits:

- No correlations with therapeutic or chemical profile of the drugs.

1.11 QUALITY CONTROL OF DRUGS OF NATURAL ORIGIN

1.11.1 Adulteration of Drugs of Natural Origin

The most effective source of raw material for the traditional systems such as Ayurveda, Chinese, Homeopathy and Unani, etc., or even in modern medicine is not other than medicinal plants. They have their genuine utility in all areas. In fact, approximately 70% of 'synthetic' medicines are derived from plants. Hence, herbal adulteration is one of the common malpractices in herbal raw material trade worldwide. Adulteration is described as substitution or disbasement of articles with other inferior quality products.

Adulteration is defined as "a practice of substituting original crude drug partially or wholly with other similar looking substances, either free from or inferior in chemical or therapeutic properties".

In general, adulteration is considered an intentional practice. However, unintentional adulterations also exist in herbal raw material trade due to various reasons, and many of them are unknown even to the scientific community.

I. Types of Adulteration

Adulteration can be broadly classified into two types.

(i) **Deliberate (Intentional) Adulteration:** Intentional adulteration is mainly encouraged by traders who are reluctant to pay premium prices for herbs of superior quality and hence are inclined to purchase only the cheaper products. This encourages producers and traders to sell herbs of inferior quality.

(ii) **Indeliberate/Unintentional (Accidental) Adulteration:** It may occur without bad intention of the manufacturers or suppliers. Sometimes in the absence of proper means of evaluation, an authentic drug partially or fully devoid of the active ingredients may enter the market.

Adulteration involves different conditions such as: (a) deterioration, (b) admixture, (c) sophistication, (d) substitution, (e) inferiority, and (f) spoilage.

(a) **Deterioration:** Impairment in the quality of a drug.

(b) **Admixture:** Addition of one article to another due to ignorance or carelessness, or by accident.

(c) **Sophisticaton:** Intentional or deliberate type of adulteration.

(d) **Substitution:** Completely substitute different substance in place of original drug.

(e) **Inferiority:** Any sub-standard drug.

(f) **Spoilage:** Deterioration due to the attack of microorganisms.

II. Types of Adulterants

Generally, the drugs are adulterated by substitution with substandard commercial varieties, inferior drugs, or artificially manufactured commodities.

The following types of adulteration are common.

1. **Substitution with substandard commercial varieties:** The adulterants here may resemble the original crude drug in morphological, chemical, or therapeutic characters, but are substandard in nature and hence are cheaper. This is the most common practice of adulteration.

   Example: Strychnous nux-blanda or *S. potatorum* in place of *S. nux-vomica*, *Capsicum annuum* in place of *C. minimum*, Indian senna is substituted with Arabian senna or dog senna, medicinal ginger is substituted with inferior varieties of African, Japanese, or Cochin ginger. *Solanum xanthocarpum* adulterated with *Solanum mammosum*.

   It can be avoided by careful selection of plant material.

2. **Substitution with superficially similar inferior drugs:** These inferior drugs may or may not be having any chemical or therapeutic value as that of original drug. Due to their morphological resemblance to the authentic drug, they are marketed as adulterants.

   Example: Belladonna leaves are substituted with ailanthus leaves, saffron is admixed with dried flowers of *Carthamus tinctorious*, and bees wax is substituted with Japan wax.

3. **Substitution with artificially manufactured substances:** It has been also observed that substances artificially prepared to resemble the original drug are used as substitutes. This practice is followed for costlier drugs.

   Examples: Compressed chicory in place of coffee, yellow coloured paraffin wax for bees wax, properly cut and shaved basswood for nutmeg.

4. **Substitution with exhausted drug:** The same drug is admixed but is devoid of any medicinally active constituents as they are already extracted out. This practice is more common in case of volatile oil containing drugs like fennel, clove, coriander, caraway, etc. Sometimes natural characters of exhausted drugs like colour, and taste are manipulated by adding other additives and then it is substituted.

   Examples: Exhausted gentian made bitter with aloes, artificial colouring of exhausted saffron, etc.

   Besides these common practices, sometimes other methods are also employed like use of synthetic chemicals to enhance the natural characteristics of natural drugs.

   Example: Addition of benzyl benzoate to balsam of peru, citral to citrus oils like oil of lemon and orange oil, etc.

5. **Presence of vegetative matter from the same plant:** Sometimes, the other miniature plants growing along with medicinal plants are admixed with the authentic drug, due to their resemblance in colour, odour, and in some cases constituents.

   Example: The lower plants like moss, liverworts, and epiphytes growing on bark portion are mixed with cascara or cinchona, The stem portions are mixed along with leaf drugs like stramonium, lobelia, and senna.

6. **Harmful adulterants:** Sometimes the waste from the market is collected and admixed with the authentic drug. This is particularly noticed in liquids or unorganized drugs.
   Examples: Pieces of amber coloured glass in colophony, limestones in asafoetida, lead shot in opium, white oil in coconut oil, cocoa butter mixed with stearin or paraffin. Addition of wheat flour to powdered ginger, with enough capsicum to restore the pungency & curcuma to maintain the colour; Rosewood in capsicum powder; powdered bark adulterated with brick powder.
   The addition of rodent faecal matter to cardamom seed is a very harmful adulteration. Synthetic chemicals are used to enhance natural character of drugs like various synthetic colorants added in powder drugs.
   Examples: Citral is added to citrus oils (like oil of lemon and oil of orange). Carcinogenic mentanil yellow in turmeric powder.
7. **Spoilage adulteration:** Substandard condition produced by microbial or other pest infestation which makes a drug unfit for medicinal preparation.
   Examples: Ativisha, vatsanabha and vacha. It can be avoided by giving more careful attention to the drying and storage conditions.
8. **Adulteration of powders:** Besides the entire drug the powdered forms are frequently found to be adulterated.
   Examples: Dextrin in ipecacuanha, powered liqourice or gentian admixed with powdered olive stones, exhausted ginger powder in powdered colocynth or ginger, red-sanders wood in capsicum.

III. Reasons for Adulteration

Some probable reasons of adulterations may include:

- Confusion in vernacular names.
- Lack of knowledge about authentic sources.
- Similarity in morphology.
- Lack of authentic plants.
- Unscientific collection.
- High price of the drug in the market.
- With the intention of enhancing profits.

IV. Examples of adulterants of some medicinal plants

Table 1.12 Examples of adulteration for few medicinal plants

S.N.	Drug Name	Genuine Source	Adulterant
1	Asoka	*Saraca asoca*	*Polyalthia longifolia*
2	Vasha	*Adhatoda vasica*	*Ailanthus excels*
3	Yashtimadhu	*Glycyrrhiza glabra*	*Abrus precatorius*
4	Sarpagandha	*Rauwolfia serpentina*	*Rauwolfia densiflora*

1.11.2 Evaluation of Crude Drugs

The identity, quality and purity of crude drugs is ensured by drug evaluation. Biochemical variation in plant drugs, effect of storage, adulterations, substitutions, etc., make it mandatory to undergo such evaluation process.

The methods currently employed in evaluating herbs are:

I. Organoleptic evaluation
II. Microscopic evaluation
III. Chemical evaluation
IV. Physical evaluation
V. Biological evaluation.

I. Organoleptic evaluation

Organoleptic evaluation means the evaluation of drugs using sensory organs. It includes colour, odour, taste, size, shape, and special features, such as touch, texture, etc. Obviously, the initial sight of the plant or extract is so specific that it tends to identify itself. If this is not enough, perhaps the plant or extract has a characteristic odour or taste.

Talka gum, which is used as a substitute for acacia gum could be identified by its colour and form. Talka gum is usually broken and also some tears are brown in colour and other colourless, whereas acacia is white to yellow in colour. Mangosteen fruits are a substitute for bael fruits and can be identified by darker rind and the wedge dshaped radiate stigmas. Cuprea bark *(Remijia pedupiculata)* differs in its morphological character with cinchona. Blood root used as an adulterant for hydrastis is dark reddish-brown in colour, whereas hydrastis is yellow in colour. *Rheum rhaponticum* are much smaller than those of the Chinese rhubarb and are easily distinguished.

Ginger and capsicum have pungent taste, whereas gentian and chirata have bitter taste. Morphological differentiation of leaves and pods of Indian senna and Alexandrian senna, sweet taste of liquorice, odours of umbelliferous fruits, disc-shaped structure of nux-vomica, conical shape of aconite, quills of cinnamon, etc., are a few examples of this organoleptic evaluation.

II. Microscopical evaluation

It is an indispensable and initial step of identification of herbs. Even though, identifying small fragments of crude or powdered herbs, and in the detection of adulterants as well as identifying the plant by characteristic tissue features can be easy with this evaluation process.

Every plant possesses a characteristic tissue structure, which can be demonstrated through study of tissue arrangement, cell walls, and configuration when properly mounted in stains, reagents, and media. Lignin stains red or pink with a drop of phloroglucinol and concentrated hydrochloric acid. Mucilage is stained pink with rhuthenium red, and N/50 iodine solution stains starch and hemicellulose blue.

The characteristic features of cell walls, cell contents, starch grains, calcium oxalate crystals, trichomes, fibres, vessels, etc., have been studied in detail.

Surinam quassia is recognized by the absence of calcium oxalate and presence of uniseriate medullary rays, crystal fibres, and wavy medullary rays of cascara bark, lignified trichomes, and plasmodesma in nux-vomica. Stone cells are absent in the frangula bark, whereas they are present in cascara. Presence of pith in rhizomes and absence in roots, warty trichomes of senna, and presence or absence of crystals of aloin indicates different varieties of aloes, glandular trichomes of mint, etc. The powder of clove stalks contains sclereids and calcium oxalate crystals, but cloves do not contain these two.

The techniques like microscopic linear measurements, determination of leaf constants and quantitative microscopy are also used in this evaluation.

Linear measurements include size of starch grains, length and width of fibres, trichomes, etc. The diameter of starch grains present in ipecacuanha assists in distinguishing its varieties. The diameter of starch grains in cassia bark distinguishes from cinnamon and detects senna stalk in powdered senna leaf. The size of the stomata in leaves of *Barosma betulina* distinguishes it from other species of barosma. The diameter of phloem fibres aids the detection of cassia in cinnamon, and the width of the vessel helps to detect clove stalks in powdered cloves. Measurements of diameter for the identification of commercial starches and for the detection in them of foreign starch are a few examples of linear measurements.

Determination of leaf constants include

(a) Stomatal number
(b) Stomatal index
(c) Vein islet number
(d) Vein termination number
(e) Palisade ratios

(a) Stomatal number is the average number of stomata per sq. mm of epidermis of the leaf. It varies with plant to plant even species to species of same plant.

Example:

Name of the drug	Stomatal number
Alexandrian senna	10–15
Indian Senna	14–20

(b) Stomatal index: It is the percentage numbers of stomata form to the total number of epidermal cells, each stoma being counted as one cell. Stomatal index can be calculated by using the following formula:

$$\text{S.I.} = \frac{S}{S+E} \times 100$$

where,

S = number of stomata per unit area

E = number of epidermal cells in the same unit area.

(c) Vein-islet number: It is defined as the number of vein islets per sq. mm of the leaf surface midway between the midrib and the margin. It is a constant for a given species of the plant and is used as a characteristic for the identification of the allied species.

(d) Veinlet termination number: It is defined as the number of veinlet termination per sq. mm of the leaf surface midway between midrib and margin. A vein termination is the ultimate free termination of veinlet.

Example

Name of the drug	Veinlet termination number
Alexandrian senna	25–29.5
Indian senna	19.5–22.5

(e) Palisade ratio: It is defined as the average number of palisade cells beneath each epidermal cell. Palisade ratio can be determined with the powdered drug.

1.11.3 Quantitative Microscopy (Lycopodium Spore Method)

This is an important technique employed in identification of crude drug when chemical and physical methods are inapplicable. Using this, one can determine the proportions of the substances present by means of the microscope, using the lycopodium spore method.

The powdered drugs with well-defined particles which may be counted, for example, starch grains or single-layered cells or tissues—the area of which may be traced under suitable magnification or the objects of uniform thickness, and the length of which can be measured under suitable magnification and actual area calculated are usually evaluated using this method.

Adulterated starchy drugs can be determined by counting the number of starch grains per mg and calculating the amount from the known number of starch grains per mg of the pure starch or starchy material.

Thus, if spent ginger is the adulterant, one knows that ginger contains 286,000 starch grains per mg, and the amount used as an adulterant can be calculated by using this figure. The percentage purity of an authentic powdered ginger is calculated using the following equation:

$$\% \text{ Purity} = \frac{N \times W \times 94,000 \times 100}{S \times M \times P}$$

where,

N = number of characteristic structures (e.g., starch grains) in 25 fields

W = weight in mg of lycopodium taken

S = number of lycopodium spores in the same 25 fields

M = weight in mg of the sample, calculated on basis of sample dried at 105°C

P = 2,86,000 in case of ginger starch grains powder.

If the material is one for which a constant is not available, it is necessary to determine one by a preliminary experiment.

III. Chemical evaluation

Chemical evaluation of crude drugs has been performed to evaluate the presence of chemicals and their quantifications. It includes (a) qualitative chemical tests, (b) quantitative chemical tests, (c) chemical assays, and (d) instrumental analysis.

The isolation, purification, and identification of active constituents are chemical methods of evaluation.

(a) Qualitative chemical tests: It includes qualitative determination or identification of various phytoconstituents presence in plant or extract, i.e., alkaloids, glycosides, tannins, saponins, terpenoids, phenolics, etc. Examples of this evaluation are:

Table 1.13 Examples of reagents for specific phytoconstituents

Tests	Phytoconstituents
Dragendoraff's reagent Hagers reagent Wagner's reagent Mayer's reagent	Alkaloids
Copper acetate	Resins, balsams, and waxes
Holphen's test	Cottonseed oil
Baudouin's test	Sesame oil in olive oil
Van Urk's reagent	Ergot
Vitali's morins test	Tropane alkaloids
Murexide test	Purine bases alkaloids

(b) Quantitative chemical tests: It is also a useful parameter for the evaluation of crude drugs by means of chemical treatments, resulted quantitative detection. It includes

(i) Acid value (for resins, balsams)
(ii) Saponification value (for balsams)
(iii) Ester value (for balsams, volatile oils)
(iv) Acetyl value (for volatile oils, etc.)

(c) Chemical assays: The process of chemical assay under chemical evaluation can provide significant chemical information about the presence or absence of assayed chemicals and also suggest the quality and purity of the drugs. It includes chemical assays for alkaloid, resin, volatile oil, glycoside, vitamins, or other constituent.

Few example, (i) assay of total alkaloid in belladonna, (ii) total alkaloid and non-phenolic alkaloid in ipecacuanha, (iii) estimation of strychnine in nux-vomica, (iv) total resin content in jalap, and (v) total vitamin A content in cod-liver oil, etc.

(d) Instrumental analysis: This method is comparatively advanced with the aid of sophisticated instruments for analysis of chemical groups or phytoconstituents present in the drug for the sake of identification and quality assurance. This method includes chromatographic and spectroscopic techniques.

Chromatographic methods include paper chromatography, thin-layer chromatography (TLC), gas chromatography (GC), high-performance liquid chromatography (HPLC), high-performance thin-layer chromatography (HPTLC), etc., where spectroscopic techniques include ultraviolet and visible spectroscopy (UV), infrared spectroscopy (IR), mass spectroscopy (MS), nuclear magnetic spectroscopy (NMR), etc.

IV. Physical Evaluation

In crude drug evaluation specially unorganized drugs, physical methods play a significant role in identification and assessment of the quality of crude drugs. It includes the solubility, specific gravity, optical rotation, viscosity, refractive index, melting point, moisture content, degree of fibre elasticity, and other physical characteristics of the herbal raw materials.

(i) Solubility: The solubility of drugs stands with a specific behavior towards solvents, which have a high impact and consideration. Such parameter is always useful especially for the examination of oils and oleoresins.

Table 1.14 Examples of drugs soluble in specific solvents

Drugs	Solvent
Colophony	Light petroleum
Balsam of Peru	Chloral hydrate Equal volume of alcohol, 90%,
Castor oil	Half its volume of light petroleum Three volumes of 90% alcohol,
Alkaloidal bases and salts	Organic solvents and polar solvents

(ii) Optical Rotation: Optical rotation is a phenomenon where one enantiomer from sample, a chiral molecule can rotate the orientation of plane-polarized light characteristically an anisotropic crystalline substance. Such substances are said to be optically active, rotates either clockwise (dextrorotatory (*d*) or (+) enantiomer) or anticlockwise (levorotatory (*l*) or (–) enantiomer) direction.

Table 1.15 Examples of drugs with different optical rotation

Drug	Optical rotations
Eucalyptus oil	0° to +10°
Honey	+3° to –15°
Chenopodium oil	+30° to –80°

(iii) Refractive Index (RI): RI states that when light travels at an angle between two different materials or mediums, their refractive indices determine the angle of transmission refraction of the light beam. RI varies based on the frequency of the light as well. This could be used as a parameter in evaluating the herbal drugs.

Table 1.16 Examples drugs with specific RI

Drugs	RI
Castor oil	1.4758 to 1.527
Clove oil	1.527 to 1.535

(iv) Specific Gravity: The ratio of the mass of a solid or liquid to the mass of an equal volume of distilled water at 4°C (39°F) or of a gas to an equal volume of air or hydrogen under prescribed conditions of temperature and pressure called, specific gravity. It is commonly known as relative density.

Table 1.17 Examples of drugs with different specific gravity

Drugs	Specific gravity (kg/m³)
Cottonseed oil	0.88-0.93
Coconut oil	0.925
Castor oil	0.95

(v) Viscosity: Viscosity is the resistance of a fluid to flow. This resistance acts against the motion of any solid object through the fluid and also against motion of the fluid itself past stationary obstacles. Viscosity of a liquid is constant at a given temperature and is an index of its composition.

Viscosity also acts internally on the fluid between slower- and faster-moving adjacent layers. Since it is constant at a given temperature, it is used as an evaluation parameter. *Example:* Pyroxylin kinematic viscosity, 1100-2450 centistokes.

(vi) Melting Point: The melting point of a solid is the temperature at which it changes its state from solid to liquid. Plant constituents have very sharp and constant melting points. As far as crude drugs are concerned, melting point range has been fixed due to mixed chemicals. The following drugs could be evaluated using this parameter; for example: 1) bees wax 62-65°C, 2) wool fat 34-44°C, 3) agar melts at 85°C, etc.

(vii) Moisture Content: The moisture content of a drug will be responsible for decomposition of crude drugs either producing chemical change or microbial growth. So the moisture content of a drug should be determined and controlled. The moisture content is determined by heating a drug at 105°C in an oven to a constant weight. Following are the examples of two crude drugs with their moisture content limit. Moisture content of digitalis and ergot should not be more than 5% w/w and 8% w/w, respectively.

(viii) Ultraviolet Light: Certain drugs fluoresce when the cut surface or the powder is exposed to ultraviolet radiation, and it is useful in the identification of those drugs. Some pieces of rhapontic, Indian, and Chinese rhubarb are very difficult to distinguish, and it is very difficult in powdered form, but examination in ultraviolet light gives such marked differences in fluorescence that the varieties can be easily distinguished from each other.

(ix) Ash Values: The ash value determination is useful for detecting low-grade products, exhausted drugs, and excess of sandy or earthy matter. Different types of ash values are used in detection of crude drugs like, total ash, acid-insoluble ash, water-soluble ash, and sulphated ash.

Total ash is useful in detecting the crude drugs that are mixed with various mineral substances like sand, soil, calcium oxalate, chalk powder, or other drugs with different inorganic contents to improve their appearance, as is done with nutmegs and ginger. The maximum temperature used for total ash should not be more than 450°C because alkali chlorides that may be volatile in higher temperatures would be lost.

Acid-insoluble ash means the ash insoluble in dilute hydrochloric acid. It is often of more value than the total ash. The majority of crude drugs contain calcium oxalate, and the quantity of calcium oxalate varies very frequently. So total ash of a crude drug also varies within wide limits for specimens of genuine drug. For example, rhubarb, total ash range from 8 to 40%.

In this case, the total ash is useless to detect earthy matter adherent to such a drug. So acid-insoluble ash would be preferable for rhubarb. The calcium oxide or carbonate, yielded by the incinerated oxalate, will be soluble in hydrochloric acid when the ash is treated with hydrochloric acid; the remaining ash is weighed, which is known as the acid-insoluble ash. By this it can detect the presence of excessive earthy matter, which is likely to occur with roots and rhizomes and with leaves which are densely pubescent, like those of foxglove, clothed with abundant trichomes secreting resin, as in henbane, and tend to retain earth matter splashed on to them during heavy rainstorms.

The water-soluble ash is used to detect the presence of material exhausted by water. Sulphated ash is done by addition of sulphuric acid in order to get sulphate salts, and the percentage ash is calculated with reference to the air-dried drug. The temperature used for this is above 600°C. The total ash and acid-insoluble ash values of Guduchi are not more than 16 and 3%, respectively. The total ash value and water-soluble ash values of ginger are 6 and 1.7%, respectively.

(x) **Extractive Values:** The extracts obtained by exhausting crude drugs with different solvents are approximate measures of their chemical constituents. Various solvents are used according to the type of the constituents to be analysed. Water-soluble extractive is used for crude drugs containing water-soluble constituents like glycosides, tannins, mucilage, etc.; alcohol-soluble extractive is used for crude drugs containing tannins, glycosides, resins, etc.; and ether-soluble extractives are used for drugs containing volatile constituents and fats.

Table 1.18 Examples of drugs with their extractive values

Extractive values	Examples
Water-soluble extractive	Aloe (NLT 25.0%), Glycyrrhiza (NLT 20%)
Alcohol-soluble extractives	Aloe (NLT 10%), Asafoetida (NLT 50%)
Ether-soluble extractives	Linseed (NLT 25%), Capsicum (NLT 12%)

(xi) **Foreign Organic Matters:** The parts of the organ or organs other than those parts of drugs mentioned in the definition and description of the drug are known as foreign organic matters. They may be insect, moulds, earthy material, animal excreta, etc. Each and every vegetable drug has own limits.

Few examples of such limits are:

Table 1.19 Examples of drugs with limitation of organic content

Drugs	Limit
Garlic	Not more than (NMT) 2%
Saffron	Not more than (NMT) 2%
Satavari	Not more than (NMT) 1%

V. *Biological evaluation*

The pharmacological or therapeutic activity, potency and toxicity of plant or plant extracts can be evaluated by various biological methods conferred as biological evaluation of crude drugs. It can provide more significant results better than physical or chemical method of evaluation of such drugs which cannot be quantified by other means.

The bioassay methods are of three types they are:

(a) In vivo (toxic, symptomatic effect)
(b) In vitro (isolated tissue or organ methods)
(c) Microbiological.

Different animals are used in in vivo assay method for evaluation of toxic (lethal dose) and symptomatic effects of crude drugs whereas, in vitro methods are used with isolated organ or tissues for evaluation of therapeutic actions, i.e., potency, toxicity and dose. Both these assays are conducted by determining the amount of drug of known potency required to produce a definite effect on suitable test animals or organs under standard conditions. Reference standards are used in certain bioassay procedures to minimize errors.

Table 1.20 Examples of animal source of drugs with therapeutic value

Therapeutic activity and assay	Animal used
Oxytocic activity (vasopressin injecton)	Guinea pigs
Depressor activity	Cat
Mydriatic effects of drugs	Cat's eye, rabbit's eye
Anthelmintic activity	Worms
Cardiac and gastrointestinal activities	Dog
Assay for oxytocic injection	Young domestic chicken
Assay for digitalis glycosides	Pigeons

Other biological activities include hepatoprotective activity, hypoglycaemic activity, anti-inflammatory activity, antiulcer activity, immunomodulatory activity, etc.

The third type is microbiological assays which are carried out to determine the effects and dose of drug in various microorganisms, best known for determination of antimicrobial potentials. Not only antimicrobial potentials it can be used for assaying of various amino acids and vitamins by using different bacteria, yeast and moulds, etc.

EXERCISE

1. Define pharmacognosy. Write the scopes of pharmacognosy.
2. Write an overview of chronological developments in pharmacognosy.
3. Define crude drugs, and describe its various sources.
4. Describe the various methods of crude drug classification and their merits and demerits.
5. Define adulteration. Describe its various types with suitable examples.
6. Describe various methods of crude drug evaluation.
7. Explain in details the biological evaluation of crude drugs.
8. Briefly describe the physical evaluation of crude drugs with suitable examples.
9. Differentiate between organised and unorganised crude drugs with suitable examples.
10. Differentiate between gums and mucilage with suitable examples.
11. Explain chemotaxonomical and serotaxonomical classification of crude drugs. Give their merits and demerits.
12. Enlist the leaf constants with suitable examples.
13. What is extractive value? Explain its significance.
14. What is ash value and its significance? Write the procedure of ash value determination.
15. Explain the method and its significance of lycopodium spore method for quantitative microscopical evaluation of crude drugs.

UNIT II

Cultivation, Collection, Processing and Storage of Drugs of Natural Origin

Objectives

- To illustrate the techniques of medicinal plant cultivation, conservation and processing of crude drugs.
- To understand the concept in genetic pattern of cultivation.
- To describe the cultivation, collection, processing and storage of drugs of natural origin.

2.1. INTRODUCTION

Crop planning is done through cultivation. Growing medicinal plants involves rigorous supervision and attention, depending on the grade of medicinal plant components needed, different growing conditions and time. It can stabilize its supply, which prevents the problem of raw material scarcity for sectors that depend on crude pharmaceuticals. The cultivation of a crude medicine assures consistent supply. The crude pharmaceuticals must be processed before being marketed. Drugs are prepared for transit and storage stability as well as to guarantee that no replacements or extraneous organic material is present. It is frequently a crucial technique for preserving the health of the soil, reducing the growth of weeds, and promoting crop growth.

2.1.1 Cultivation of Drugs of Natural Origin

The quality improvement of plants may happen with cultivation process. Cultivation helps in the selection of plant species, plant varieties or hybrids which have desired phytoconstituents. Controlled environmental growth might be the reason of altered phytochemicals in plant varieties. Even though, obtain better plant products, cultivation also eases the process of collection and further processing steps as compared to wild varieties. Cultivated plants offer maximum secondary metabolites. Hence, cultivation of medicinal plants provides sustainability of raw materials to the medicine industries which turns rapid industrialization in the country. Not only economic growth, it also promotes medicinal plant research as well.

The Advantages of Cultivation of Medicinal Plants as Follows

1. Quality and purity of medicinal plants can be ensured. Highest crude drug quality can be obtained by maintaining operational uniformity throughout the process of cultivation. Furthermore, the contamination of crude drugs can be conveniently avoided by keeping the cultivated plants weeds free.

For example, adequate quantity of fertilizers and proper irrigation would maximize the quality of rhizomes during cultivation.

Medicinal crop with maximum content of volatile oil and other constituents is the collaborative result of systematic cultivation. The best relevant examples are ginger, turmeric and liquorice.

2. Cultivated plants are therapeutically and economically more sound in terms of yield and therapeutic potentials. High yield and therapeutic qualities are maintained in cultivated plants once the crude drugs collection for market is done by skilled and experienced personnel only.

   For example, collection of latex from poppy capsules and oleo resins from *Pinus* species, collection of tea leaves from tea plants, etc.

   Retention of green colour of senna leaves during processing and minimization of cardiac glycosides deterioration in freshly collected leaves of digitalis, etc.
3. Sustainable supply of raw medicinal plant materials would be ensured with cultivation of medicinal plants. It is a method of crop planning which would further regularize its supply chain. As a result, the herbal based industries do not struggle for raw materials in industrial process.
4. In the way of promoting industrialization, and economic boost, the medicinal and aromatic plants cultivation also hold the vital role. For examples:
   - Coffee and cocoa cultivation in Kerala has given rise to several cottage and small scale industries.
   - Cinchona cultivation in West Bengal has led to the establishment of the cinchona-alkaloid factory near Darjeeling.
   - Cultivation of poppy by government owned opium factory at Ghaziabad is an eloquent testimony.
5. Another advantageous part of medicinal plant cultivation is the application of modern technological aspects such as mutation, polyploidy and hybridization, etc., in modern-day cultivation process.

2.1.2 Collection of Drugs of Natural Origin

The most important step after cultivation of medicinal plant is collection process. This process holds the key for quality retention in medicinal harvested materials. Collection of plant materials depends upon individual expertize of collector even also drugs are collected from wild source. Cultivated medicinal drugs should be collected scientifically when they contain maximum amount of phytoconstituents. Very important aspect of plant collection is the collecting season at which the amount, and nature, of the active constituents would be in high node. Even though, phytoconstituents keep on changing more or less throughout the year.

For example, rhubarb is collected only in summer seasons because no anthraquinone derivatives would be present in winter season but anthranols are converted to anthraquinones during summer.

Another most important aspect in collection process is the age of the plant. Because it not only governs the total amount of active constituents produced in the plants but also adopts the proportions of the constituents of the active mixture.

For example, a young plant of peppermint contains high proportion of pulegone which can be replaced by menthone and menthol over the age.

Percentage of alkaloids in datura species reduces as the plant ages.

Some interconversions in plant metabolites may happen during day and night. The alteration of chemical composition of few secondary plant metabolites also varies throughout the day and night. That's the reason; the time of collection of plant materials is very essential parameter in collection process. During collection process, special attention has to be given for rejection of discoloured drugs or drugs which were affected by any kind of insects.

Table 2.1 Collection of various parts of medicinal plants

Parts of plants	Time of collection	Examples
Leaves	Just before the flowering season	Vasaka, Digitalis,
Flowers	Before expand fully	Clove, Saffron
Underground organs	Aerial parts of plant cells die	Liquorice, Rauwolfia
Fruits	After their full maturity or ripe	Fennel, Coriander
Barks	Spring season	Cinnamon, Cinchona
Unorganized drugs	As soon as they oozes out	Resins, Latex, Gums

Not only the time or sessional variation can impact the phytochemicals in medicinal plants but the collection methods also have high impact in quality retention of medicinal plants. For example, barks are usually separate from the wood during this spring season and should be collected by using three techniques. They are:

1. **Felling technique:** Where bark is peeled off after cutting the tree at base.
2. **Uprooting technique:** Underground roots are dug out and barks are collected from branches and roots.
3. **Coppicing technique:** Plant is cut one meter above the ground level and barks are removed.

2.1.3 Harvesting Drugs of Natural Origin

Medicinal plant harvesting is an essential step of medicinal plant cultivation process. Such operation reflects the economic gain of crude drugs. Most importantly, this stage is specific for the type of drug to be harvested and specifies pharmacopoeial standard which has to be achieved. Proper harvesting of medicinal plants can be achieved with skilled workers. The selection of accurate plant part for harvestment is more advantageous in crude drugs other than genuineness but simultaneously rejection of similar appearance drugs at the site of collection is strongly recommended.

The harvesting of medicinal plant parts may be done by two ways based on the type of plant parts to be harvest. It includes:

Physical method
Mechanical method, however, both are laborious and less economical.

1. ***Physical method:*** Certain plant parts like digitalis leaves, tea leaves, vinca leaves, senna leaves, etc., cannot be harvested by mechanical method because of its specific selective parts which is only possible by physical means. The beating plant with bamboos is used in case of clove buds.
2. ***Mechanical method:*** On the other hand, underground drugs like roots, rhizomes, tubers, etc., are harvested by mechanical devices, such as diggers or lifters, whereas, all aerial parts of medicinal plants are harvested by the help of binders.
   Moreover, flowers, seeds and small fruits are harvested by the device called seed stripper. The brushing technique has been applied for cochineal insects which are collected from branches of cacti. Agar producing seaweeds are harvested by long handled forks. Mowers are utilized for harvesting peppermint and spearmint plants, whereas fennel, coriander and caraway plants are uprooted and dried. Fruits are separated by winnowing process after drying. Sometimes, reaping machines are also used for their harvesting.

2.1.4 Drying of Drugs from Natural Origin

Pre-marketing of medicinal crude drugs has to undergo processing for acquisition of pharmaceutical elegance and better shelf-life for long storage. It includes several processes or treatments, depending upon the chemical nature and source (i.e., animal or plant) of crude drugs.

Removal of moisture from crude drugs is generally termed *drying*. This process improves the quality of crude drugs and makes them microorganisms growth resistant. It can prevent the spoilage of crude drugs by inhibiting partially enzymatic reactions. It also facilitates the mechanical approaches like pulverizing or grinding process of crude drugs.

Usually, some crude drugs required some special methods to attain specific pharmacopeial standards. For example:

Slicing and cutting into smaller pieces is done for the drugs like glycyrrhiza, squill and calumba to enhance drying process. Moreover flowers are dried in shade for retention of natural colour and volatile principals (volatile oils).

Basically, the drying method can be finalized for crude drugs depending upon the type of chemical constituents present on it and heat source or energy utilization. The former being done under the influence of solar energy or wind and the later by the application of artificial heat under controlled conditions of temperature, humidity and air flow.

Drying can be of two types:

1. Natural drying method
2. Mechanical or artificial drying method

(1) Natural drying methods

Natural drying may be either direct exposure to sunlight or sun-drying or indirect or sun-drying. For retention of natural colour of the crude drugs like the leave of digitalis, clove, senna, etc., or in case of retention of volatile principles in the drugs like peppermint, eucalyptus, etc., preferred drying in shed drying process.

On the other hand, if the contents of the drugs are quite stable to the temperature and sunlight, the drugs can be dried directly in sunshine like gum acacia, seeds, fruits, etc.

Different types of natural drying of drugs:

(a) Air drying

(b) Sun drying

(a) Air Drying: Air drying of crude drugs is done by hanging it on roof of shade houses or spreading as thin layers on floor. When sunlight causes discolouration or warping/ shrivelling shade dry it in specialized shade houses. While drying in shade houses or drying frames stirring or turning has to be done frequently to avoid mould formation. For getting adequate air circulation the drying frames should be located at a sufficient height above the ground and sufficient space has to be provided in between two shelves of frames. This method of drying is purely weather dependent, even pre-harvest as well as post-harvest weather conditions can affect the quality of dried produce and its drying behaviour.

For example, high quality caraway oil contains high carvone and low limonene content in shade dried caraway leaves. In *Salvia officinalis*, the phytochemicals like 1,8-cineole and camphor found decreases, where β-thujone and β-pinene content increases but, trans-caryophyllene concentration remains constant even after drying. When *Rosemarinus officinalis* air dried, phytochemicals, i.e., α-pinene, limonene, camphor, etc., decreases but camphene and β-pinene concentration increases significantly.

(b) Sun Drying: This method is suitable for those crude drugs that are not adversely affected by excessive sunlight. Sun drying is usually done by spreading the collected crude drugs as thin layer on floor or in drying frames under open sun. This method is exclusively weather dependent even more; the raw materials can get damaged by birds, insects, pathogens, wind-blown debris, etc., while drying. Volatalisation may hamper the quality of drying materials too. Also, uniform drying is not always possible by sun drying which favours microbial growth and production of aflatoxins (fungal toxin). Sun drying requires more space and labour as well as time up to days or even weeks.

(2) Mechanical / Artificial Drying

Rapid process of moisture removal or drying of crude drugs by artificially. Different types of artificial drying are:

(a) By oven; i.e., tray dryers

(b) Vacuum dryers

(c) Spray dryers

(d) Tunnel dryer

(e) Fluidised bed dryers

(f) Microwave dryer

(g) Infrared radiation dryer

(a) Tray dryers (Oven): Thermo-stable and negligible or lowest contents of volatile principles drugs or which need deactivation of enzymes are dried in conventional tray dryers. This process is facilitated with instrumentation (hot air oven) where hot air of the desired temperature is circulated through the dryers and quick removal of water content form drugs takes place. For example, various parts of the plant like belladonna roots, cinchona bark, tea and raspberry leaves and gums, etc., are dried by adopting this method.

(b) **Vacuum dryers:** Thermo-labile crude drugs which are sensitive to higher temperature are preferably dried by this process.

Examples: Tannic acid and digitalis leaves are dried by vacuum drying.

(c) **Spray dryers:** This method is comparatively more expensive than other previously mentioned methods. Certain drugs are highly sensitive to atmospheric conditions. Even though, they cannot withstand the temperature of vacuum drying. Such drugs are preferred dried by spray drying method. The technique is followed for economically important plant or animal constituents, rather than the crude drugs for quick drying.

Examples: Papaya latex, pectin, tannins, etc.

(d) **Tunnel Dryer:** Tunnel dryers are composed of a few elongated cabinets. The tray or carts containing raw crude drugs which can be dried are passed through the cabinet of tunnel dryer and hot air is blown opposite to these trays under controlled conditions (temperature, humidity, and air flow).

The standard optimized drying parameters for complete drying of mint leaves for commercial production are 0.26 mm layer thickness and a temperature of 45-65°C for a period of 4 to 6.5 hours.

(e) **Fluidised Bed Dryer:** This equipment is more sophisticated . Heated air is blown up from the bottom of a cylindrical cabin through the crude drugs which is contained in it, with just enough force to suspend the particles in a gentle bowling motion. The heated air is actually introduced through a porous plate that supports the raw material and the moist air is exhausted at top and is a continuous process. This method is applicable for more economically important plant or animal constituents, rather than the crude drugs.

Example: Mint.

(f) **Microwave Dryer:** Microwave dryer is a new addition to the existing drying techniques. Microwaves are a form of electromagnetic energy with frequencies that lie between 300 MHz and 300 GHz, generated by magnetrons under the combined force of an electric and a magnetic field perpendicular to each other. During microwave drying, the water molecules of the product to be dried readily absorb this energy, which is converted to heat. Thus, the water vaporizes and diffuses through the product to the surface. Microwave drying is more efficient than conventional hot air drying and 95-98% faster.

Example: Drying of Aswagandha roots (microwave power of 6W, 60°C).

(g) **Infrared Radiation Dryer:** It works on the principle of infrared radiation. Hot bodies such as quartz, silica, etc., are able to emit infrared rays when heated to a high temperature and can penetrate the crude drugs, vapourise the moisture and make the produce dried.

Like the microwave dryer it has a cabinet to hold the raw material and infrared radiation is projected from the heat source arranged above the trays of the product.

Infrared drier provides significantly higher amount of essential oil in peppermint when compared to microwave drying. Microwave and infrared radiation drying are confined for small-scale production of dried crude drugs.

2.1.5 Garbling (Dressing)

It is the next step forward after drying of crude drugs towards the preparation for market. When the non-desired substances are necessary to remove from the crude drugs, i.e., dirt, foreign organic parts of the same plant, not constituting drug substances, etc., there the process of garbling is anticipated. The extraneous matter or foreign organic matter is removed by several ways and practicable at the site of the preparation of the crude drugs. Non-removal of such extraneous matter from crude drugs will lead compromise in the quality and create obstacle to pharmacopoeial standard of limits.

Examples:

(a) In lobelia, stramonium, the excessive stems and in cloves, stalks are needed to be removed.
(b) Drugs constituting rhizomes need to be separated carefully from roots and rootlets and also stem bases.
(c) Pieces of bark should be removed by peeling as in gum acacia.
(d) Pieces of iron must be removed with the magnet in case of castor seeds before crushing.

2.1.6 Packing of Crude Drugs

Appropriate packing of crude drugs is always desired to retain the morphological and chemical nature of drug.

Even special consideration is continually essential to retain its ultimate use and effects of climatic conditions during transportation and storage.

Few crude drugs and their packing considerations are described below.

Table 2.2 Crude drugs packed with the different packaging material

Name of crude drugs	Packaging
Aloe	Packed in goat skin
Colophony and balsam of Tolu	Packed in kerosene tins
Asafoetida	Stored in well closed containers to prevent loss of volatile oil
Cod liver oil	Should be stored in such containers, which will not have effect of sunlight
Senna, vinca	Pressed and baled
Cinnamon bark	Packed one inside the other quill, so as to facilitate transport and to prevent volatilization of oil from the drug

Packing of costly and moisture sensitive drugs like digitalis, ergot and squill has to pay special attention as they are very susceptible to microbial contamination. Hence, the chemicals which absorb excessive moisture (desiccating agents) from the drug are incorporated in the containers to counter this problem. Auto-oxidation may be prevented during packing of colophony once it is packed in big masses. Cinnamon bark, which is available in the form of quills, is packed one inside the other quill, so as to facilitate transport and to prevent volatilization of oil from the drug.

In case of some organized drugs like roots, seeds, etc., may not need special packing attention. They can be packed in gunny bags, while in some cases bags are coated with polythene internally.

2.1.7 Storage of Crude Drugs

The knowledge about physical and chemical properties of crude drugs is useful in preservation process during storage conditions. The quality of drugs can be retained with proper preservation methods.

Generally, in well closed and possibly filled containers is advised for crude drug storage. Such containers must be stored in the premises which are water-proof, fire-proof and rodent-proof.

Natural crude drugs usually absorb the moisture in storage (extent up to of 25% of their weight) which makes them highly sensitive against microbial contamination or microbial growth. It not only bulk the drug also impairs the quality of crude drugs. It decomposes the drugs by initiating enzymatic degradation in active constituents on crude drugs. The best example is digitalis leaves and wild cherry bark. Few more examples are listed below with their cause of degradation of bioactives.

Table 2.3 Examples of drugs which causes bioactive degradation

Crude drugs	Causes of bioactive constituents degradation
Gentian and ergot	Mould infestation due to excessive moisture.
Ergot, cod liver oil and digitalis	Destruction of active chemical constituents due to direct sun-light containing radiation.
Squill, when stored in powdered form	Hygroscopic and forms rubbery mass on prolonged exposure to air.
Colophony powder form	Rapidly oxidized in normal conditions.

Entire form or mass of colophony can be stored for long time without degradation but when the same is stored in powdered form, it rapidly oxidizes in normal conditions. Even colophony in powdered form loses solubility in ether. As like colophony, powdered ergot containing fixed oil also shows rancidity on storage. It can be prevented if ergot is defatted with lipid solvent prior to storage. Sain benzoin can be added during storage of lard (purified internal fat of the abdomen of the hog).

Storage containers play a crucial role in drug storage. Atmospheric oxygen induces oxidation to several drugs during storage. Hence, such drugs should be filled completely in well closed containers. Nowadays, inert gas like nitrogen can be used for replacement of atmospheric oxygen during storage of drugs to avoid oxidation.

For example,storage of shark liver oil, papain, etc., small quantities of crude drugs could be readily stored in air-tight, moisture-proof and light-proof containers such as tin, cans, covered metal tins, or amber glass containers, etc. Wooden boxes and paper bags should not be used for storage of crude drugs.

Protection from living infecting things is also as important as its physico-chemical degradation. Different types of infectious living things like insects, nematodes, worms, moulds, mites, etc., may infest the crude drugs during storage.

List of infectious organisms and their biological names are given below.

Table 2.4 Examples of organism with biological source

Name of the pest	Biological name
Coleoptera	*Stegobium paniceum, Calandrum granarium*
Lepidoptera	*Ephestia kuehniella, Tinea pellionella*
Archnida or mites	*Tyroglyphus farinae, Glyophagus domesticus*

Such pest infestation can be prevented or minimized by proper drying of crude drugs or pre-treatment with suitable fumigants (methyl bromide, carbon disulphide, hydrocyanic acid, etc.) before storage. Currently, some special techniques are adopted for better storage of crude drugs such as liming of the ginger, coating of nutmeg, etc.

One of the most important aspects in drug storage is temperature. Temperature alteration leads to decomposition of the chemical constituents in crude drugs by accelerating several chemical reactions within. Hence, most of the drugs are vulnerable to temperature change. Such drugs need to be preserved at refrigerated temperature in well closed containers. Even though, low temperature also inhibits the growth of microorganisms in the stored materials.

2.1.8 Factors Influencing the Cultivation of Medicinal Plants

Cultivated plants are more advantageous than the wild grown plants in various aspects of quality. Certain essential factors play a commendable role behind the overall growth and development of plants. Even though, the nature, quality and quantity of plant secondary metabolites also depend on such factors.

Such affecting factors include:

1. Altitude
2. Temperature
3. Rainfall
4. Length of day, day light
5. Atmosphere humidity
6. Soil and soil fertility
7. Fertilizers and pests
8. Pests and pests control, etc.

1. **Altitude:** The altitude / elevation from sea level is one of the important factors influencing cultivation of medicinal plants. With the increase in altitude, the temperature and atmospheric pressure decreases while the wind velocity, relative humidity and light intensity increases. Thus, as the climatic conditions change with height, they also produce changes in the vegetation pattern. Short wave solar radiation increases with altitude while air temperatures usually, but not always, falls. For many hours of the day at high elevation the maximum solar radiation may indeed be well above the saturation levels for photosynthesis of C_3 plants (C_3 plants include the cereals barley, oats, rice, and wheat, alfalfa (lucerne), cotton, Eucalyptus, sunflower, soybeans, sugar beets, potatoes, tobacco, chlorella, etc., nearly about

85% of plant species on the earth). The direct observation includes the bitter principles of *Gentiana lutea* and Pyrethrum increases with high altitude and the alkaloids and oil contents of thyme and peppermint of *Aconitum nacelles* and *Lobelia inflate* gradually decrease, etc.

Table 2.5 Examples of plants grows in different altitude

Plant	Altitude
Tea	9500-1500 metres
Cinnamon, cardamom	500-1000 metres
Saffron	Up to 1250 metres
Eucalyptus	1000–2000 metres
Coffee	1000–2000 metres
Clove	Up to 1250 metres
Cinchona	1000–2000 metres

2. **Temperature:** Plant growth, metabolism and the yield of plant secondary metabolites are deeply controlled or affected with temperature. Each plant species has adapted its own natural environment for best growth with a considerable range of temperature. Many common plants grow better in temperate regions during summer, but they lack in resistance to withstand frost in winter. The sudden decrease in temperature causes the formation of the ice crystals in intercellular spaces of the plant. As a result, water comes out of the cells and ultimately plants die due to drought and desiccation. The ice crystals also cause mechanical injury to the cells, temperature stimulates the growth of seedlings. Water absorption decreases at low temperatures. The rate of photosynthesis is affected by change in temperature. The rate of respiration increases with increase in temperature.

Table 2.6 Examples of plants require optimum temperature

Plant	Optimum temperature (°F)
Cinchona	58-73°F
Coffee	55-70°F
Tea	75-90°F
Cardamom	50-100°F

3. **Rainfall:** Rainfall is required for proper measurement for development of plants and falls under the most important factor influencing cultivation of medicinal plants. Some cases like Xerophytic plants do not require irrigation or rainfall (example, aloes).The annual rainfall throughout the year and water holding soil capacity are considerable aspects. Difference in rainfall leads to variation in plant constituents . On one side, excessive rainfall could cause a reduction in the secondary metabolites by leaching water soluble substances from the plants and on the other side lack of rainfall influences morphological and physiology of plants.

Rainfall and snowfall have a large effect the climate condition. The minerals in the soil get dissolved in water and are then absorbed by plants.

Examples: Glycoside and alkaloids producing plants on continuous rain can lead to a loss of water-soluble substance from leaves and root by leaching.

4. **Day length and day light:** For plants, light is the only external source of energy which influences the process of photosynthesis, opening and closing of stomata, plant movements, seed germination, flowering, vegetative growth, etc. The day length has a well proven effect over the metabolites production in medicinal plants. The plants that are kept in long day conditions may contain more constituents as compared to the plants kept in short day. The amount and intensity of the light, both are required for development of plants. Even the type of radiation too has an effect over the development and metabolites of plants.

   For example, peppermint produces menthone, menthol and traces of mentho-furan in long day conditions and only mentho-furan in short day condition. Dry sunny weather increases the proportion of glycosides in digitalis and alkaloids in belladonna plant, even the same was observed in stramonium and cinchona too.
5. **Atmosphere humidity:** The atmospheric humidity generally presents in the form of water vapours and the clouds and fog are the visible forms of humidity. The evaporated water vapour from earth surface is the major sources of atmospheric humidity. The major effect of humidity on plant life and climate is transpiration. Evaporation of water, its condensation and precipitation depends upon relative humidity and humidity affects structure, form and transpiration in plants.
6. **Soil and soil fertility:** Surface layer of the earth is defined as soil which is formed by the climate factors like weathering of rocks, plants and microorganisms. The soil for cultivation of medicinal plants should contain appropriate amounts of nutrients, organic matter and other elements to ensure optimal medicinal plant growth and quality. Soil also provides mechanical support, along with water and essential foods (macro- and micro-elements) for the development of plants. Optimal soil conditions, including soil type, drainage, moisture retention, fertility and pH, are dictated by the selected medicinal plant species and/or target medicinal plant parts.

   The soil is basically made up of five components, i.e.,

   (i) Mineral matter
   (ii) Soil air
   (iii) Soil water
   (iv) Humus
   (v) Soil organisms, etc.

   Soil influences seed germination, capacity of plant to remain erect, form, vigour and woodiness of the stem, depth of root system, number of flowers on a plant, drought, frost, etc.

   The water holding capacity of water is generally influenced by the soil particle size and also same is used to differentiate the soil types, ranging from clay, sand, gravel, etc. The type and amount of minerals play a vital role in medicinal plants cultivation.

Table 2.7 Different types of soil with particle size

Type of soil	Particle size (in mm)
Fine clay soil	Less than 0.002
Coarse clay or silt soil	0.002-0.02
Fine sand	0.02-0.2
Coarse sand	0.2-2.0

Even though, some plants are capable enough to determine their own soil pH range for their best growth. In this context, the contribution of various soil microbes should be taken into consideration which grow well at certain pH and show symbiotic action.

For example, calcium favours the growth of certain plants whereas with some plants it does not produce any effects. Nitrogen containing soil increases production of alkaloidal content in some medicinal plants.

Soil Fertility is defined as the capacity of soil to provide adequate quantity and balanced proportion of nutrients to plants. It gets lost in case of cropping done without fortification of soil with plant nutrients. It also diminishes through leaching and erosion.

Soil fertility can be maintained by addition of animal manures, nitrogen-fixing bacteria or by application of chemical fertilizers.

7. **Fertilizer and manures:** To keep the soil fertility, fertilizer and manures have a vital role in medicinal plants cultivation.

The fertilizers are two types:

1. Biological origin fertilizer.
2. Synthetic fertilizers/chemical fertilizer

1. Biological origin fertilizer: Soil is generally poor in organic matter and nitrogen. The substances of biological origin used as fertilizer, manures are thus selected if these could provide the elements required for fortification of soil. They are two types.

(i) Manures: Manure is material, which is mixed with soil. These supply almost all the nutrients required by the crop plants. This results in the increase in crop productivity. Castor seed cake, poultry manures, neem and *karanj* seed cakes vermicompost, etc., are examples of manures. Oil-cake and compost normally consist of 3-6% of nitrogen, 2% phosphates and 1-1.5% potash. Bone meal, fish meal, biogas slurry, blood meal and press mud are the other forms of organic fertilizers.

Manures are three types:

(a) **Farmyard manure:** This is a mixture of cattle dung and remaining unused parts of straw and plant stalks fed to cattle.

(b) Composited manure: This is a mixture of rotten or decomposed and useless parts of plants and animals.

(c) Green manures: It is an herbaceous crop ploughed and mixed with the soil while still green to enrich the soil. The plants used as green manure are often quick growing. These add both organic as well as nitrogen to the soil. It also forms a protective soil cover that checks soil erosion and leaching. Thus, the crop yield increases by 30-50%.

(ii) Biofertilizer: It can be defined as biologically active products or bacteria, algae and fungi which are useful in bringing about soil nutrient enrichment. These mostly include nitrogen fixing microorganisms. Some of the biofertilizers are mentioned below.

(i) Legume: Rhizobium symbiosis
(ii) Azolla: Anabaena symbiosis.
(iii) Free-living bacteria.
(iv) Loose association of nitrogen-fixing bacteria.
(v) Cyanobacteria (blue-green algae).
(vi) Mycorrhizae.

2. **Synthetic fertilizers/Chemical fertilizers:** Plants during metabolic process towards synthesizing various biocompounds need essential sixteen macro- and micro-nutrient elements. Macro-nutrients are categorized into two types. Primary nutrients, i.e., nitrogen, phosphorus, potassium and magnesium, calcium and sulphur are required in small quantities and hence, they are known as secondary nutrients.

   Trace elements like copper, manganese, iron, boron, molybdenum, zinc are also necessary for plant growth are known as micronutrients. Carbon, hydrogen, oxygen and chlorine are provided from water and air. Every element performs some specific function in growth and development of plants. Their deficiency is also characterized by certain symptoms. Some examples of such chemical fertilizers are urea and potash.

8. **Pests and pest control techniques:** Pests are the undesired plant or living species which cause huge loss or hamper medicinal plants cultivation.

Various types of pest include:

(a) Microorganisms
(b) Insects
(c) Non-insect weeds, etc.

(a) Microorganisms: Microbial infections due to the presence of various microbes are one of the important factors in medicinal plants growth. The causative microbs includes fungi, bacteria and viruses.

For example, Armillaria root rot, a fungal infection caused by *Armillaria mellea,* belongs to the family of Marasmiaceae characterized by weak, shorter shoots. Such infected plants become nonproductive and have short longevity (dies within two to four years).

Another example is Summer Bunch Rot, which is also a fungal disease in which masses of black, brown, or green spores develop on the surface of infected berries. *Aspergillus niger, Alternaria tennis, Botrytis cinerea, Cladosporium herbarum, Rhizopus arrhizus, Penicillium* sp., etc., are known for such infection. Some more fungal diseases and causative fungus are mentioned below.

Table 2.8 Examples of causative fungus

Causative microorganism	Diseases
Fomitopsis pinicola	Red-belted fungus
Pythium pinosurn	Pythium rhizome rot
Septoria digitalis	Leaf spot
Phywphthora cinnamomi	Little leaf
Agrobacterium tumefaciens	Crown gall

Pierce's disease is caused by bacterium *Xylella fastidiosa*. In this infection plant leaves become slightly yellow, margins are dry and eventually plants die.

Some viral infectious diseases cause necrosis of leaves, petioles and stems of medicinal plants and hampers the natural healthy growth of plants. Such viruses are tobacco mosaic virus, mosaic virus, cucumber mosaic virus, tobacco ring spot virus, yellow vein mosaic, etc.

Controlling techniques: There are various methods to control such microbial diseases such as chemical fumigation of soil, use of fungicide or bactericide, pruning, proper water and fertilizer management, heat treatment of planting stock, cut and remove the infected parts, genetic engineering (fungi and bacteria resistant plant), etc.

(b) Insects: Other insects like ants (*Linepithema humile, Formica aerate, Formica perpilosa, Tetramorium caespitum*, etc.) spoil the soil by making nests and they feed honey dew secreted in plants. Branch and Twig Borer *(Melalgus confertus)* burrow into the canes through the base of the bud or into the crotch formed by the shoot and spur cause the twist and break stems of infected plants. The click beetle *(Limonius canus)* can feed on buds. Leafhoppers *(Erythroneura elegantuhi, Erythroneum variabilis)* remove the contents of leaf cells that appear as pale yellow spots.

Controlling techniques: Various methods are used for controlling the insect population for the benefit of plant cultivation. Such techniques include tilling the soil, collection and destruction of eggs, larvae, pupae and adults of insects, trapping the insects, use of insecticides, etc.

(c) Non-insect pests: Non-insect pests are basically divided into two categories, i.e., vertebrate and invertebrate pests. The premier one or vertebrates are those pests who disrupt the plants such as monkeys, rats, birds, squirrels, etc., and the former one are non-vertebrates like webspinning spider mites *(Tetranychus pacificus, Eotetranychus willamettei, Tetranychus urticae*, etc.*)* induce leaves discolouration and yellow spots.

Another category of pests are nematodes *(Meloidogyne incognita, Xiphinema americanum, Criconemella xenoplax*, etc.) which revise giant cell formation on plant, interrupt nutrients and water uptakes, and also interfere in plant growth.

Controlling techniques: Preventive measures can control such pest influence like construction of concrete warehouses, traps, biological methods, use of rodenticides, etc.

(d) **Weeds:** The influence of weeds in cultivation field highly impacts the growth and yield of medicinal plants. Weeds generally compete for the basic essential requirements such as water, nutrients, and sunlight with the growing plants. As a result, the desired plants suffer insufficiency of such vital elements which causes low yield. Hence, weed control may enhance the plant growth and optimize the yield.

The soil texture and its nutrient contents (organic matter) influence the weeds development. Like annual species such as puncturevine, crabgrass, horseweed, *Panicum* spp., etc., or perennials like johnsongrass, nutsedge, bermudagrass are more widespread on light-textured soil whereas curly dock, field bindweed, and dallisgrass are more common on heavy-textured soils.

Controlling techniques: Soil characteristics are important for weed management. The weeds can be controlled by use of low rates of herbicides which are active against germinating weed seeds (pre-emergent herbicides) or on growing plants (post-emergent herbicides) or both combined.

Miscellaneous Factors

(i) **Air Pollution:** Air pollution also influences the growth of plats to some extant. The air pollutants cause mortality and stunt in growth of medicinal plants. Even though, some deciduous and coniferous trees are very sensitive to certain pollutants, observe leaf injury as the first sign of pollution effect. Furthermore, spots between the veins, discolouration of leaf margin, tip burns are common symptoms of such pollution effect which also influences the host sensitivity and genetic characteristics in future.

(ii) **Herbicides:** Unwanted herbs are removed from cultivation area by using various herbicides to provide uninterrupted nutrition supply to the desired plant for optimized growth. But misapplication of herbicides can often damage non-target plants too. Through the exact amount of such damage is still unclear. Herbicides induce growth abnormalities (cupping or twisting of foliage), foliage yellowing or browning, defoliation or death. The herbicide injuries are variable in their symptoms may be due to their distinct mode of action, dosage, time of exposure, plant species or other environmental conditions.

2.2 PLANT HORMONES AND THEIR APPLICATIONS

Plant hormones or phytohormones are the biological substances which act as intercellular messengers in plant's life cycle. It includes overall growth regulations in plant including germination of seeds, rooting, flowering, ripening of fruits, foliage and even death. The hormone levels may change over the lifespan and also depend upon season and environment.

Such growth regulators are widely utilized in industrialized agriculture process to improve productivity. It allows synchronization of plant development. In this context, fruit ripening can be controlled with manipulating the desired atmospheric ethylene levels and allowing commercial plants to be ripened in storage during and after transportation. After all, it makes the harvesting process much more efficient and effective. On the other hand, growth regulators induce or suppress rooting of seedlings simultaneously in promotion of cell division in plant cell cultures.

Over all, the right combination of growth regulators is always vital to achieve the desired cellular behavioural characteristics and the productive development of plants. Plant growth regulators have greatest impact on plant tissue culture techniques to obtain therapeutically valuable *secondary metabolites*.

Characteristics of Plant Growth Regulator

Plant growth regulators can be of a diverse chemical composition such as gases (ethylene), terpenes (gibberellic acid) or carotenoid derivatives (abscisic acid). They are also referred to as plant growth substances, phytohormones or plant hormones. Based on their action, they are broadly classified as follows:

- **Plant growth promoters:** They promote cell division, cell enlargement, flowering, fruiting and seed formation. Examples are auxins, gibberellins and cytokinins.
- **Plant growth inhibitors:** These chemicals inhibit growth and promote dormancy and abscission in plants, for example, abscisic acid. Ethylene can be a promoter or an inhibitor, but is largely a plant growth inhibitor.

Classification of Plant Growth Regulator

The plant growth regulators are classified into two major classes, i.e., natural and synthetic. The natural regulators are also known as endogenous regulators and the synthetics are called the exogenous regulators.

Five major classes of plant hormones are:

1. Auxins
2. Cytokinins
3. Gibbereilins
4. Abscisic acid
5. Ethylene

Currently, more active biomolecules or regulators are being searched and found some new families of regulators. One of them is polyamines (putrescine or spermidine).

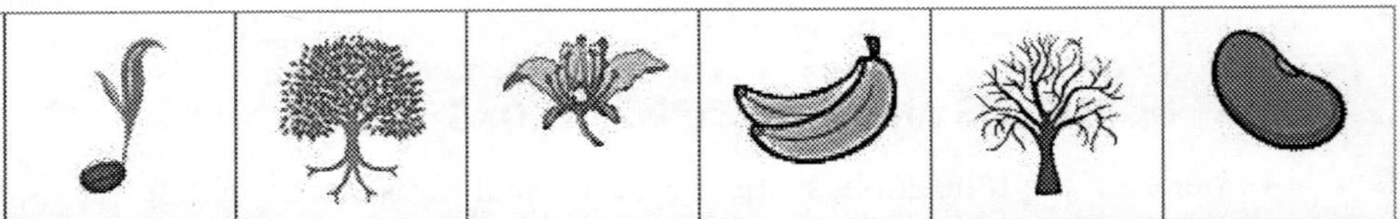

	Germination	Growth to Maturity	Flowering	Fruit Development	Abscission	Seed Dormancy
Gibberelin	✓	✓	✓	✓	×	×
Auxin	×	✓	✓	✓	×	×
Cytokinins	×	✓	✓	✓	×	×
Ethylene	×	×	✓	✓	✓	×
Abscisic acid	×	×	×	×	✓	✓

Fig. 2.1 Plant hormones and their physiological effects

1. *Auxins*

Auxins are plant hormones basically involved in plant-cell elongation, apical dominance, and rooting. The term 'auxin' derives from the Greek word 'auxein' which means 'to grow'. Generally, compounds are considered auxins if they are able to induce cell elongation in stems and otherwise resemble indoleacetic acid (well known natural auxin) in physiological activity.

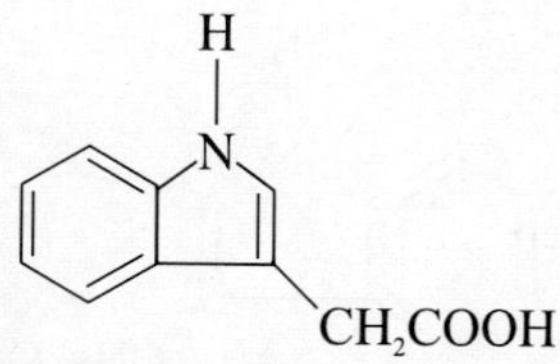

Fig. 2.2 Indole acetic acid

Discovery

The first growth hormone 'auxin's discovery goes to the observations of Charles Darwin and his son, Francis Darwin. They observed that the growth and bending of coleoptile (protective sheath) in canary grass is directed by the source of light. This phenomenon is popularly known as 'phototropism'. Their observations were described in the book *The Power of Movement in Plants* dated back in 1880. Even more such observations showed that the coleoptile tip was the site responsible for the bending. Salkowski discovered indole-3-acetic acid (IAA) in fermentation media in 1885. The isolation of the same product from plant tissues could not be found in plant tissues for almost 50 years. Finally, in 1926, the isolation of the first auxin was succeeded by F. W. Went from the coleoptile tip of oat seedlings. Later on, Kogl and Haagen-Smit, purified the compound auxentriolic acid (auxin A) from human urine in 1931 and isolated some other compounds similar in structure and function to auxin A from urine. In 1954 a committee of plant physiologists was set up to characterize the group of auxins.

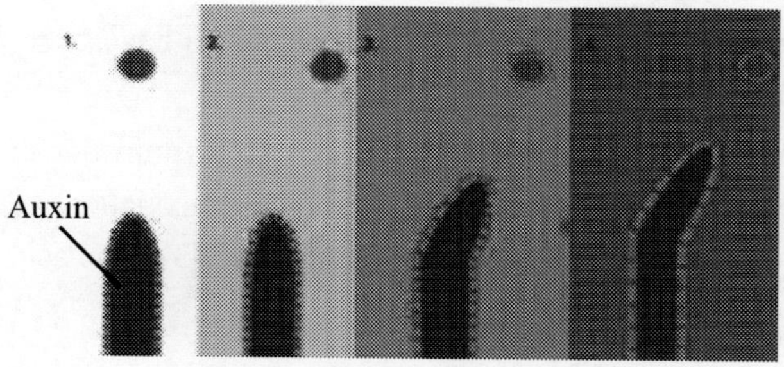

Fig. 2.3 Physiological changes of auxins

Table 2.9 Different types of auxin

Endogenous or natural	Exogenous or synthetic
Indole-3-acetic acid (IAA)	Indole-3-butyric acid (IBA)
Indole butyric acid (IBA)	α-napthyl acetic acid (NAA)
indole-3-acetonitrile (IAN)	2-napthyloxyacetic acid (NOA)
phenyl acetic acid (PAA)	1-napthyl acetamide (NAD)
4-chloroindole-3-acetic acid	5-carboxymeth-yl-N, N-dimethyl dithiocarbamate, 2,4-dichlorophenoxy acetic acid (2,4-D)

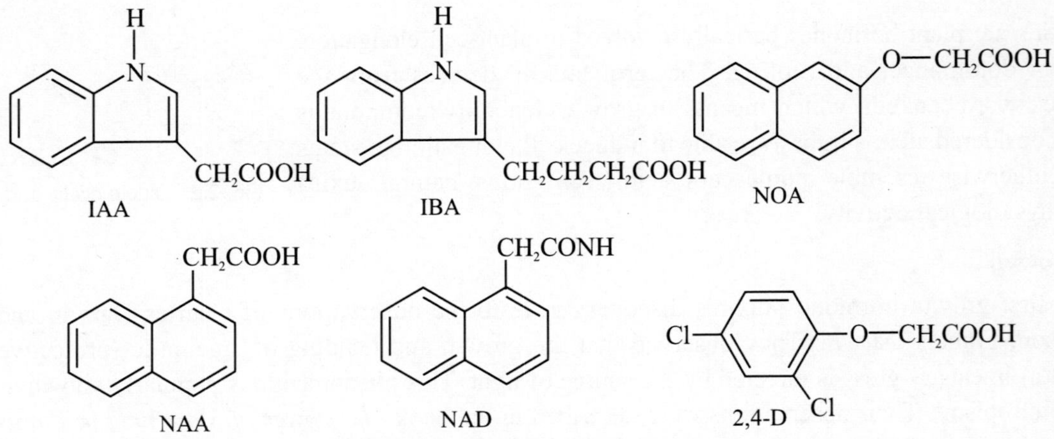

Fig. 2.4 Structure of natural growth regulators

Occurrence and Production

Auxins are basically produced in meristematic tissues of shoot and root tips, young leaves, mature root cells and small amounts in mature leaves and transported throughout the plant. The production of IAA is likely to be more in day as compared to night. Ethylene has direct or indirect detrimental effect in enhancing the synthesis of auxin.

Structurally IAA is similar to the amino acid tryptophan and it is well proven that the amino acid tryptophan is the origin of IAA. So far three mechanisms have been proposed to explain such conversions.

- Tryptophan is converted to indolepyruvic acid through a transamination reaction. Indolepyruvic acid is then converted to indole acetaldehyde by a decarboxylation reaction. The final step involves oxidation of indoleacetaldehyde resulting in indole-3-acetic acid (IAA).

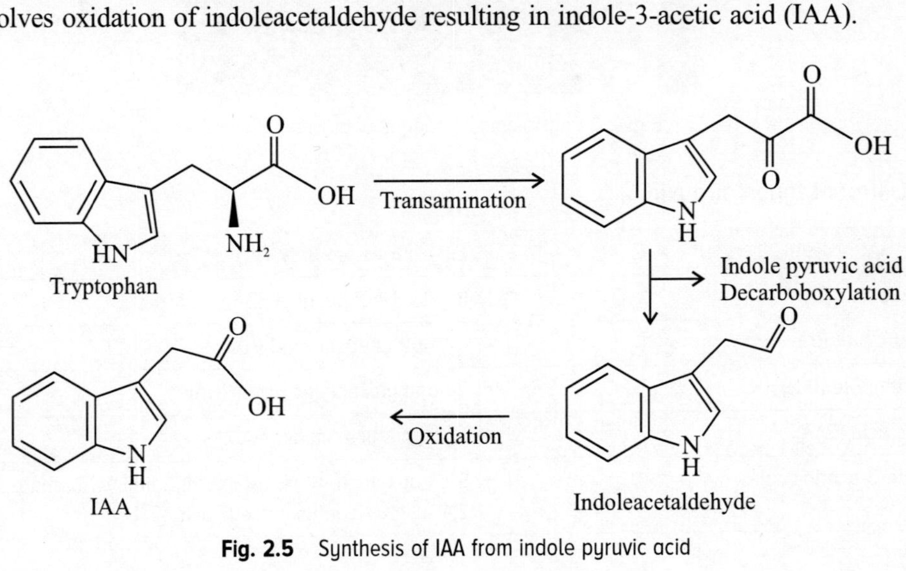

Fig. 2.5 Synthesis of IAA from indole pyruvic acid

- Tryptophan undergoes decarboxylation resulting in tryptamine. Tryptamine is then oxidized and deaminated to produce indoleacetaldehyde. This molecule is further oxidized to produce indoleacetic acid.

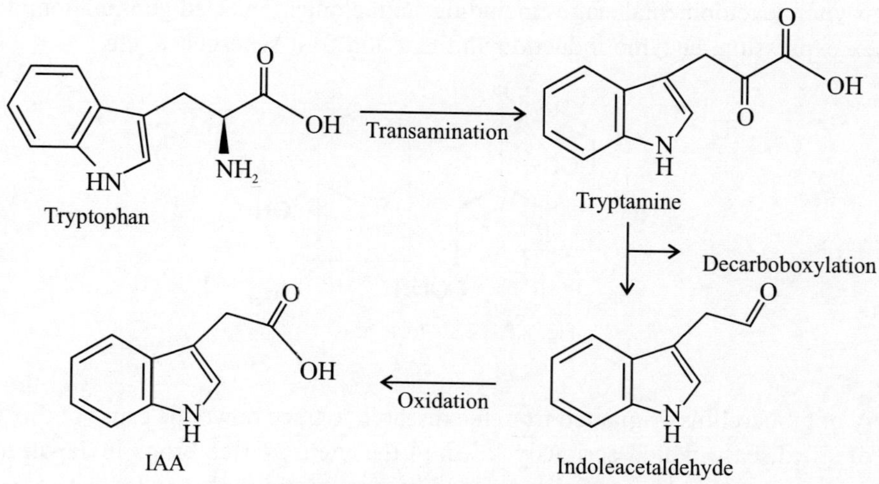

Fig. 2.6 Synthesis IAA from tryptamine.

- IAA can be produced via a tryptophan-independent mechanism. This mechanism is poorly understood, but has been proven using tip (-) mutants. Other experiments have shown that, in some plants, this mechanism is actually the preferred mechanism of IAA biosynthesis.

Effects of auxins

- Stimulate cell elongation process.
- Suppression of apical bud, i.e., suppress the growth of lateral buds. Apical dominance is the inhibiting influence of the shoot apex on the growth of axillary buds.
- Differentiation of vascular tissue (xylem and phloem) is stimulated by IAA.
- Promote flowering in plants like pineapple.
- Help to initiate rooting in stem cuttings and lateral root development in tissue culture (adventitious rooting).
- Prevent dropping of fruits and leaves too early.
- Promote natural detachment (abscission) of older leaves and fruits.
- Control xylem differentiation and help in cell division.

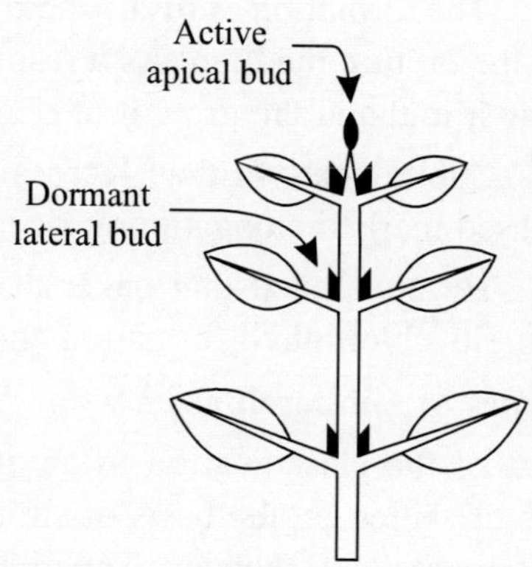

Fig. 2.7 Effect of auxins during growth

Applications

1. Used for plant propagation.
2. To induce parthenocarpy, i.e., the production of fruit without prior fertilization.
3. 2,4-D is widely used as a herbicide to kill dicotyledonous weeds.
4. Used by gardeners to keep lawns weed-free.

2. *Gibberellins*

Gibberellins are basically a group of diterpenoid acids, act as plant growth regulators on higher plants in their vital developmental stages including stem elongation, seed germination, dormancy, flowering, sex expression, enzyme induction and leaf and fruit senescence, etc.

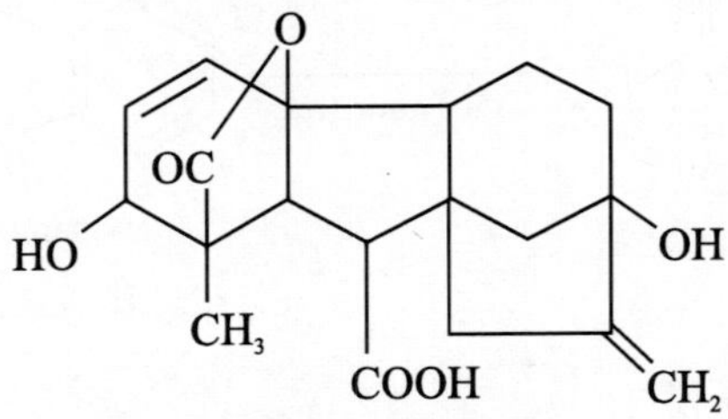

Fig. 2.8 Gibberellic acid

Discovery

The discovery of gibberellins originated from the research to trace down the cause of the 'bakanae' (foolish seedling) disease which seriously lowered the yield of rice crops in Japan and other Asian countries, characterized by pale yellow, elongated seedlings with slender leaves and stunted roots. The disease is caused by the fungal pathogen *Gibberella fujikuroi.* The final breakthrough was found in 1934, when Yabuta isolated a crystalline compound from the fungal culture filtrate which was inhibiting the growth of rice seedlings. The structure of the inhibitor was found to be 5-n-butylpicolinic acid or fusaric acid.

The formation of fusaric acid in culture filtrates was suppressed by changing the composition of the culture medium. As a result, a noncrystalline solid was obtained from the culture filtrate that stimulated the growth of rice seedlings. This compound was named gibberellin by Yabuta.

Subsequently, Eiichi Kurosawa (1926) found that culture filtrates from dried rice seedlings caused marked elongation in rice and other sub-tropical grasses.

He concluded that bakanae fungus secretes a chemical that stimulates shoot elongation, inhibits chlorophyll formation and suppresses root growth.

Types of Gibberellins

Unlike the classification of auxins which are classified on the basis of function, gibberellins are classified on the basis of structure as well as function. All gibberellins are derived from the entgibberellane skeleton. The gibberellins are named GA_1. GA_n in order of discovery. Gibberellic acid was the first gibberellin to be structurally characterized as GA_3. There are currently 136 GAs identified from plants, fungi and bacteria. Over the past 20 years by using modern analytical techniques many more gibberellins have been identified.

Production and occurrence

Produced in the roots, embryo and germinating seeds. The level of gibberellins goes up in the dark when sugar cannot be manufactured and will be reduced in the light. It is released in mature cells (particularly root) when they do not have enough sugar and oxygen to support both themselves and released by all cells when they are experiencing conditions which would normally cause a mature root cell to produce GA.

Gibberellins are diterpenes synthesized from acetyl CoA via the mevalonic acid pathway. They all have either 19 or 20 carbon units grouped into either four or five ring systems. The fifth ring is a lactone ring as shown in the structures above attached to ring A. Gibberellins are believed to be synthesized in young tissues of the shoot and also the developing seed. It is not clear whether young root tissues also produce gibberellins. There is also some evidence that leaves may also contain them.

The gibberellins are formed through the pathway, three acetyl CoA molecules are oxidized by two NADPH molecules to produce three CoA molecules as a side product and mevalonic acid. Mevalonic acid is then phosphorylated by ATP and decarboxylated to form isopentyl pyrophosphate. Four of these molecules form geranylgeranyl pyrophosphate which serves as the donor for all GA carbon atoms.

Functions of gibberellins

1. Stimulates stem elongation by stimulating cell division and elongation.
2. GA controls internode elongation in the mature regions of plants. Dwarf plants do not make enough active forms of GA.
3. Flowering in biennial plants is controlled by GA. Biennials grow one year as a rosette and after the winter, they bolt (rapid expansion of internodes and formation of flowers).
4. Breaks seed dormancy in some plants that require stratification or light to induce germination.
5. Stimulates α-amylase production in germinating cereal grains for mobilization of seed reserves.
6. Juvenility refers to the different stages that plants may exist in. GA may help determine whether a particular plant part is juvenile or adult.
7. Stimulates germination of pollen and growth of pollen tubes.
8. Induces maleness in dioecious flowers (sex expression).
9. Cause parthenocarpic (seedless) fruit development or increase the size of seedless fruit (grapes).
10. Delay senescence in leaves and citrus fruits; may be involved in phytochrome response.

3. Cytokinins

Cytokinins are compounds with a structure resembling adenine which promote cell division and have other similar functions to kinetin. They also regulate the pattern and frequency of organ production as well as position and shape. They have an inhibitory effect on senescence. Kinetin was the first cytokinin identified and so named because of the compounds ability to promote cytokinesis (cell division). Though it is a natural compound, it is not made in plants, and is therefore usually considered a 'synthetic' cytokinin. The common naturally occurring cytokinin in plants today is called zeatin which was isolated from corn.

Cytokinins have been found in almost all higher plants as well as mosses, fungi, bacteria, and also in many prokaryotes and eukaryotes. There are more than 200 natural and synthetic cytokinins identified. Cytokinin concentrations are more in meristematic regions and areas of continuous growth potential such as roots, young leaves, developing fruits, and seeds.

Haberlandt (1913) and Jablonski and Skoog (1954) identified that a compound found in vascular tissues had the ability to stimulate cell division. In 1941, Johannes van Overbeek, discovered that the milky endosperm from coconut and other various species of plants also had this ability. The first cytokinin was isolated from herring sperm in 1955 by Miller and his associates. This compound was named kinetin because of its ability to promote cytokinesis (cell division). The first naturally occurring cytokinin was isolated from corn in 1961 by Miller and it was later called zeatin. Since that time, many more naturally occurring cytokinins have been isolated and the compound was common to all plant species in one form or another.

The naturally occurring cytokinins are zeatin, N^6 dimethyl amino purine, isopentanyl aminopurine. The synthetic cytokinins are kineatin, adenine, 6-benzyl adenine benzimidazole and N, N′-diphenyl urea.

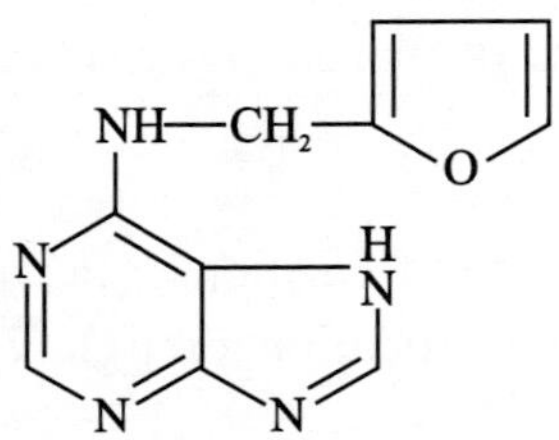

Fig. 2.9 Kinetin

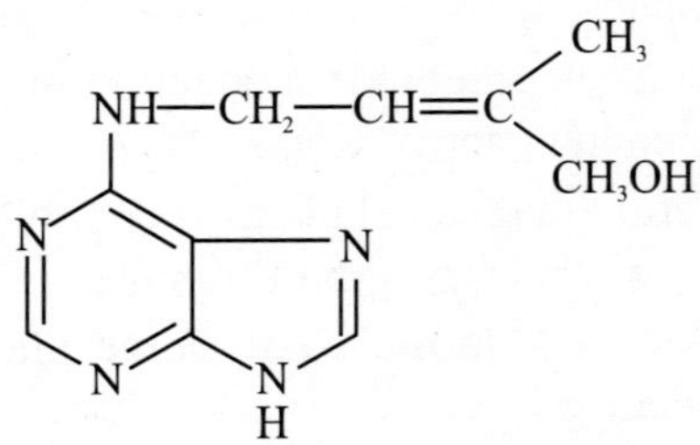

Fig. 2.10 Zeatin

Production and occurrence

Produced in root and shoot meristematic tissue, in mature shoot cells and in mature roots in small amounts. It is rapidly transported in xylem stream. Peak production occurs in daytime and their activity is reduced in plants suffering drought. It is directly or indirectly induced by high levels of gibberlic acid.

Cytokinin is generally found in meristematic regions and growing tissues. They are believed to be synthesized in the roots and translocated via the xylem to shoots. Cytokinin biosynthesis happens through the biochemical modification of adenine. They are synthesized by following pathway.

A product of the mevalonate pathway called isopentyl pyrophosphate is isomerized. This isomer can then react with adenosine monophosphate with the aid of an enzyme called isopentenyl AMP synthase. The result is isopentenyl adenosine-5′-phosphate (isopentenyl AMP). This product can then be converted to isopentenyl adenosine by removal of the phosphate by a phosphatase and further converted to isopentenyl adenine by removal of the ribose group. Isopentenyl adenine can be converted to the three major forms of naturally occurring cytokinins.

Other pathways or slight alterations of this one probably lead to the other forms.

Occurence

Cytokinins occur largely due to the enzyme cytokinin oxidase. This enzyme removes the side chain and releases adenine. Derivatives can also be made but the difficulties are with pathways, which are more complex and poorly understood.

Functions of cytokinin

1. Stimulate cell division (cytokinesis).
2. Stimulate morphogenesis (shoot initiation/bud formation) in tissue culture.
3. Stimulate the growth of lateral (or adventitious) buds release of apical dominance.
4. Stimulate leaf expansion resulting from cell enlargement.
4. May enhance stomatal opening in some species.
6. Promotes the conversion of etioplasts into chloroplasts via stimulation of chlorophyll synthesis.
7. Stimulate the dark germination of light-dependent seeds.
8. Delays senescence.
9. Promotes some stages of root development.

4. Ethylene

It is a group of plant growth regulators which are extensively used in fruit ripping and fruit and flower production. It is a small unsaturated hydrocarbon, flammable colourless gas denoted by the formula C_2H_4. It has sweet and musky odour.

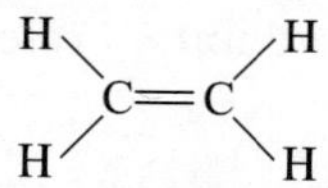

Fig. 2.11 Ethylene

Discovery

Ethylene has been practicsed since Egyptian periods where theyused gas figs to stimulate ripening. Russian scientist Dimitry Neljubow (1901), showed that the activity of ethylene in abnormal plant growth. Doubt (1917) discovered that ethylene stimulated abscission. Ethylene evolved from stored apple inhibited the growth of potato shoots enclosed with them was demonstrated in 1932. Gane (1934) reported that plants synthesize ethylene. Crocker (1935) proposed that ethylene was the plant hormone responsible for fruit ripening as well as inhibition of vegetative tissues.

Production and occurrence

Ethylene is generally found in germinating seeds and nodes of stems, tissues of ripening fruits, response to shoot environmental, pest, or disease stress and in senescent leaves and flowers. Ethylene production is directly induced by high levels of auxin, root flooding and drought.

Ethylene is produced in all higher plants and is produced from methionine in essentially all tissues. Production of ethylene varies with the type of tissue, the plant species, and also the stage of development.

The mechanism behind ethylene production in plant initiated by amino acid methionine and it possess three steps.

ATP and water are added to methionine resulting in loss of the three phosphates and S-adenosyl methionine (SAM). 1-amino-cyclopropane-l-carboxylic acid synthase (ACC-synthase) facilitates the production of ACC from SAM. Oxygen is then needed in order to oxidize ACC and produce ethylene. This reaction is catalyzed by an oxidative enzyme called ethylene forming enzyme.

Functions of ethylene

1. Production stimulated during ripening, flooding, stress, senescence, mechanical damage, and infection.
2. Regulator of cell death programmes in plants (apoptosis). Stimulates the release in dormancy.
3. Stimulates shoot and root growth and differentiation.
4. Regulates ripening of climacteric fruits.
5. Stimulates leaf and fruit abscission.
6. Flowering in most plants is inhibited by ethylene. Mangos, pineapples and some ornamentals are stimulated by ethylene.
7. Induction of femaleness in dioecious flowers. Stimulates flower opening.
8. Stimulates flower and leaf senescence.

5. *Abscisic Acid*

It is the naturally occurring enantiomer of abscisic acid. It is an important sesquiterpenoid plant hormone which acts as a regulator of plant response to environmental stress such as drought and cold.

It is called 'abscisin II' originally because it was thought to play a major role in abscission of fruits. Abscisic acids generally play mostly inhibitory roles in plant besides have many promoting functions.

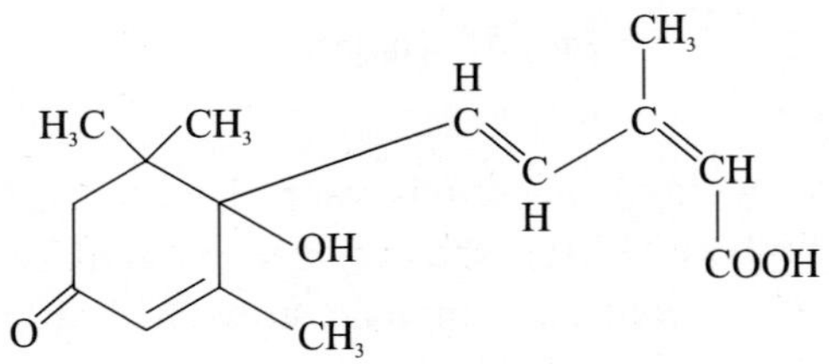

Fig. 2.12 Abscisic acid

Discovery

Frederick Addicott (1963) and his associates identified abscisic acid. Two compounds were isolated and named as abscisin I or and abscisin II or abscisic acid (ABA). The discovery was confirmed with the similar findings by Philip Wareing and Van Steveninck in the same time.

Production and occurrence

ABA is partially produced via the mevalonic pathway in chloroplasts and other plastids. Because it is synthesized partially in the chloroplasts, it makes sense that biosynthesis primarily occurs in the leaves.

The production of ABA is by stresses such as water loss and freezing temperatures. The biosynthesis occurs indirectly through the production of carotenoids.

Breakdown of these carotenoids occurs by the following mechanism: Violaxanthin (forty carbons) is isomerized and then split via an isomerase reaction followed by an oxidation reaction. One molecule of xanthonin is produced from one molecule of violaxanthonin and it is not clear what happens to the remaining byproducts. The one molecule of xanthonin produced is unstable and spontaneously changed to ABA aldehyde. Further oxidation results in ABA.

Functions of Abscisic acid

1. Stimulates the closure of stomata (water stress).
2. Involved in abscission of buds, leaves, petals, flowers, and fruits.
3. Production is accentuated by stresses such as water loss and freezing temperatures.
4. Involved in bud dormancy.
5. Prolongs seed dormancy and delays germination (vivipary).
6. Inhibits elongation of plant parts.
7. Implicated in the control of elongation, lateral root development, and geotropism, as well as in water uptake and ion transport by roots.
8. Promotes the metabolism of ripening.
9. Promotes senescence.
10. Reverse the effects of growth stimulating hormones.

6. Others

(a) Polyamines (PAs)

Polyamines (Pas) are low molecular weight aliphatic nitrogenous bases containing two or more amino groups effective in relatively high concentrations (5 to 500 mg/L). It has great impact on flowering and plant regeneration.

Examples: Spermine, spermidine and putrescine.

Spermine and spermidine bind to the phosphate backbone of nucleic acids during genetic processes and gene expression. The interaction is mostly based on electrostatic interactions between negatively charged phosphates of the nucleic acids and the positively charged ammonium groups of the polyamines.

Production and occurrence

Spermine and spermidine are derivatives of 1,4-diaminobutane or putrescine. L-ornithine is the precursor of such putrescine synthesis with the influence of ornithine decarboxylase (ODC).

Spermine and spermidine are derivatives of putrescine (1,4-diaminobutane) which is produced from L-ornithine by action of ODC (ornithine decarboxylase). Spermidine is a triamine structure that is produced by spermidine synthase (SpdS) which catalyses monoalkylation of putrescine (1,4-diaminobutane) with decarboxylated S-adenosylmethionine (dcAdoMet) 3-aminopropyl donor. The putrescine with the 3-aminopropyl donor yields the symmetrical tetraamine spermine when induced akylation of both amino groups.

(b) Brassinosteroids

Brassinosteroids (BRs) are the naturally occurring polyhydroxy steroids. It was named after the first one identified, brassinolide, which was isolated from rape in 1979. They appear to be widely distributed in the plant kingdom.

Brassinosteroids are the new class of plant growth substances which have an effect at extremely low concentrations, both in bioassays and whole plants.

Functions of brassinosteroids

1. Promote shoot elongation at low concentrations.
2. Strongly inhibit root growth and development. Promote ethylene biosynthesis and epinasty.

3. Interfere with ecdysteroids (moulting hormones) in insects.
4. Enhance xylem differentiation.
5. Decrease fruit abortion and drop.
6. Enhance resistance to chilling, disease, herbicide, and salt stress.
7. Promotion of germination.
8. Promote changes in plasmalemma energization and transport, assimilate uptake.
9. Increase RNA and DNA polymerase activities and synthesis of RNA, DNA, and protein.

2.3 POLYPLOIDY, MUTATION AND HYBRIDIZATION IN MEDICINAL PLANTS

2.3.1 Polyploidy

Plant species with three or more genomes are known as polyploidy. The basic set of chromosomes undergoes multiplications.

For example, in chrysanthemum basic set is x = 9. Its species and hybrids show multiples of 9, such as 18, 27, 36, 45. In nicotiana and solanum basic set is x = 12 and multiples of somatic chromosome numbers are 24, 48 and 72 and in triticum it is x = 7 and multiples are 14, 21, 42.

Also among fruit plants, such as banana – *Musa sapientum* (3x = 33) and mango – *Mangifera indica* (40), polyploidy is quite frequent. On the other hand, rye, barley and beet, the diploid is maintained (14 in rye and barley, 18 in beet).

Types of Polyploidy

There are four different types, namely:

(i) Auto-polyploidy,
(ii) Allopolyploids,
(iii) Segmental allopolyploids
(iv) Autoallopolyploids.

(i) Auto-polyploidy: Auto-polyploidy occurs when the same genome is duplicated, i.e., the same basic set of chromosomes is multiplied. For instance, if a diploid species has two similar sets of chromosome or genomes (AA), an auto-triploid will have three similar genomes (AAA) and an auto- tetraploid will have four such genomes (AAAA).

Auto-triploids are known in watermelon, banana, sugar beet, tomato, grapes, and auto-tetraploids are common in rye, corn, red clover, snapdragon and *Allium tuberosum.*

(ii) Allopolyploids: Polyploidy may also result from doubling of chromosome number in hybrid which is derived from two or more distinctly different species. This brings two (or more) different sets of chromosome in hybrid. The doubling of chromosomes in the hybrid, which gives rise to a polyploidy, is called an allopolyploid.

An allopolyploid in which a sterile hybrid (AB) originating out of the combination of two different species, undergoes duplication of chromosome set, is known as amphidiploid (AABB).

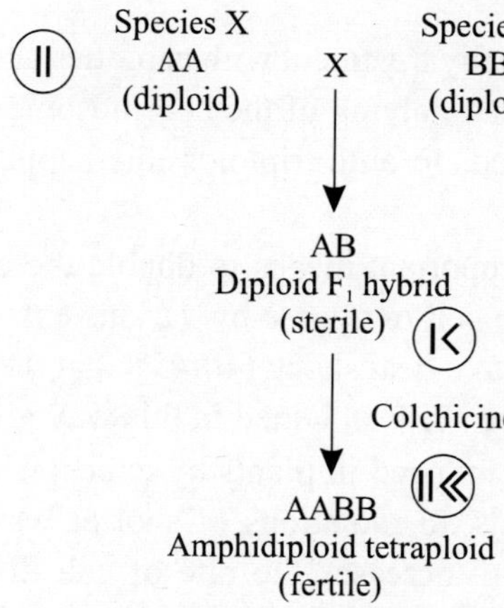

Fig. 2.13 Amphidiploid (AABB).

Raphanobrassica is a classic example of amphidiploidy. A cross between *Raphanus sativus* ($2n = 18$) and *Brassica oleracea* ($2n = 18$) to produce F_2 hybrids which were completely sterile.

This sterility was due to lack of chromosome pairing, since there is no homology between genomes from *Raphanus sativus* and *Brassica oleracea*. Among these sterile hybrids certain fertile plants were found. On cytological examination, these fertile plants were found to have $2n = 36$ chromosomes, which showed normal pairing into 18 bivalents.

(iii) Segmental Allopolyploids: In some allopolyploids the different genomes that are present are not quite different from one another, i.e., having partial homology with each other. Consequently, in these polyploidy, chromosomes from different genomes do pair together to some extent and multivalents are formed. This means that segments of chromosomes and not the whole chromosome is homologous.

Such allopolyploids are called segmental allopolyploids (Stebbins). These chromosomes which are partially homologous and not completely homologous with each other are sometimes also described as homologous chromosomes. It is also believed that most of the naturally occurring polyploidy are neither true autopolyploidy nor true allopolyploids.

Example: Solanum tuberosum is the best example of segmental allopolyploid.

(iv) Auto-Allopolyploids: When autopolyploidy is combined with allopolyploidy, autoallopolyploids are produced (AAAA6B). Polyploidy of this type are possible from hexaploid level upward as observed in *Nicotiana tabacum* and *Solanum nigrum*. Autoallopolyploids have importance in the evolution of certain plant species.

Induction of Polyploidy

For induction of polyploidy two basic strategies are adopted

(i) Prevention of the halving of the chromosome number at meiosis.

(ii) Suppression of chromosome separation at mitosis.

Both methods have yielded positive results. Under the influence of various agents the chromosomes may divide, but the daughter halves fail to separate and remain in the same cell.

By different external agents, especially treatment with narcotics and high or low temperatures, meiosis may be disturbed and the normal halving of the chromosome number does not occur. In this way unreduced gametes are formed. In auto-triploids this happens spontaneously, because meiosis is always irregular.

(a) **Temperature treatment:** An important means to double the chromosome number is the treatment of ordinary vegetative cell or zygote by various external agents. One method is to expose the fertilized egg cell to a heat shock (40-45°C) at the time of its first division. A low but regular percentage of the seeds obtained in this way gives rise to auto-tetraploids.

(b) **Radiation:** Polyploidy may be induced in plants by exposing their certain parts, such as vegetative buds and flower buds, to radiations of shorter wavelengths, ultraviolet rays, X-rays, gamma-rays. Irradiation increases the rate of cell division and also causes the multiplication of chromosome number (somatic doubling of chromosomes).

(c) **Injury:** When the meristematic zones of a plant are injured, the cells at the points of injury grow rapidly and form a callus. Callus growth is enhanced by a chemical substance named coumarin which also brings about somatic doubling of chromosomes. Vegetative buds generally developing from callus tissue are polyploidy in nature. From injured parts of tomato plants, it is possible to produce tetraploid plants.

(d) **Regeneration *in-vitro*:** Polyploidy is a common feature in the cells of cultured tissue in vitro. Some of the plants regenerated from the callus or suspension culture may be found to be polyploidy. Polyploidy has been developed from callus cultures of nicotiana, datura, rice and several other species.

(e) **Chemical treatment:** A number of chemicals are now known which induce polyploidy in plants. Important among them are colchicine, 8-hydroxyquinoline, nitrous oxide, chloral hydrate, some narcotics and alkaloids, veratin sulphate, acenaphthane, and gammexane (hexachlorocyclohexane). Colchicine ($C_{22}O_6N$) is the best chemical for this purpose.

Colchicine is obtained from the extract of seeds and corms of *Colchicum autumnale*, *Colchicum luteum* and *Gloriosa superba* of family Liliaceae.

Method of Application of Colchicine

Colchicine treatment is done in one of the following ways:

(a) **Seed treatment:** The dry or soaked seeds are soaked in aqueous solution of colchicine of different strength in shallow container to facilitate aeration (generally, solutions of 0.05 to 0.5% concentrations are used). Colchicine treatment is given for a definite period which is different for different seeds.

After the seeds are soaked in colchicine solution for a desired period, they are washed thoroughly in water and then sown. Treatment of dry seeds gives better result than soaked seeds in some cases.

(b) **Seedling treatment:** Seedlings may be treated in young stage. During treatment, the shoot tips are dipped in 0.2% colchicine solution and root tips are covered with cotton soaked in water. The treatment may be given from 3 to 24 hours and in some cases the treatment should be repeated on 2nd and 3rd days.

(c) Treatment of growing buds of shoot: In some cases, growing plants are treated with 0.1 to 0.5% solution of colchicine which is applied with a brush or a dropper. Sometimes cotton soaked in the aqueous solution of colchicine is applied over the growing point of plant. The treatment is repeated once or twice daily for a few days. Alternatively, 0.2 to 0.5% colchicine solution is mixed with lanoline paste and is smeared on the shoot apex. This treatment may be repeated 2-3 times daily for a week.

Role of Polyploidy

Some of the important roles played by polyploidy are described below.

(a) Role of Polyploidy in Plant Breeding: Many important crop plants like wheat, oat, sugarcane, cotton, tobacco as well as many fruits and vegetables are the polyploidy of various degrees. One of the important effects of polyploidy is the changes in the blooming season of the induced polyploidy. As such, interspecific hybrids can be obtained of such species which otherwise remain isolated by seasonal isolation and different blooming season.

By artificial polyploidy induction, disease resistance and other desirable characteristics have been incorporated into some commercial crop plants. For example, *Nicotiana tabacum* is susceptible to TMV whereas *N. glutinosa* appears to be resistant.

The two tobacco species when crossed, the hybrids were found to be resistant but totally sterile. When the chromosomes were doubled it was possible to secure a fertile polyploidy resistant to the virus. Many polyploidies are selected and cultivated because of their larger size, vigour and ornamental value. Several varieties of apples, pears and grapes have produced giant fruits which are of much economic value.

(b) Role of Polyploidy in Evolution: Polyploidy combined with interspecific hybridization provides a mechanism by which new species may arise in nature and play a role in evolution. Allopolyploidy can produce new species by combining new characters and stable in evolution.

Origin of some of the economically important plants like rice, wheat, cotton, tobacco is important in this aspect. The chromosome number of rice (*Oryza sativa*) is $2n = 24$. It is an example of typical secondary allopolyploids with basic chromosome number $x = 5$.

(c) Media of Conservation of Characters: Polyploidy plays an important role in conserving the characters. A recessive mutation in order to be expressed in an autotetraploid, all four genes must be in recessive condition which is a time requiring process. Thus the characters in a polyploidy plant could be conserved.

(d) Polyploidy and Geographical Distribution: The polyploidy plants can cope with diverse geographical areas than a diploid. Hence, the geographical distributions of polyploidy plants are greater than diploids. Autopolyploidy cannot produce new species, but they can colonize a new environment easily. As allopolyploids contain different genomes, they can withstand different environmental conditions.

Both these, power of colonization and coping with a diverse environment of the polyploidy plants, help their wide geographical distribution.

2.3.2 Mutation

The term 'mutation' was introduced by Hugo De Vries, a Dutch botanist and also rediscovered of Mendel's laws of heredity.

Mutation is defined as sudden, hereditary change in the genetic makeup of an organism. Mutation is of two types: gene mutations or point mutations and chromosomal mutations.

Gene mutations include changes in the structure or composition of genes whereas chromosomal mutations or chromosomal aberrations involve changes in the structure or number of chromosomes.

Since gene consists of a few segments of DNA, gene mutations include changes in the number or arrangement of nucleotides. Thus, gene mutations alter or modify the expressions of a particular gene. Sickle cell anaemia, chloroph-ll deficiencies in plants and albinism (loss of pigment) are caused by gene mutations. Naturally occurring mutations are known as spontaneous mutations. In 1910, Morgan found a few white eyed Drosophila in a population of nor mal red eyed Drosophila. In Drosophila many mutant forms such as white eye, black body, vestigial wings arose through spontaneous mutations.

Mutations caused by mutagenic agents like X-ray, ultraviolet rays, mustard gas, formaldehyde, caffeine, phenol, etc., are known as induced mutations. In contrast to spontaneous mutations, the frequency of induced mutations is high.

Causes of Gene Mutations

Since gene mutations or point mutations involve changes in the number of nucleotides in a DNA segment or cistron, it is otherwise known as the frame shift mutation. Addition or insertion of one or more nucleotides or deletion of one or more nucleotides changes the sequence of amino acids during protein synthesis. If a nucleotide pair (= nitrogenous base pair) is substituted (substitution mutations) by another pair it will also produce gene mutations.

These substitutions are caused either as:

(i) transitions or (ii) transversions

(i) Transitions: In transition, a purine is replaced by another purine and a pyrimidine is replaced by another pyrimidine, i.e., $A = T$ is replaced by $G = C$ or vice versa.

(ii) Transversions: In transversion, a purine is replaced by a pyrimidine or a pyrimidine by a purine, i.e., $C = G$ is replaced by $G = C$ or $A = I$ is replaced by $T = A$.

Examples of Gene Mutations

The earliest record of gene mutations dates back to 1791, when Seth Wright observed a lamb with unusually short legs in his flock of sheep. This short legged or Ancon sheep could not gel over the low stone fence and damage the crop in the nearby fields. Wright thought that it would be worthwhile to have a whole flock of these short legged sheep for this reason.

In the successive generations, this character was transferred and a line was developed where all sheep had short legs. This trait resulted from a recessive mutation and the short legged individuals were homozygous recessive. This gene mutation was discovered at a time when the science of genetics did not even have its birth.

The scientific study of mutations started in 1910, when T.H. Morgan started his work on fruitfly, Drosophila melanogaster, and reported white eyed male individuals among normal red eyed females. Later it was found that the gene for this character was found on sex chromosome.

The human blood disease sickle cell anaemia is another example of point mutation. It is caused due to abnormal haemoglobin S which is an insufficient oxygen carrier. It has been observed that the abnormal haemoglobin differs from the normal one only in its two P polypeptide chains (haemoglobin 2 alpha and 2 beta chains) which contain amino acid valine instead of glutamic acid at the position sixth.

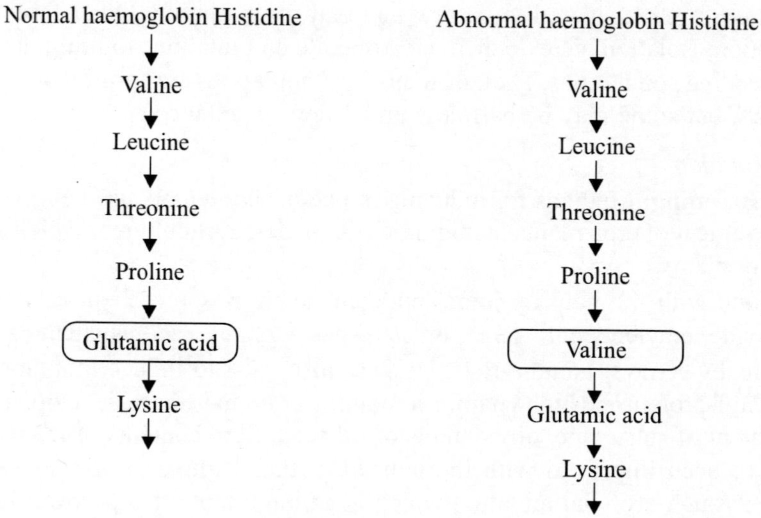

Fig. 2.14 Transition

Minor change involving two nucleotides in DNA brings substitution in amino acid and thus producing profound change preventing synthesis of normal haemoglobin. Thalassemia, phenyl ketonuria, alcaptonuria and many other human diseases are caused by simple base substitution in the nucleotide that prevents synthesis of normal protein. Gene mutations although cause minute change in the base pairing, its impact is largely felt by the organisms bearing such mutant gene.

Types of Mutations

Generally, mutations are harmful or deleterious and do not produce visible effects. Less than 20% mutations are lethal. The mutant genes when present in homozygous condition cause death of the organism. Mutant genes are mostly recessive to the normal gene. These genes produce their effects only in homozygous condition hence remain undetected for a period of time. It means that the mutation rate is actually much higher than the frequency of visible or detectable mutations.

(i) Forward and Reverse Mutations: A mutation from wild type (original type) to a new type is known as forward mutation. The mutated gene may mutate back to the wild type. It is known as reverse mutation.

(ii) Somatic and Gametic Mutations: Mutations occurring in somatic or non-reproductive cells are called somatic mutations, these are not heritable and are lost with the death of the mutant organism. Mutations occurring in germ cells or gametes produce gametic mutations which are heritable.

(iii) Spontaneous and Induced Mutations: Spontaneous mutations occur in natural conditions and have a very low frequency. Under experimental or artificial conditions induced mutations are caused. Any physical or chemical agent which introduces mutation in an organism is a mutagen or mutagenic agent. H.J. Muller (1927) induced mutations in Drosophila by X-rays and observed that the frequency of mutations is directly proportional to the amount of X-ray.

Role of Mutation in Evolution

At present mutations are considered to be raw material for evolution. Other forces of evolution like natural selection, isolation, genetic drift, etc., operate on mutations to bring divergence in the naturally inter-breeding populations. Though, majority of mutations are harmful or disadvantageous to their possessors, but some may be harmless and a few advantageous.

Applications of Mutation

(i) In Plant Breeding: Methods for inducing mutations are widely used all over the world in the improvement of crop plants including food, fodder, horticulture, medicinal or industrial commodity plants.

This is done with the help of some mutagens such as some chemicals and radiations. Nitrous oxide, ethylene, colchicine, mustard gas, etc., are used as chemical mutagens.

Irradiations by X-rays, gamma-rays, etc., are also used to induce mutations. Many high yielding, high protein and high vitamin containing crops have been developed by irradiation. Sugar content of sugarcane, oil contents of oil seed, fibre contents of many fibre yielding plants have been improved with the help of artificial mutation. Some insect pests are sterilized through artificial mutation which is an important attempt towards pest control.

(ii) In Animal Breeding: Breeding of useful animals through mutation may lead to more healthy and disease-resistant animal varieties. However, induced mutants have rarely been tried for this purpose although a number of mutant varieties of animals have also been found beneficial.

Short legged Acorn breed of sheep described in the earlier paragraph belongs lo this category. Now certain mutant varieties of cattle, horses, pigeon and cats have been selected and interbred to maintain their races. Some new breeds of sheep have been developed in USA, Australia and New Zealand.

(iii) In Microorganisms: It is easy to induce mutations in microorganisms like bread mould: *Neurospora* (a unicellular fungus) and intestinal bacterium, *Escherichia coli,* than the higher plants and animals. Haploid microorganisms have just one copy of each gene. In them, each and every mutation is expressed in the same generation and thus easy to locate mutation. Development of better varieties of yeast, Penicillium and some other microorganisms may increase commercial production of alcohol, antibiotics, acids and solvents.

Mutagens: Mutation inducing agents are known as mutagens.

Types of Mutagens

1. Chemical Mutagens

They are chemicals which induce mutation. Example of some of the chemical mutagens are given below.

Table 2.10 List of chemical mutagens

Class of chemicals	Mutagen
Acridines	Ethyleneimine
Mustard	Nitrogen mustard, Sulphur mustard
Nitrosamines	Diethylnitrosamine, Diethylsulphonate
Epoxide	Ethyleneoxide, Diepoxybutane
Alkyl sulphonates	Diethylsulphonate, Methylmethanesulphonate
Others	Nitrous acid, Hydroxylamine

2. **Physical Mutagensi**
   (i) **Radiations as Mutagens:** Radiation is the most important among the physical mutagens. Radiations damaging the DNA molecules fall in the wavelength range below 340 nm and photon energy above 1 electron volt (eV). Radiation induced damage can be categorized into the three broad types: lethal damage (killing the organisms), potentially lethal damage (can be lethal under certain ordinary conditions) and sub-lethal damage (cells do not die unless radiation reaches to a certain threshold value). The effect of damage is at molecular level.
   (ii) **Ultraviolet (UV) Radiation:** UV radiation causes damage in the DNA duplex of the bacteria and phages. The UV rays are absorbed and cause excitation of macromolecules. The absorption maxima of nucleic acid = (280 nm) and protein (260 nm) are more or less similar. The DNA molecule is the target molecule for UV rays but not the proteins. However, absorption spectrum of RNA is quite similar to that of DNA.
   (iii) **X-Rays:** The X-rays cause breaking of phosphate ester linkages in the DNA. This breakage occurs at one or more points. Consequently, a large number of bases are deleted or rearranged in the DNA molecule. The X-rays may break the DNA either in one or both strands. If breaks occur in both strands, it becomes lethal. The DNA segment between the two breaks is removed resulting in deletion. Since both the X-rays and UV rays bring about damage in DNA molecule, they are used in sterilization of bacteria and viruses.

2.3.3 Hybridization of Medicinal Plants

Plant hybridization refers to a process of interfering with the natural plant breeding process. It is generally the deliberate breeding of two different varieties within the same species of plant and is something called selective breeding. The male pollen is artificially transferred to the female pistil and a seed is formed. Selective breeding or plant hybridization is usually undertaken in order to combine positive characteristics of two different plant varieties. The merits of hybrid varieties of plants are therefore supposed to outweigh the merits of either plant "parent."

Advantages of Selective Breeding

Hybrid plants are usually more vigorous and faster growing than other plants. This can be great for those working in agriculture as they can reap greater crops and make more money.

These plant types are also more resistant to many diseases and afflictions, which affect parent plants. Fungi, bacteria and viruses can otherwise wipe out whole crops. Disease is such a problem for plants that some selective breeding is done for the purpose of creating strains that are more disease resistant.

In a similar vein, hybrid plants can be less susceptible to problematic growing conditions. Plants can be bred to be more tolerant of little water or extremes of temperature. Many seeds sold for home gardens are selectively bred to make them easier to grow, essentially.

For plants that are not being grown for food, selective breeding can be useful in creating uniformity. The plants will, therefore, be perceived as more attractive. Plants can even be selectively bred to produce more visually appealing characteristics, such as bigger or more bright coloured flowers.

Selective breeding is also a much safer way of manipulating plants than through genetic modification, commonly known as GMO. It's more a process of speeding up evolution, rather than overriding it entirely.

Potential Problems

One of the main problems people have with selective breeding is that it can contribute to loss of variety. This gives little room for evolutionary expansion in plants in the future.

Some criticize selective breeding as it does not take into account genetic mutation. It can only maximize good traits, rather than removing bad. Therefore, in the future, the whole species of plant can end up with the same bad trait, which can lead to species wipe-out. A depression in gene diversity can actually cause genetic mutation, too.

Hybridization may be of following types

(i) **Intra-varietal hybridization:** The crosses are made between the plants of the same variety.

(ii) **Inter-varietal or intraspecific hybridization:** The crosses are made between the plants belonging to two different varieties.

(iii) **Interspecific hybridization or intragenric hybridization:** The crosses are made between two different species of the same genus.

(iv) **Introgressive hybridization:** Transfer of some genes from one species into the genome of the other species is known as introgressive hybridization. The crosses between different species of the same genus or different genera of the same family are also known as distant hybridization or wide crossing. Such crosses are called distant crosses.

Role or applications of plant hybridization

1. Improves water use efficiency in plants.
2. To increase nutrient use efficiency in plants specially nitrogen and phosphorus.
3. Increase weed competitiveness in plants.
4. Produce the tolerance of mechanical weed control.
5. Development of pest/disease resistance.
6. Induce early maturity in plants for avoidance of particular stresses.
7. Produce abiotic stress tolerance like drought, salinity, etc.

8. Increase the yield of crops and medicinal entity.
9. Develop high nutritional value for forage crops.
10. Developments of resistance and new medicinal and commercial food crops traits for environmental stressors.

2.4 CONSERVATION OF MEDICINAL PLANTS

Conservation is defined as 'sustainable development support for protection and utilization of biological resource in the way of protect from diminish world's genetic verities and species or destruction from imperative habitats and ecosystems.

Generally, it involves a combined activity, i.e., collection, propagation, characterization, evaluation, disease indexing and elimination, storage, distribution, etc. There are two methods for the conservation of plant genetic resources, namely, in situ and ex situ conservation.

A. In Situ Conservation

'Conservation of natural ecosystem and habitats conditions of living species along with recovery, maintenance of viable species' population and protection of surroundings of domesticates or cultivated species where distinctive properties developed' is defined as in situ conservation.

Most medicinal plants are endemic species, and their medicinal properties are mainly because of the presence of secondary metabolites that respond to stimuli in natural environments, and that may not be expressed under culture conditions.

The objective of in situ conservation in worldwide focused on establishing protected areas and captivating an ecosystem-oriented approach rather than species oriented. The success of in situ conservation depends on certain rules, regulations, and potential compliance of medicinal plants within their growth habitats.

Two potential approaches for in situ conservation include the following.

1. *Natural reserves*

The major cause for the loss of medicinal plant resources in recent times is due to the degradation and destruction of habitats of medicinal plant species. Hence, natural reserves are created to protect the areas of important wild resources and to restore biodiversity. Currently, more than 12,700 protected areas have been established as natural reserves around the world which covering around 8.81% of the total earth surface accounting for 13.2 million sq. km area.

2. *Wild nurseries*

A wild nursery is broadly established for species-oriented cultivating and domesticating of endangered medicinal plants. It is a protected area, natural habitat, or a place that is only a short distance from where the plants naturally grow.

B. Ex Situ Conservation

It is defined as 'conservation outside the native habitat and generally used to safeguard the viable plant populations in danger of destruction, replacement or deterioration'.

Ex situ conservation of plants involves three potential approaches, namely:

1. Field gene banks
2. Seed bank
3. In vitro storage

1. *Field gene bank*

It has been created to provide easy access to conserved material for use and they run the risk of destruction by strategies using the tools of biotechnology are increasingly being applied towards conservation of plant genetic resources. These include:

(a) In vitro conservation
(b) In vitro propagation and re-introduction of plants to their natural habitats.
(c) Molecular marker technology, etc.

2. *Seed banks*

It is the most efficient and effective method of conservation for orthodox seeds. It is nothing but the effective and compact method of seed storage. The seeds are placed in packets and stored in medium-term storage facilities (maintained at 0°C to 5°C temp. and 15% to 20% relative humidity). Most of the material is also kept in long-term storage facilities (held at colder temperatures, –20 to –180°C). Most seed samples are expected to remain viable for 20 to 30 years in medium-term storage and for up to 100 years in long-term storage depending upon the species, the initial seed quality and specificity of storage environment and general state of infrastructure.

3. *In vitro storage*

Some in vitro techniques have been developed for storage of vegetative propagated and recalcitrant seed producing species. In general, they fall under two categories.

(i) Slow growth procedures: Where germplasm accessions are kept as sterile plant tissues or plantlets on nutrient gels, provide short- and medium-term storage options.

(ii) Cryopreservation: Viable freezing of biological material and their subsequent storage at ultralow temperatures (–196ºC) using liquid nitrogen is defined as "cryopreservation". In this method, with the help of cryo-protectant the viable biological materials (vegetative growing parts) can be conserved for highest duration of time (more than 30 years). The use of liquid nitrogen, either by itself or as a source of nitrogen gas, is based on the following unique combination of features: it includes its chemical inertness, relatively low cost, non-toxic, non-flammable and moreover readily available.

Germplasm Technique for Conservation

Germplasms are basically the living genetic resources like seeds or tissues which are maintained for the purpose of breeding, preservation, and research. These resources include seed banks, trees growing in nurseries, gene banks, etc. Germplasm collections can range from collections of wild species to elite, domesticated breeding lines that have undergone extensive human selection. Maintenance of biological diversity and food security, the most important step is germplasm collection.

Disadvantages of Germplasm

1. Some crops do not produce viable seeds.
2. Some seeds remain viable for a limited duration only and are recalcitrant to storage.
3. Seeds of certain species deteriorate rapidly due to seed-borne pathogens.
4. Some seeds are very heterozygous, not suitable for maintaining true to type genotypes.

EXERCISE

1. Describe the advantages of cultivation of medicinal plants.
2. Describe the various methods for collection of crude drugs and their significance.
3. Explain briefly the harvesting and drying process of natural crude drugs.
4. Explain the significance and techniques of crude drug packaging and storage conditions.
5. Describe the various factors affecting cultivation of medicinal plants.
6. Briefly explain the various plant hormones and their biological role in plant growth.
7. Define polyploidy, its types, and applications with suitable examples.
8. What is mutation? Explain various types of mutation with their applications.
9. Explain the role of hybridization in the development medicinal plants.
10. What is in situ conservation? Explain two potential approaches in in situ conservation of medicinal plants.
11. Explain various approaches of ex situ conservation of medicinal plants.
12. Explain germplasm technique for conservation of medicinal plants and its disadvantages.
13. Define mutagen and describe types of mutagens with suitable examples.
14. Describe the method of application of colchicine in polyploidy induction in medicinal plants.
15. Describe the strategic approaches for polyploidy induction in medicinal plants.
16. Write short notes on:
    (a) Poly amines, and (b) Brassino steroids
17. Describe auxins and cytokinins, their chemistry, physiological effect, and applications.
18. Explain the mechanism of synthesis of IAA.
19. Write a short note on fertilizers and manures in medicinal plant cultivation.
20. Explain various mechanical processes of drying of medicinal plant materials.

UNIT III

Plant Tissue Culture

Objectives

- To discuss the concept and techniques of plant tissue culture.
- To describe the requirements, maintenance and applications of plant tissue culture.
- To explain the concept and applicability of edible vaccine.

3.1 INTRODUCTION

Tissue culture is one of the major areas of biotechnology. A group of techniques which is formally known as Biotechnology shares two things in common, i.e., manipulation of living cells, cellular molecules and best applications in our lives. The major techniques of biotechnology include genetic engineering, cell culture, tissue culture, bioprocessing, protein engineering, etc.

Plant tissue culture, is defined as "a technique of producing a large number of plants from small pieces of plant selected from known desirable agriculture qualities in relatively short periods of time under controlled conditions."

Plant tissue culture techniques can create entire crop population with premium qualities from a single elite specimen plant. The specimen tissue piece (explant) may be taken from shoot tip, leaf, lateral bud, stem or root tissue of the mother plant and established and multiplied under in vitro' conditions, providing the optimum prerequisite for plant growth.

Inoculated explants undergo various stages of growth such as initiation, multiplication and rooting of explant tissue for producing a cell into a full-fledged plant. These ready plantlets are then hardened in climatically controlled greenhouses or poly houses. Depending on the species, the plants become ready for plantation in the field.

3.1.1 History of Plant Tissue Culture

Guttlieb Haberlandt, a German botanist first proposed the concept of totipotency in plant cell or tissue and regeneration of plant via totipotencyin the year 1902. He is regarded as the father of plant tissue culture.

During his experiments, the tissue of Lamium Purouream and *Eichhornia crassipes*, the epidermal cells of *Ornithogalum* genus and epidermal hairs of *Pulmonaria mollissima* were used. All the plant parts were grown on a particular salt solution containing sugar such as sucrose. He observed an obvious cellular growth in those plant parts even more the cells found viable for 1 month. However, unfortunately none of the cells were divided. The reason behind such outcome might be the plant parts which were highly differentiated cells and leak of growth hormones which was necessary for inducing division in mature cells. The other important milestones in the history of plant tissue culture have given below.

Table 3.1 Milestones in the developments of plant tissue culture

Year	Name of the scientist	Contribution in the area of plant tissue culture
1940	Hanning	Excised nearly mature embryos of some plants like *Raphanus sativus* and successfully grew them to maturity on mineral salts and sugar solution.
1941	Van Overbeck	Demonstrated the stimulatory effect of coconut milk, similar to embryo sac fluid, on embryo development and callus formation in Datura plant.
1963 1965	Raghavan and Torrey Norstog	Development of synthetic media for the culture of younger embryos.
1925-1929	Laibach	Demonstrated the practical application of embryo culture in the field of plant breeding. He isolated embryos from nonviable seeds of a particular plant and reared them to maturity on a nutrient medium.
1922	Robbins and Kotte	Reported some success with growing isolated root tips.
1934	White	Success in continuously growing tomato root tips.
1939-1950	Street	Understand the role of vitamins, implant growth and shoot-root relationship.
1934 1939	Gautheret White Nobecourt	Successfully cultured cells of Salix, Nicotianahybrid and carrot on synthetic media. Demonstrated that growth regulators and vitamins relationship with callus formation.
1944 1951 1955	Skoog Tsui Miller	Demonstrated the induction of divisions in isolated, mature and differentiated cells by using synthetic as well as natural compounds.
1953	Muir	Developed a technique of growing single cells into liquid medium in case of *Tenetes erecta* and *Nicotiana tabacum*.
1957	Skoog and Miller	Showed that changing the relative concentrations of the two substances in the medium could regulate the organ differentiation.
1958-59	Reinert and Steward	Embryo formation from carrot tissue.
1946	Ball	Successfully raised whole plants of Lupinus and Tropaeolum by culturing shoot tips.
1952	Morel and Martin	Recovered virus-free Dahlia plants from infected individuals by culturing their shoots.
1966	Guha and Maheshwari	Demonstrated the possibility of raising large number of plantlets from pollen grains of Dhatura.
1972	Carlson	Produced the first somatic hybrid between two plants by fusing their protoplasts.

Contd...

1971	Takebe	Regenerated tobacco plants from isolated mesophyll protoplasts.
1971	Carlson	Obtained protoplast fusion between *Nicotiana glauca* and *Nicotiana longsdorffii* and developed first interspecific somatic hybrid.
1978	Melchers	Developed intergenic hybrid between potato and tomato called Pomato.
1983	Chilton	Produced transformed tobacco plants from single cell transformation and gene insertion.
1984	Horsh	Developed transgenic tobacco by *Agro bacterium* mediated gene transfer.

3.1.2 Basic Concepts of Tissue Culture

Basic concepts of plant tissue culture are totipotency, differentiation, redifferentiation and dedifferentiation.

(i) **Totipotency:** A single matured and differentiated plant cell retains the ability to change a meristematic state and differentiates into a whole plant if it has retained an intact membrane system and a viable nucleus. Such phenomenon is called cellular totipotency. The cell or group of cells having this capacity is known as totipotent cell.

(ii) **Differentiation:** It is the process of biochemical and structural changes of plant cell where cells become specialized in form and function. Example is formation of callus.

(iii) **Redifferentiation:** It is the further process of differentiation of cells which are already differentiated into another type of cell. As an example, when the cells of callus which have the ability to form a whole plant in further differentiation in a nutrient medium, the phenomenon is called redifferentiation.

(iv) **Dedifferentiation:** It is a process of reversion of mature cells to the meristematic state leading to the formation of callus, called dedifferentiation.

Generally both the process, i.e., redifferentiation and dedifferentiation are the inherent capacities of living plant cells or tissue which is expressed as totipotency.

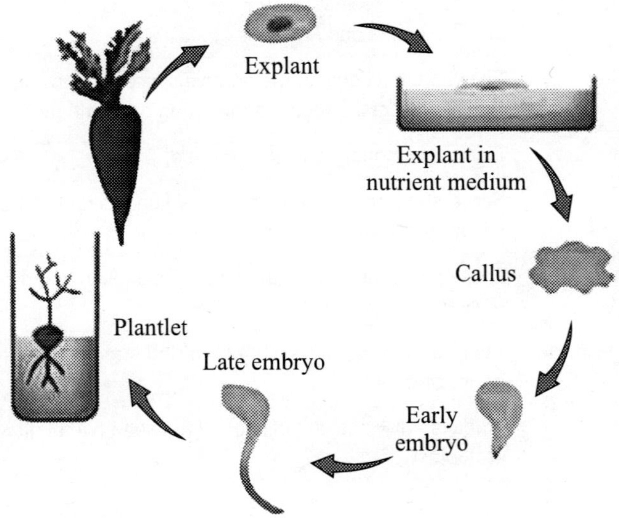

Fig. 3.1 Sequence of dedifferentiation and differentiation in plant tissue cultures

3.1.3 Plant Regeneration Pathway

From the explants, plants can be regenerated by somatic embryogenesis or organogenesis.

(i) **Somatic embryogenesis:** Formation of embryos directly from the callus tissue is known as somatic embryogenesis. Such embryos are called embryoids. Basically, in vitro cells directly from pre-embryonic cells which differentiate into embryoids. It provides potential plantlets which after hardening period can establish into plants. Somatic embryoids can be used in synthetic seeds development.

(ii) **Organogenesis:** The process for morphological changes in the callus leading to the formation of plant organs such as shoot, roots, etc., is known as organogenesis. It can be induced in vitro by introducing plant growth regulators in the MS medium. Auxin and cytokinins induce shoot and root formation. Generally, the ratio of these two hormones can determine plant development as shown below.

Concentration of plant growth regulator	Outcome
↑ Auxin and ↓ Cytokinin	Root development
↑ Cytokinin and ↓ Auxin	Shoot development
Auxin = Cytokinin	Callus development

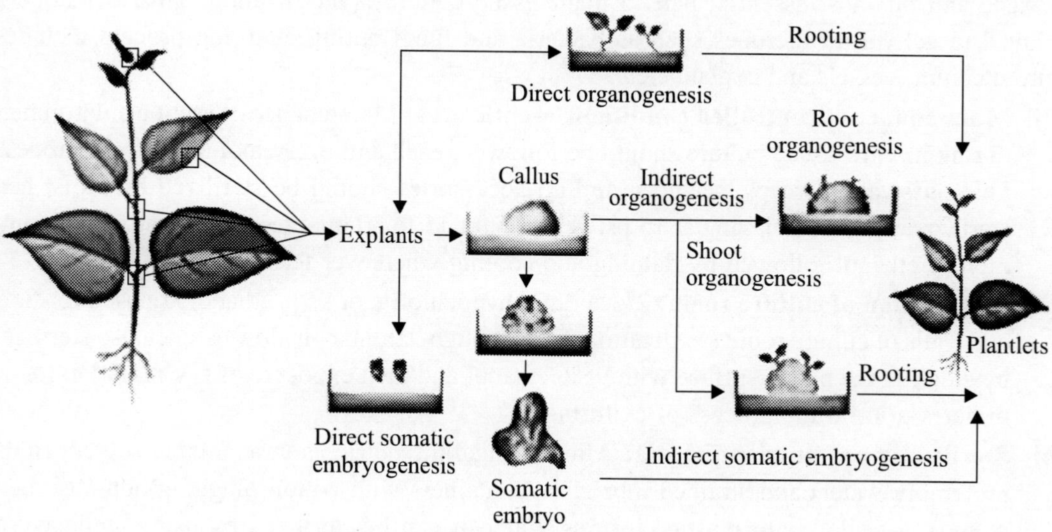

Fig. 3.2 Plant regeneration pathways

3.1.4 General Steps Involved in Plant Tissue Culture (PTC)

This technology is based on three fundamental principles:

- The plant part or explant (the tissue taken from a selected plant) must be selected in the plant body.
- Explant isolated from the plant body and sterilized.

- The explant must be maintained in controlled physically (environmental) and chemically defined (nutrient medium) conditions.

The practical approach of PTC is described below.

1. Laboratory Facilities

The laboratory for plant tissue culture should contain the following facilities:

- Separate area of washing glassware and proper place for drying ovens (hot air oven).
- Preparation room for tissue culture media well equipped with autoclave, electronic balance and pH meter.
- Transfer area sterile room with laminar air-flow bench and a positive pressure ventilation unit called high efficiency particulate air (HEPA) filter to maintain aseptic condition.
- Culturing facility for growing the explant, inoculated into culture tubes at 22-28°C with illumination of light 2400 lux, with a photoperiod of 8-16 hours and a relative humidity of about 60%.

2. Techniques Involved in PTC

1. Sterilization

The basic and far most essential part in plant tissue culture is sterilization. This technique is employed to get rid of microbes such as bacteria and fungi during culturing process includes, culture medium, vessels and explants, etc.

(i) **Maintenance of controlled conditions/aseptic area:** Maintenance of aseptic environment during in vitro tissue culture should be followed, each and every tool used in the process, i.e., glassware, forceps, scalpels, and all accessories should be sterilized by moist heat sterilization by autoclaving at 15 psi (121°C) for 15 to 30 minutes or alternatively dipping in 70% ethanol followed by flaming and cooling whereever feasible.

(ii) **Sterilization of culture room:** 2% sodium hypochlorite or 95% ethanol are used for floor and walls of culture room sterilization. Even though, laminar air-flow cabinet also sterilized by clearing the bench surface with 95% ethanol and then exposure of UV radiation for 15 minutes prior to the process of culturing.

(iii) **Sterilization of nutrient Media:** Aftermixingallthe nutrients in a suitable solvent (most preferably water) and strained into glass containers with cotton plugging(non-absorbent cotton) or sealed with plastic closures. Later, it can be sterilized by using autoclave at 15 psi (121°C) for 15 minutes. Membrane filtration or millipore filter (with 0.2 mm pore diameter) are widely used in sterilization of plant extracts, vitamins, amino acids and hormones just before addition to sterilized nutrient medium in laminar airflow chamber under sterile condition.

(iv) **Surface Sterilization of Explants:** The plant partor explant should be surface sterilized by first exposing the material in running tap water and then treating it in surface sterilization agents like 0.1% mercuric chloride, 70% ethanol under aseptic conditions inside the flow chamber of laminar air.

2. Media Preparation

Medium alone is not capable enough to maintain optimum growth of all plant tissues. But this is also true that the success of tissue culture lies in the composition of the growth medium. Specific plant growth regulators and culture conditions (like temperature, pH, light and humidity) play the main role in tissue development. However, suitable nutrient medium is prepared and used as per requirements of culture. As per requirement, medium may be solid or semisolid or liquid in nature. For solidification, a gelling agent such as agar (a complex mucilaginous polysaccharide obtained from marine algae (seaweeds)) can be added in various concentrations on the basis of requirement.

In plant tissue culture, commonly used media is MS nutrient medium (Murashige and Skoog, 1962). It has well balance carbon sources and other suitable essential growth regulators such as vitamins hormones, etc.

Apart from MS media, other media formulations available for plant tissue culture are:

Name of the media	Contributor
B5 medium White medium Nitsch's medium	Gamborg.et.al., 1968 White, 1943 Nitsch & Nitsch, 1969

Table 3.2 Composition of MS (Murashige and Skoog) medium

Macronutrients	
Ammonium nitrate (NH_4NO_3)	1650.0 mg/L
Potassium nitrate (KNO_3)	1900.0 mg/L
Calcium chloride ($CaCl_2$ $2H_2O$)	440.0 mg/L
Magnesium sulphate ($MgSO_4$ $6H_2O$)	370.0 mg/L
Potassium dihydrogen phosphate (KH_2PO_4)	170.0 mg/L
Micronutrients	
Manganese sulphate ($MnSO_4$ $4H_2O$)	22.3 mg/L
Zinc sulphate ($ZnSO_4$ $4H_2O$)	8.6 mg/L
Boric acid (H_3BO_3)	6.2 mg/L
Potassium iodide (KI)	0.83 mg/L
Minor nutrients	
Sodium molybdate (Na_2 MO_4 $2H_2O$)	0.250 mg/L
Cupric sulphate ($CuSO_4$ $5H_2O$)	0.025 mg/L
Cobaltous chloride ($CoCl_2$ $6H_2O$)	0.025 mg/L

Contd.

Iron stock	
Na EDTA	37.25 mg/L
Ferrous sulphate ($FeSO_4$ $7H_2O$)	27.85 mg/L
Vitamins	
Glycine	2.0 mg/L
Nicotinic acid	0.5 mg/L
Pyridoxin HCl	0.5 mg/L
ThaiamineHCl	0.1 mg/L
Growth Hormones	
IAA	1.30 mg/L
Kinetin	0.4-10.0 mg/L
Myo-inositol	100.0 mg/L
Sucrose	30.0 g/L
Solidifying agent	
Agar	8.0 g/L

3. **Culture Conditions**

   3.1 pH: The pH of medium is normally adjusted in between 5.6-6.0 for the best results.

   3.2 Temperature: The cultures should be incubated normally at constant temperature of 25°C ± 2°C for optimal growth.

   3.3 Humidity and light intensity: The cultures require 50-60% relative humidity and 16 hours of photoperiod by the illumination of cool white fluorescent tubes of approximately 1000 lux.

   3.4 Aeration: Aeration to the culture can be provided by shaking the flasks or tubes of liquid culture on automatic shaker or aeration of the medium by passing with filter-sterilized air.

4. **Induction of Callus**

Sterile segment of explant nearly about 1-2 cm basically selected from leaf, stem, tuber or root is inoculated in the sterilized MS nutrient medium. The medium has been supplemented with auxins and incubated at 25°C ± 2°C in an alternate light and dark period of 12 hours. It will facilitate the process of cell division and soon the upper surface of explant develops into an undifferentiated proliferated cell mass, commonly known as callus.

5. **Embryogenesis**

Post-callus development, the callus cells further undergo cellular differentiation process and produce somatic embryos or embryoids. These embryoids are sub-cultured to produce plantlets via this in vitro cultivation method.

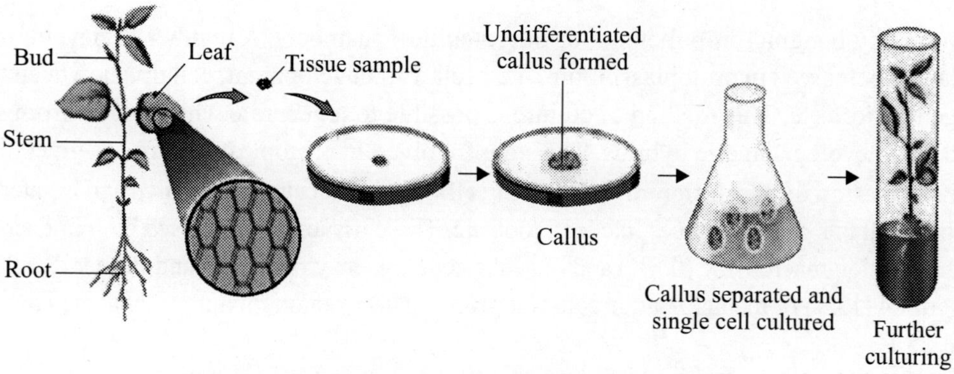

Fig. 3.3 Basic steps involved in plant tissue culture

6. Hardening

Hardening is the process of gradual exposure of in vitro developed plantlets in humid chambers in diffused light for acclimatization. It will enable the plantlets to grow under normal field conditions with greater adoptability. In this case, the plantlets developed by in vitro method are exposed to hardening period and followed by transferred to greenhouse or hardening chamber and lastly to normal environmental conditions in field for further developments.

3.1.5 Types of Plant Tissue Cultures

Based on the explants some other plant tissue culture types are given below.

1. *Organ culture*

(a) **Vegetative organ culture:** In this type of culture, vegetative parts or organ of the plant such as shoot, leaf, root or other parts can be used as an explant. Various methods are employed for vegetative organ culture, such as plasma clot method, raft method, grid method, agar gel method, etc. For preservation of the structural and functional properties of an organism, this culture method is commonly used. Example: shoot culture, leaf culture, root culture, stem culture, etc.

(b) **Reproductive organ culture:** This method is deployed with various reproductive parts or organs of plant, i.e., embryos, anthers, ovaries, pollen, etc., act as an explant cultivated on culture media. Example: pollen culture, anther culture, embryo culture.

2. *Meristem culture*

This type of culture deals with the apical meristemitic cells (ability to enlarge, stretch and differentiate into other types of cells as they mature) from angiosperm and gymnosperm shoots which are cultured to produce plants that found to be significantly resistant from disease and contamination. For this reason, meristem culture is often preferred as the lack of vascular tissues ensures that contamination and spread of disease is limited.

3. *Protoplast culture*

Protoplast cells are defined as the cells without a cell wall, but bounded by a cell membrane or plasma membrane. Culturing of such protoplast cells is known as protoplast culture which could be performed by hanging-drop method, or micro-culture chambers. A number of developmental phases can be perceived in protoplast culture, i.e., cell wall development, cell division even whole plant regeneration, etc. This method of culture is possible to regenerate whole plants from single cells and also develop somatic hybrids. The steps involved in protoplast culture are given below.

(i) Preparation and isolation of protoplast cell: Protoplast cells are prepared and isolated from the small bits of plant tissues like leaf, root, etc. These tissues are processed by immersing into the solution macrozyme (0.5%) and onozuka cellulase enzymes (2%)) and further dissolved in sorbitol (13%) or mannitol at the constant pH 5.4. This reaction mixture is incubated overnight at 25°C.

After incubation, protoplast cells are obtained by a gentle teasing of cells and transferred to sucrose solution (20%) for retention of viability. The final isolation of pure protoplast cells isobtained from debris of cell walls by centrifugation process.

(ii) Protoplast cell fusion: The fusion of protoplast cells is done with the use of a suitable fusogen (a glycoprotein that facilitates the fusion of cell-to-cell membranes) like polyethylene glycol (PEG).

The isolated protoplast cells are incubated in PEG (25-30%) with Ca^{++} ions. The protoplast cells show agglutination (clumps of cells) and fusion. The process of fusion may be possible with different other method also like electrofusion.

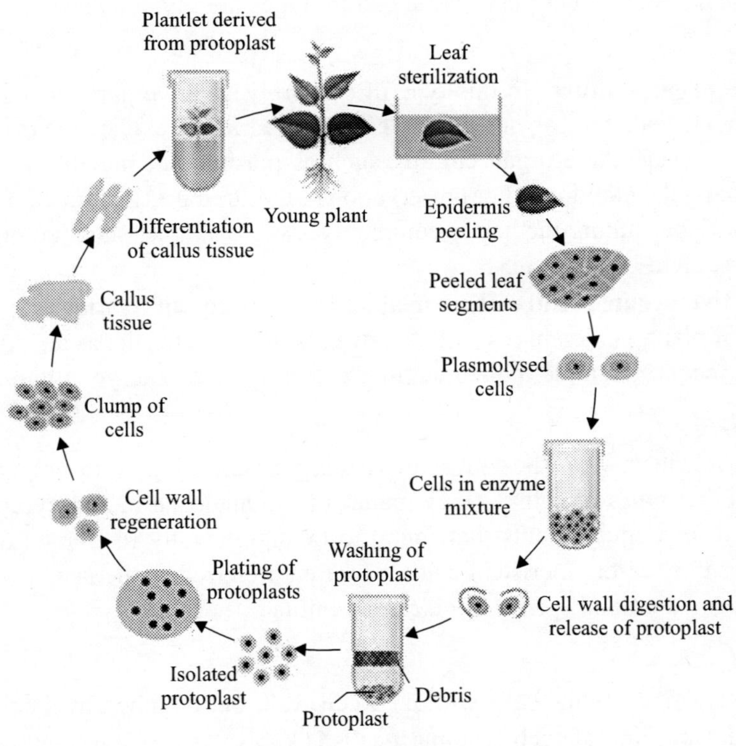

Fig. 3.4 Protoplast culture

(iii) Protoplast cell culture: Protoplast cell culture generally is preformed with MS liquid medium by applying droplet, plating or micro-drop array techniques. The cellular viability of protoplast is tested with fluorescein diacetate before the cell culture.

The fused protoplast cells are cultured by incubating in continuous light 1000-2000 lux at 25°C. Initiation and formation of cell wall occurs within 24-48 hours and moreover the first cell division occurs in the newly generated cells between 2 and 7 days in incubation culture conditions.

(iv) Selection of somatic hybrid cells: The fusion product of protoplasts without nucleus of different cells is called a cybrid (cells or plant containing nucleus of one species but cytoplasm from both the parental species), obtained by spontaneous or mechanical fusion method, generally known as somatic hybridization. Fused cybrids are further propagated for regeneration of desired characteristic plants.

4. Cell culture

4.1 Callus culture: An undifferentiated cell mass (callus) generated from any part of the plant material which is cultured under in vitro conditions. In such type of culture no specific section of the plant part or organ is being used.

4.2 Cell suspension culture: The growing of cells including the culture of single cells or small aggregates of cells in vitro in liquid medium is known as cell suspension culture. The cell suspension is prepared by transferring a portion of callus to the liquid medium and agitated using rotary shaker instrument. The cells are separated from the callus tissue and used for cell suspension culture for further propagation.

There are two types of cell suspension cultures.

A. Batch cell suspension culture

B. Continuous cell suspension culture

Each of these cultures has its own advantages and all types are used.

A. Batch cell suspension culture

Batch culture is a type of cell suspension where the cell material grows in a finite volume of agitated liquid medium. These cultures are maintained continuously by subculturing. Batch cultures are most commonly maintained in conical flasks incubated on orbital platform shakers at the speed of 80-120 rpm. It is a closed system, with no additions or removal of nutrient and waste products during the period of incubation.

Types of batch suspension culture

1. **Slow rotating cultures:** In this culture, single cells and cell aggregates are grown in a specially designed flask, the nipple flask. Each nipple flask possesses eight nipple-like projections, having a capacity of 250 mL. They are loaded in a circular manner on the large flat disc of vertical shaker. When the flat disc rotates at a speed of 1-2 rpm, the cells within each nipple of the flask are alternatively bathed in the culture medium and exposed to air.

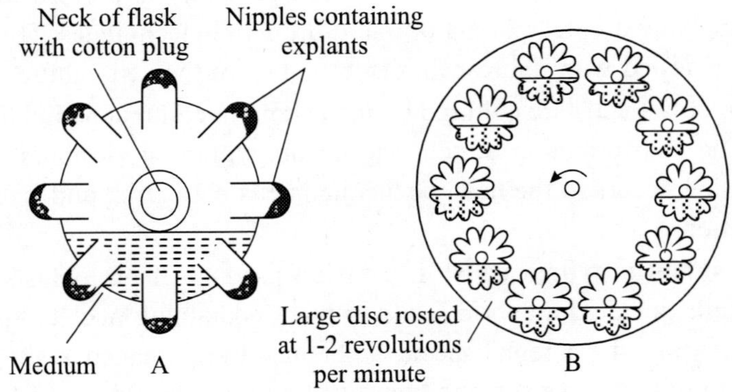

Fig. 3.5 Nipple flask

2. **Shaker suspension cultures:** It is a very effective system. In this method, single cells and cell aggregates in fixed volume of liquid medium are placed in conical flasks. These flasks are then mounted with the help of clips on a horizontal large square plate of an orbital platform shaker. The square plate moves in a circular motion at the speed of 60-180 rpm.

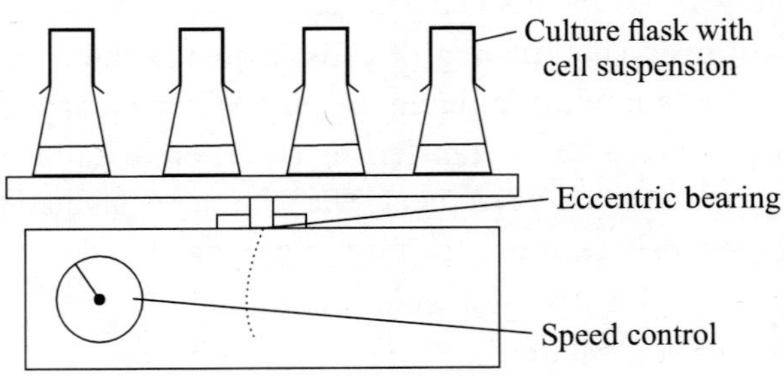

Fig. 3.6 Shaker suspension cultures

3. **Spinning suspension cultures:** In this culture system, large bottles are used, usually bottles with the capacity of 10 L. A large volume of cell suspension is cultured in 10 L bottles, with the bottles spinning in a spinner at 120 rpm at an angle of 45°.
4. **Stirred suspension culture:** This system is used for large-scale batch culture. In this method, the large culture vessel (round-bottom flask) is not rotated but the cell suspension inside the vessel is kept dispersed continuously by bubbling sterile air through the culture medium. Internal magnetic stirrer is used to agitate the culture medium safely. The magnetic stirrer revolves at 200-600 rpm.

B. Continuous cell suspension culture

In continuous culture system, the old liquid medium is replaced continuously by the fresh liquid medium to stabilize the physiological states of the growing cells. In this system, nutrient depletion does not occur due to the continuous flow of nutrients and the cells always remain in the steady growth phase. Continuous culture is further divided into two types:

1. In closed type continuous cell suspension culture, the used medium is replaced with the fresh medium, hence, the cells from used medium are mechanically retrieved and added back to the culture and thus, the cell biomass keeps on increasing.

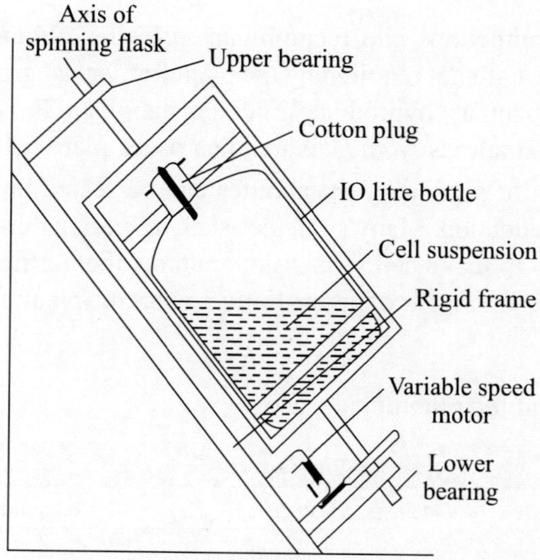

Fig. 3.7 Stirred suspension culture

2. In open type continuous cell suspension culture, both the cells and used medium are replaced with fresh medium thus maintaining culture at constant and submaximal growth rate.

Open continuous cell suspension culture is of two types.

(i) Chemostat: In this system, culture vessels are usually cylindrical or circular in shape and possess inlet and outlet pores for aeration and the introduction and removal of cells and medium. Such a system is maintained in a steady state. Thus in a steady state condition the density, growth rate, chemical composition and metabolic activity of the cells remain constant. Such continuous cultures are ideal for studying growth kinetics and the regulation of metabolic activity in higher plants.

(ii) Turbidostats: A turbidostatis a continuous culturing method where the turbidity of the culture is held constant by manipulating the rate at which medium is fed. In this system, the cells are allowed to grow up to certain turbidity, when the predetermined volume of culture is replaced by fresh culture. The turbidity is measured by the changes of optical density of medium. An automatic monitoring unit is connected with the culture vessel and such unit adjusts the medium flow in such a way as to maintain the optical density or pH at chosen, present level.

4.3 Importance of cell suspension culture: Such systems are capable of contributing significant information about cell physiology, biochemistry, metabolic events, etc. It is important to build up an understanding of an organ/embryoid formation starting from a single cell.Mutagenesis studies maybe facilitated by cell suspension culture to produce mutant cell clone from which mutant plants can be raised.

4.4 Applications of cell suspension culture on plant metabolite production: Cell suspension culture can be useful for the production of secondary metabolites like alkaloids, flavonoids, terpenoids, phenolic compounds and recombinant proteins. Secondary metabolites are chemical compounds that are not required by the plant for normal growth and development but are produced in the plant as 'byproducts' of cell metabolism. For example, biosynthesis and isolation of indole alkaloids from Catharanthusroseus plant cell culture.

The process of production of secondary metabolites can be scaled up and automated using bio-reactors for commercial production. Many strategies such as biotransformation, elicitation and immobilization have been used to make cell suspension cultures more efficient in the production of secondary metabolites. Few examples of industrially important plant secondary metabolites are listed in Table 3.3.

Table 3.3 Plant constituents and their therapeutic uses

Secondary metabolites	Plant source	Therapeutic use
Quinine	*Cinchona officinalis*	Antimalarial
Codeine	*Papaver sominiferum*	Antitussives
Capsaicin	*Capsicum annum*	Rheumatic pain
Vincristine	*Catharanthus roseus*	Anticancer

The advantages and disadvantages of cell suspension culture are tabulated below.

Table 3.4 Advantage vs disadvantage of cell suspension culture

Advantages	Disadvantages
(i) The nutrients can be continually adjusted. (ii) This system can be scaled for large-scale production of the cells. (iii) A whole plant can be regenerated from a single plant cell.	(i) The productivity of suspension cultures decreases over extended subculture periods. (ii) Slow growth and low productivity of plant cells. (iii) Cells may get damaged by shear conditions.

3.1.6 Nutritional Requirements for Culture Media

The success of any culture technique either cell, tissue or organ depends on the choice of nutrients and growth regulators. Usually, various media and growth regulating hormones are used in plant tissue culture techniques with assured reproducible results.

Most number of plant cells are cultured in well-defined medias. But some exceptional cases need additional complex ingredients such as coconut milk or tomato juice, etc. However, the choice of a medium and ingredients are strictly focused on the purpose and the species or type of plant and its developmental stage.

Nutritional Compositions

The plant tissue culture media must be enriched with the essential macro- or micro-elements, carbon source, vitamins and growth regulators.

(i) **Macro-elements (inorganic nutrients):** Macronutrients act as source of nitrogen, potassium, phosphorus, sulphur, calcium, magnesium, etc., like essential nutrients which

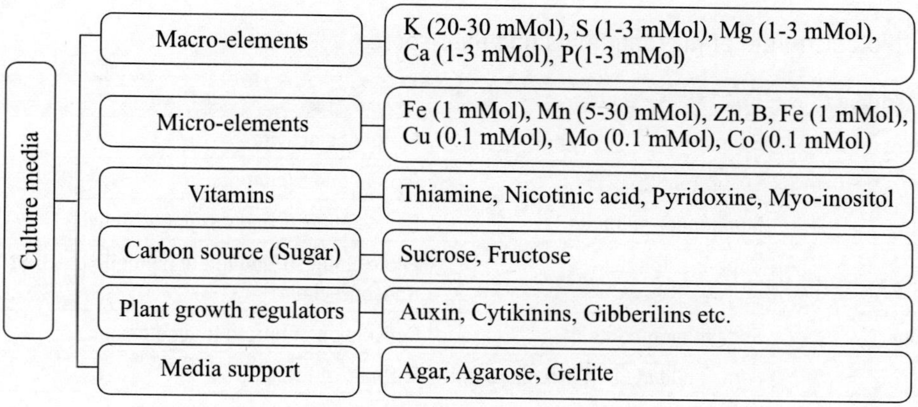

Fig. 3.8 Nutritional requirements in culture media

are required for healthy plant development and growth. For example, such nutrients required in higher quantity, such as the tolerated level of sodium and potassium ions are up to 50-60 nM. They provide both anions and cations for plant cells. Nitrogen is provided in the form of nitrate salt. Even more, some media contains both ammonia and nitrate as source of nitrogen. Interestingly, it has been observed that, the alteration of pH in media depends on the source nitrogen, i.e., elevation of pH with nitrate and decrease with ammonium. Phosphates provide phosphorus and also act as buffer in media.

Macronutrients have structural and functional rolesin protein synthesis, cell wall synthesis, enzyme co-factors and membrane integrity.

Table 3.5 Biological role of macronutrients and their source

Macro nutrients	Source	Role
Nitrogen	Amino acid, organic acids, casein hydrolysate	Helps in synthesis complex organic molecule
Potassium	Cytoplasm (100-200 mM) and chloroplast (20-200 mM)	Maintaining the ion balancing, osmotic pressure, osmotic regulation of cells and activation of many enzymes
Calcium	Calcium chloride, calcium nitrate	Strength to cell wall, cell and root multiplication, enzyme co-factor
Phosphorus	Sodium hydrogen phosphate, potassium hydrogen phosphate	Energy metabolism, essential element for DNA and RNA
Magnesium	Magnesium sulphate	Enzymatic reactions and ATP synthesis
Sulphur	Magnesium sulphate, potassium sulphate	Enhance protein and chlorophyll synthesis

(ii) Micro-elements (inorganic nutrients): As like macronutrients, several micronutrients or trace elements are essential for the growth of plant cells, tissues and organs. Various micronutrients and their source and role have been described below.

Table 3.6 Biological role of micronutrients and their source

Micro nutrients	Source	Role
Boron	Boric acid	Enzymatic activity
Zinc	Zinc sulphate	Protein and tryptophan
Manganese	Manganese sulphate	Photosynthesis and enzymatic activity
Copper	Copper sulphate	Photosynthesis and intermediate in electron transport chain
Molybdenum	Sodium molybdate	Conversion of nitrate to ammonium
Iron	Ferric sodium EDTA (Na_2Fe EDTA)	Enzyme co-factor

Apart from the above-mentioned nutrients, iodide, has been used to stimulates cell growth. Iron is added in a chelated form either as an EDTA salt or as agricultural chelates, e.g., sequestrene 330 Fe.

(iii) Carbon sources: Carbon is the main backbone of any living structure. But most of the laboratory cultures cannot have sufficient capacity of photosynthesise enough sugars, for cellular growth. For that the carbon source is essentials to supply. Majorly, sucrose in the range of 20-30 g/L is used to the medium. A like sucrose, the use of glucose is less often, even fructose used occasionally. This is because; compared to other sugars, sucrose is readily taken up in the media within 1-2 days and converted to starch granules within the cells. Even though, m-inositol (a beneficial component for cell wall metabolism) has also been used in certain media as source of carbon.

(iv) Vitamins: In vitro cultures require thiamine, pyridoxine, nicotinic acid and myoinositol,etc. like vitamins which enhance the effects of growth and development of plant cells. All these vitamins are stable during autoclaving. Other vitamins like biotin, pantothenic acid, folic acid, choline chloride, p-aminobenzoic acid, riboflavin, vitamin B_{12} and ascorbic acid are added at 1 mg/L or less in some instances, especially when cells or protoplasts are cultured.

(v) Plant growth regulators: In vitro tissue culture also requires essential plant growth regulators either phytohormones (naturally occurring plant hormones) or synthetic hormones. Most of the synthetic hormones have similar structural analogs of the natural hormones and bind to the same receptors.

Plant growth regulators such as auxins, cytokinins, gibberellins and abscisic acid, etc. are used frequently in plant tissue culture whereas auxins and cytokinins have their more solo uses among all.

(a) Auxins

Auxins facilitate cell elongation, apical dominance and adventitious root formation in culturing plant cell. Callus induction, organogenesis and somatic embryogenesis in plant tissue culture generally initiated by auxins with cytokinins or other plant growth regulators (PGRs). Natural and synthetic auxins are generally used in tissue culture:

(i) Natural ones: Indole-3-acetic acid (IAA), Indole-3-butyric acid (IBA)

(ii) Synthetic ones: 1-Naphthalene acetic acid (NAA), 2,4-Dichloro phenoxy acetic acid (2,4-D)

(b) Cytokinins

Cytokinins promote cell division and are used for initiation of culture or for long-term growth. The more commonly used cytokinin is kinetin, since it induces development and multiplication of shoot bud. The other more commonly used cytokinins are the synthetic kinetin (6-furfural laminopurine) and 6-benzyl aminopurine (BAP). Most of the cytokinins except zeatin and its derivatives can be autoclaved with the media and are used in the range of 1-50 μm.

(c) Gibberellins

Gibberellins cause stem elongation, flowering, breaking of dormancy of seeds, parthenocarpic development of fruits, etc., in whole plants. However, only GA_3, gibberellic acid and GA_{417} are used in plant tissue culture. Gibberellins, in plant tissue culture inhibit induction of organogenesis, especially adventitious root formation.

(d) Abscisic acid (ABA)

ABA regulates closure of stomata and cause bud and seed dormancy. In plant tissue culture, ABA promotes maturation and germination of normal somatic embryos.

(vi) Media support system: Both liquid and semisolid media can be used depending on the culture. Most of the media used in plant tissue culture need semi-solid media. Agar-agar obtained from the sea weed is the most commonly used gelling agent. Some important gelling agents are: agar, agarose, and gelrite

Agar is a complex mixture of related polysaccharides built up from the sugar, galactose, obtained from red algae (*Gelidium amansii*). It contains natural polymer fractions, agarose, which gives strength to the gel and the highly charged anionic polysaccharides agaropectins which give agar its viscosity. Agar is used at varying concentrations from 0.8 to 1%. Agarose commonly preferred over agar for protoplast culture. In the other hand, gelrite can be used as an alternative to agar not only because of its lower cost but also its low concentrations (0.1-0.2% is sufficient).

(vii) Other organic additives: They do not promote growth but act as nutrients. Complex ingredients like coconut milk, yeast extract, fruit juices and casein hydrolysates are among the few. They provide amino acids, vitamins, growth regulators, etc., which can enhance plant cell growth. Some examples are listed below.

Table 3.7 Organic additives enhance the plant cell growth

Name of the organic additives	Role in PTC
Mannitol, sorbitol or combinations	Increase osmolarity of media
Citric acid, fumaric acid, malic acid or succinic acid	Maintain pH
Auxins (IAA, NAA, IBA and 2,4-D), Cytokinins (BAP and Kinetin)	Dissolved in minimum quantity of 0.1 N NaOH or ethyl alcohol

3.1.7 Growth and Maintenance of Plant Cell Culture

After callus induction, the callus is grown further on a new medium, which is referred to as sub-culturing. During subculturing the callus tissue shows sigmoid growth pattern on a particular media. The time interval for subculturing is calculated according to the growth pattern of the particular tissue type and genotype of the plant.

When the callus growth reaches to the stationary phase of growth then it needs to be cultured on to a fresh medium. Callus tissue from different explants of different plant species may be different in structure and growth habit: white or coloured, soft (watery) or hard, friable (easy to separate the cells) or compact.

3.1.7.1 Growth Curve of Plant Cells

It is an 'S' shaped curve of growth obtained in tissue or cell culture plotted against time. It is also called 'sigmoid'curve. This curve mainly shows four phases of growth. It includes:

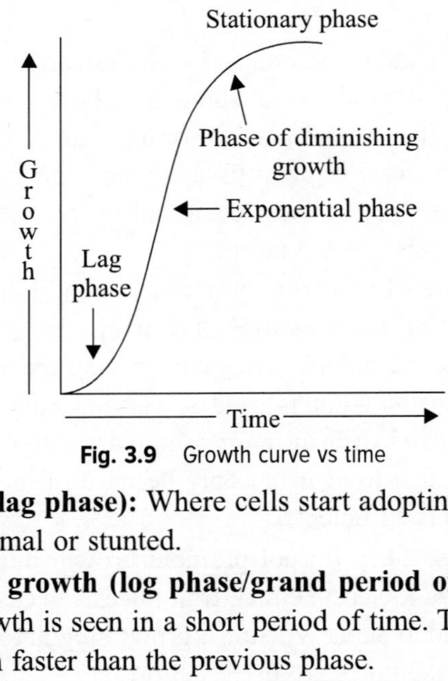

Fig. 3.9 Growth curve vs time

1. **Initial slow growth (lag phase):** Where cells start adopting the environment, as a reason growth becomes minimal or stunted.
2. **The rapid period of growth (log phase/grand period of growth/exponential phase):** Where maximum growth is seen in a short period of time. The number of cell division and multiplication is much faster than the previous phase.
3. **The diminishing phase:** This is the junction between log and stationary phase where growth will be slow and becomes steady.
4. **Stationary/steady phase:** Where finally growth stops and cells stay for long.

3.1.7.2 Assessment of Growth Parametersin Callus and Suspension Culture

Assessment of growth parameters in the different types of cultures plays an important role in evaluating the growth kinetics of plant cell and tissue culture.

3.1.7.2.1 Measuring growth in callus cultures

The growth index of the callus culture is measured by fresh and dry weight measurement.

Harvested tissue is carefully weighed on the balance to avoid tissue desiccation for the fresh weight measurements. On the other hand, tissues either lyophilized or dried (microwave oven drying, 60°C) until the constant weight achieved in case of dry weight measurement.

3.1.7.2.2 Measuring growth in cell suspension cultures

The measurement of growth in cell suspension culture can be achieved by different ways. It includes the following.

(i) **Fresh cell weight and dry cell weight:** It is a more precise measurement of cell growth than the sole culture volume. But both require the manipulation of samples in non-sterile conditions.

(ii) **Settled cell volume (SCV) and packed cell volume (PCV):** Both the volumes are measured after compacting the suspension by centrifugation. SCV is the percentage of the total volume of suspension occupied by the cell mass, whereas, PCV is the total volume of suspension occupied by the cell mass.

(iii) **Cell number/mL of media:** Cell counting is done by pipetting 1 mL of the suspension culture and counting the total number of cells under the microscope.

(iv) **Culture cell density:** After the complete disaggregation of the cell, the culture cell density is estimated. This disaggregation of cells can be achieved by incubating them with an 8% chromium trioxide solution, or with hydrolytic enzymes, such as cellulase and pectinase.

(v) **Protein and/or DNA content:** Protein or DNA content can be determined by using ethidium bromide or propidium for cell staining method. Stained cells in excited state cells emit reddish orange fluorescence.

(vi) **Medium conductivity:** Once biomass is gained, the ionic concentration of the culture medium started decreasing inversely. By using an electroporator medium conductivity has been determined by applying an electromagnetic field.

(vii) **Oxygen and mass transfers:** Factors like viscosity, density, cell buoyancy, and aggregation directly affect the solubility of oxygen and mass transfers.

(viii) **Cell viability:** Fluorescein diacetate, a staining reagent, is widely used to check cellviability in media.

(ix) **Osmolarity:** Osmotic pressure and ionic strength of culture medium influence the membrane transport pH, extracellular enzymes, and secondary metabolite production.

3.1.7.2.3 Evaluation of growth efficiency

(i) **Growth index (GI):** The ratio of the total mass transferred and final volume accumulated during propagation of the culture is known as growth index (GI) which is represented as follows:

$$GI = \frac{Fm - Im}{Fm}$$

where, GI is growth index, and Fm and Im represent the final and initial masses, respectively (either as fresh or dry weight).

(ii) **Specific Growth Rate (SG):** The rate of increased biomass of a cell population per unit of biomass concentration in called specific growth rate (SG). It occurs between the lag and stationary phases in the sigmoid curve where cell growth follows a straight line equation as follows:

$$\ln Fm = Sgt + \ln Im$$
$$Sg = \ln Fm - \ln Im/t$$

where, Sg is the specific growth rate, Fm is the biomass (or cell density) at time *t*, and *Im* is the initial biomass (or cell density).

(iii) Doubling Time (TD): This is the time consumed by the particular concentration of the cells to double from their initial concentration, e.g., TD of microorganism (hours) > plant cell (days). Among all the plant tissue cultures the fastest doubling time is reported for tobacco cells (15 h). TD is represented as follows: TD = ln 2/Sg, where Sg represents the specific growth rate.

Maintenance of cell culture

Generally, maintenance of callus tissue growth needs growth hormones in order to grow as long as they are maintained through serial subcultures. But it has been observed also that the callus tissue in some plant species may become habituated after prolonged culture.

Table 3.8 Advantages and disadvantages of plant tissue culture

Advantages	Disadvantages
Molecular to mass level of work can be performed. The tedious and laborious work such as weeding, spraying, watering, etc., can be skipped in plant tissue culture.	Requires lot of expensive and specialized procedures, facilities, and advance skills.
For rejuvenation of plant material and cultures, can be preserved for long .	Plants produced are dependent on nutritional sources in contrast to field plants.
Production is independent on season and can continue throughout the year.	It is not obligatory to have callus within a short time. Sometimes callus will not appear for months and for some plants callus does not appear.
It is the best technique for the introduction of temporal characteristics and studying the effects of several mutagens and to attempt immobilization of cells, for biotransformation or biochemical reactions.	Plantlets are initially small and have undesirable characteristics.
It may provide a continuous, reliable source of phytopharmaceuticals and could be used for the large-scale culture of plant cells.	Plants do not function autotrophically in culture and have to undergo a transitional phase before independent growth.
Plant tissue culture can produce a large number of clones (with desirable characteristics), draught resistant, flood resistant, disease-free plants, plants of high nutritional value, and high quality plants with improved yields of secondary metabolites (also used to study biogenesis of secondary metabolites).	Chances of producing genetically aberrant plants may be increased.
The process offers uniform biomass available all the time, synthesis of medicinal compounds difficult or impossible to synthesize chemically, independent of soil conditions and change in climatic conditions.	Plantlets are more susceptible to contamination and water loss in the external environment, since they are grown at a high relative humidity.

This means that the callus tissue is able to grow on a standard maintenance medium or basal medium which is devoid of growth hormone. This property of callus tissue is called habituation.

3.1.8 Applications of Plant Tissue Culture in Pharmacognosy

1. Micro-propagation

It is the process where we regenerate whole plant through tissue culture. In this propagation, a single explant initiates the formation of callus mass and gradually generates the large number of plantlet in very short period of time in restricted spaces. Again, it is possible to make a large number of callus pieces from the original stock culture during subculturing.

Hundreds of plantlets can be possible to develop on each of these callus pieces. Hence, the most obvious advantage of micro-propagation is the numerical one. Suspension cultures can also be used to exploit this numerical advantage even faster than callus tissues.

2. Clonal Propagation

It is also a type of micro-propagation. The cultured plants raised from tissue culture are derived asexually and also multiply within culture vessel by asexual means. A sexual reproduction, on the otherhand, gives rise to plants which are genetically identical to the parent plant. Multiplication of genetically identical copies of a cultivar by asexual reproduction is called clonal propagation and a plant population derived from a single donor plant in tissue culture constitutes a clone. So, the variability that can arise from sexual reproduction and seed formation in a crop plant is omitted. Clonal multiplication of cultivar is very important in horticulture and silviculture.

3. Production of Genetically Variable Plants

The chromosomal instability in the cultured cells plays an important role in polyploidization of cells and genetically variable plants can be raised from such polyploidized cells by subsequent micro-propagation. Thus, tissue culture is proving to be rich and novel source of variability with a great potential in crop improvement without resorting to mutation or hybridization. Variants which have been selected through tissue culture are known a scalliclones (from callus culture) or protoclones (from protoplast culture). Such variant plants may show some useful characters such as resistance to a particular disease, herbicide resistance, stress tolerance, etc.

4. Plant Pathology and Plant Tissue Culture

There have been many valuable contributions of plant tissue culture to problems concerning plant pathology. One outstanding success is the virus eradication by apical meristem culture and the second success of tissue culture in plant pathology is the result of its application to the problems of plant tumors, especially crown gall. The apical meristem culture is the only way to obtain a clone of virus-free plant which can be multiplied vegetatively under controlled conditions that would protect them from the chance of reinfection. The elimination procedure of virus can usually be improved by combining it with heat therapy of the host plant or the culture.

5. Plant Breeding, Plant Improvement and Plant Tissue Culture

Embryo culture is now routinely used in recovery of hybrid plants from distant crosses. Some examples are recovery of hybrids from *Hordeum vulgare* × *Secale cereale*, *Triticum aestivum* ×

Agropyron repens, *H. vulgare* × *Triticum* species. In case of triticale, a rare hybrid between triticum and secale develop viable seeds. By embryo culture, 50-70% hybrid seedlings have been obtained. It is also useful for propagation of orchids; shortening the breeding cycle and overcoming seed dormancy. In meristem culture, shoot apical meristem along some surrounding tissue is grown in vitro. It is used for clonal propagation and recovery of virus free plants and is potentially useful in germplasm exchange and long-term storage of germplasm through freeze preservation.

Anther and pollen culture have a potential application in plant breeding and plant improvement programme for the production of haploid as well as homozygous diploid plant. All-yearround rapid clonal propagation using plant tissue culture techniques has highlighted possibilities for new plant improvement techniques. Protoplast culture and somatic hybridization is a promising line for plant breeding and plant improvement techniques. But, at present, a technique for selection and multiplication of somatic hybrid and regeneration of hybrid plants is limited to a few classical plant species. So it is expected that in near future it would be possible to use this technique for a wide variety of plant species.

6. *Production of Useful Biochemicals*

A surprising number of cell cultures have been found that do produce specialized biochemicals found in the intact parent, including alkaloid such as nicotine, atropine, ephedrine, caffeine and codeine and their precursors and derivatives. Production of cardiac glycosides and other steroids, benzoquinones, latex, phenolics, anthocyanins, organic acids, anti-tumour agents, antimicrobials and various flavours and odours have also been reported.

7. *Preservation of Plant Genetic Resources or Gene Conservation Banks*

Conventionally, germplasms are stored in the form of seeds because they occupy a relatively small space and can be stored for many years. But there are a number of important species, particularly root and tuber crops, which are normally propagated vegetatively. It is now possible with modern tissue culture techniques to provide a germplasm storage procedure which uniquely combines the possibilities of disease elimination and rapid clonal multiplication. In addition, the possibility of using liquid nitrogen freezestorage techniques for the preservation of cell, tissue and apical meristem is being studied. The advantages of this technique are that cell division and normal cellular reactions are totally arrested at the very low temperature of liquid nitrogen (–196°C), which means that there should be a high level of genetic stability and that the chemical reaction responsible for cellular damage will not occur.It has already been shown to be successful with a range of cell cultures, e.g., carrot cell and sycamore suspension cells and meristem tips from a number of crop plants including asparagus, tomato and potato. Plant tissue or meristems of such plants have been successfully recovered from liquid nitrogen and grown into normal, mature fertile plants.

8. *Tissue Culture in Biotechnology*

Cell suspension culture in liquid medium is a relatively young field of biotechnology. This technology involves large-scale culture of isolated plant cell under condition which induces them to synthesize the natural secondary metabolites characteristic of parent plants from which they were obtained. In recent years, the technique of callus culture and cell suspension culture has also been viewed, particularly from the viewpoint for the study of biosynthesis and metabolism of steroids and cardiac glycosides. To increase the synthesis of natural compounds or new compounds by higher plant cells culture as a result of mixing or feeding transformable precursors in the culture medium.

9. Modification of cellular genetics

It can be achieved by mutagenesis and selection of cell lines in cell suspension culture, Transplantation of foreign genetic material in protoplasts by means of genetic engineering and Somatic hybridization by the fusion of distantly related plant proplast just to widen the genetic diversity of hybrids.

10. Production of Self-fertilizing and self-pesticides plant

Self-fertilizing plants are those plants which provide their own usable nitrogen. Some plants rely on a few types of bacteria and cyanobacteria to fix atmospheric nitrogen into a biologically useable form. Genetically engineered plants that contain the bacterial genes for nitrogen fixation could grow well even in nitrogen-poor soil. Genetic engineers are also developing plants that produce their own pesticides which can kill the pest even in one bite. In 1986, the first of such genetically engineered plants successfully passed a field test.

Sixteen important applications of plant tissue culture

1. The use of plant cells to generate useful products and or services constitutes plant biotechnology.
2. In plant biotechnology, the useful product is a plantlet. The plantlets are used for various purposes.
3. All the cells in callus or suspension culture are derived from a single explant by mitotic division.
4. Therefore, all plantlets regenerated from a callus/suspension culture generally have the same genotype and constitute a clone. These plantlets are used for rapid clonal propagation.
5. Genetic variation present among plant cells of a culture is called soma clonal variation.
6. A gene that is transferred into an organism by genetic engineering is known as transgene.
7. An organism that contains and expresses a transgene is called transgenic organism.
8. The transgenes can be introduced into individual plant cells. The plantlets can be regenerated from these cells.
9. These plantlets give rise to the highly valuable transgenic plants.
10. Mutagens are added to single cell liquid cultures for induction of mutations.
11. Tolerance to stress like pollutants, toxins, salts, drought, flooding, etc., can also be obtained by providing them in culture medium in increasing dosage. The surviving healthy cells are taken to solid medium for raising resistant plants.
12. Weedicides are added to culture initially in very small concentrations.
13. Dosage is increased in subsequent cultures till the desired level of weedicide resistance is obtained.
14. The resistant cells are then regenerated to form plantlets and plants.

15. Both apical and axillary meristems are free from virus even if the whole plant is infected by it. Virus-free plantlets are obtained by using meristem culture to grow new plants.
16. Embryos which normally do not survive inside seeds can be grown in tissue culture to form new plants. It is useful in interspecific hybridization.

3.2 EDIBLE VACCINE

Induction of selected or desired genes into plants and manufacture the altered protein for various infection prophylaxes or prevention are known as edible vaccine. Such vaccine encoded with the microbial antigen (bacterial or viral pathogens) expressed in plants in a form in which they retain native immunogenic properties. Initially, edible vaccines were used in preventing infectious diseases but currently it also been applied for the prevention of autoimmune diseases and cancer.

3.2.1 Concept of Edible Vaccines

The concept behind edible vaccine was to introduce the desired gene into the plant which can further encode the protein in plant edible parts. This process was developed by Arntzen in 1990s.

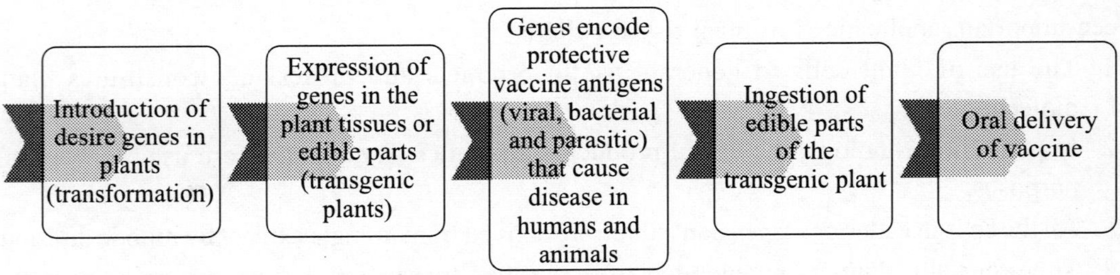

Fig. 3.10 Concept of edible vaccine

The nonpathogenic coat protein of a specific virus or bacteria is used for transformation. The best advantageous part of edible vaccines is its easyscaled-up process and lesser contamination. It is estimated that, the population of China could be vaccinated by edible vaccines which require just 40 hectares of land for production. Even though, contamination chance with plant pathogens to humans is very low or insignificant.

Edible vaccines against various diseases such as measles, cholera, foot and mouth diseases, and hepatitis B, C, and E are produced in plants like banana, tobacco, potato, etc.

Table 3.9 Examples of edible vaccines

Name of vaccine	Vector	Clinical conditions	Causative agents
Rabies	Tobacco	Rabies	Rabies virus
Hepatitis B	Potato, tobacco	Hepatitis B	Hepatitis B virus
Gastroentritis	Maize	Gastroentritis	Corona virus
HIV	Tomato	AIDS	HIV virus
Cholera	Potato	Cholera	Vibrio cholera

Mechanism of action of edible vaccines

Activation of mucosal immune system (MIS) is the prime mechanism of edible vaccines. MIS is the first line of defence in human body even though, the initial infection of pathogenic microorganism happens in this mucosal membrane. This mucosal lining basically found in digestive tract, respiratory tract, and urino-reproductive tract.

The gut mucosal layer composed of M cells and macrophages where the pathogenic antigen can enter via multiple ways. In natural conditions such macrophages are usually activated by interferon gamma and further fragmented peptides to the helper T cells resulted in production of antibodies.

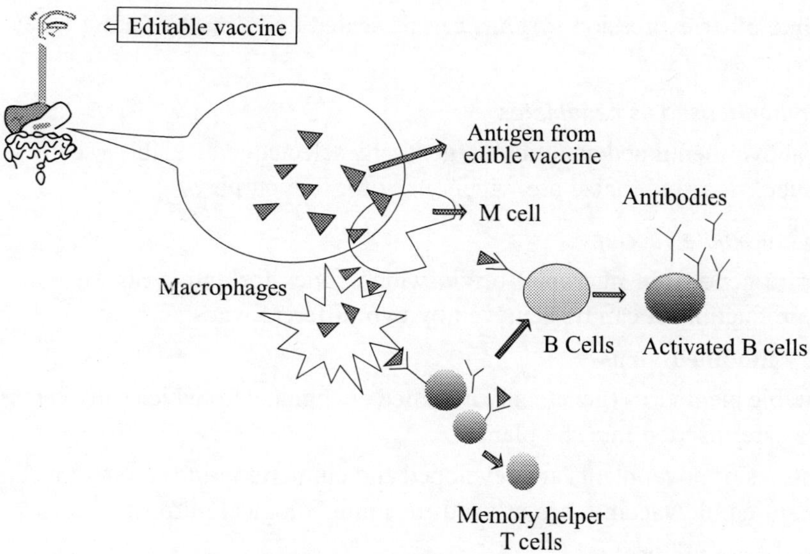

Fig. 3.11 Mechanism of action of edible vaccines

Antigens are transported to T cells via M cells. APC surface containing antigenic epitopes with the help of T cells activates B cells for antibody production. Such activated B cells migrate into mesenteric lymph nodes and get matured into plasma cells and ultimately reaches into the mucosal membranes to secrete immunoglobulin A or IgA. IgA forms secretory IgA with proper modulations and transported to lumen. Production of secretory IgA is another complex event since 50% of secretory IgA (sIgA) in gut lumen is produced by B1 cells in the lamina propria in a T-cell-independent fashion. These sIgA are poly-reactive and usually recognize the foreign antigens. In the lumen, the sIgA neutralizes the invading pathogen by reacting with the specific antigenic epitopes.

The furthermost problem associated with oral vaccines is the development of tolerance in the gut.

3.2.2 Method for Production of Edible Vaccine

(I) Selection of a candidate plant

Candidate plants are those plants that are most suitable for edible vaccine production. There are a number of factors that make a plant a good edible vaccine candidate.

- Must have long shelf life. The plant or the edible part of the plant has to be stored for a long time without degradation. Cereals such as rice, maize, and wheat are great examples of such plants.
- Must grow quickly. Fruits or vegetables that usually are produced on trees are considered bad candidates as they take a long time to grow and mature, whereas plants such as tobacco and tomato have fast growth time.
- Easy transformation. Plants on which considerable research has been carried out and transformation techniques optimized are good candidate plants.

Plants, unlike other expression systems can be scaled up to need, making it easily available to the masses.

(II) Plants commonly used as candidates

Plants with the above-mentioned qualities are generally selected to be edible vaccines. Plants such as tomato, tobacco, rice, and maize are widely used for this purpose.

(III) Production of edible vaccine

Isolation of desire gene from microbial origin which codes for antigen is the foremost step in edible vaccine production. It can be achieved by two different ways.

A. Genetically modified virus

Selection of suitable plant virus (genetically modified or engineered) which can express the desired proteins/peptides are inserted into the plant.

Huge quantities of novel plants are developed and chimeric virions are removed and purified and resultant plant edible vaccines are utilized for immunological purpose.

B. Insertion of gene via vector

The desired gene of interest is integrated with plant vector by transformation. A variety of techniques havebeen used to introduce transgene into plant cell. These could be grouped into following categories.

1. **Agrobacterium mediated gene transfer:** Agrobacterium tumefaciensisa plant pathogen responsible for crown gall disease in plant. Such bacterium is co-cultured with the plant or tissue culture for transformation of bacterial plasmid to plant cell. The suitable gene construct is inserted into the T region of a disarmed Ti plasmid of Agrobacterium, i.e., vector. This technique is well adopted specially in dicotelydenous plants like potato, tomato and tobacco, etc. The major drawback of this method is slow process or time consuming and low yield.
2. **Biolistic method:** It is an instrumental technique where gene containing DNA coated metal (e.g., gold, tungsten) particles are fired at the plant cells using gene gun or particle gun. Those plant cells that take up the DNA are then allowed to grow in new plants, and are cloned to produce large number of genetically identical crop. This method is quite attractive because DNA can be delivered into cells of plant which makes gene transfer independent of regeneration ability of the species. But the chief limitation of this method is high instrumental cost.

3. **Electroporation:** In this method, induction of genetic materials (DNA) into the cell by exposing them to high voltage electrical pulse for a brief period of time to induce transient pores in the cellular plasma lemma. The cell wall presents an effective barrier to DNA therefore, it has to be weakened by mild enzymatic treatment so as to allow the entry of DNA into cell cytoplasm.

3.2.3 Applications of Edible Vaccines

(a) Malaria

Three antigens are currently being investigated for the development of a plant based malaria vaccine, merozoite surface protein (MSP) 4 and MSP 5 from Plasmodium falciparum, and MSP 4/5 from *Plasmodium yoelli.*

(b) Hepatitis B

The hepatitis B surface antigen (HbsAg) is used as a vaccine against Hepatitis B. The HbsAg subtype was cloned into CaMv plasmid and the regenerated plants from the transformed cells were shown to produce HbsAg. Furthermore, expression of the antigen was found to be higher in roots of the transgenic potato than in leaf tissues.

(c) Measles

Measles is a highly contagious viral disease caused by the Paramyxo virus. Recent studies report expression of the Paramyxovirus surface protein haemagglutinin in tobacco, potato, rice and lettuce with satisfying results.

(d) Stopping Autoimmunity

Several cell proteins are identified which can elicit autoimmunity in people predisposed to Type I diabetes. The development of plant based diabetes vaccine in potato was attempted.The development of transgenic potato and tobacco plants showed increased levels of IgG, an antibody associated with cytokines that suppress harmful immune response. Feeding of the vaccines helped to suppress the autoimmune attack and to prevent the delay of high blood sugar.

Other Potential Domains

(a) **Cancer therapy:** Soybean has been genetically engineered to make monoclonal antibody (BR-96) as a vehicle for targeting doxorubicin for breast, ovarian, colon and lung tumours.

(b) **Birth control:** TMV has been designed to express protein (ZB3 protein). When injected, resulting antibodies were able to prevent fertilization of eggs (pre-clinically).

(c) **Chloroplast transformation:** The chloroplast genome is maternally inherited; so following chloroplast transformation, the protein would not be present in pollen, thereby reducing the risk of transmission of the transgene to neighboring crops or weed species by crosspollination. It may also result in accumulation of significantly greater quantities of transgenic protein.

(d) **Recombinant drugs/proteins:** Apart from vaccines and antibodies, plants are also being modified by engineered virus inoculation to produce enzymes; drugs such as albumin, serum protease and interferon, which are otherwise difficult or expensive to produce, for example, glucocerebrosidase (hGC) production in tobacco plants for treating Gaucherís disease.

Other novel compounds include an anti-viral protein that inhibits the HIV virus in vitro, trichosanthin (ribosome inactivator) and angiotensin-I (antihypertsensitive drug). Transgenic plantderived biopharmaceutical hirudin (an antithrombin) is now commercially produced. Food crops are being increasingly used to produce pharmaceuticals and drugs.

Advantages of Edible Vaccine

(a) Edible vaccines are effective as a delivery vehicle for immunization because adjuvants that enhance the immune response are not required.
(b) Edible vaccine can elicit mucosal immunity, which is not observed in traditional vaccines.
(c) Edible vaccines are also cost effective in availability, storage, preparation, production, and transportation.
(d) Vaccines produced by biotechnological methods are stable at room temperature, unlike traditional vaccine, which needs cold chain storage, which multiplies the yearly cost to preserve vaccines.
(e) Seeds of transgenic plants could be dried as there is less moisture content in seeds and the plants with oil or their aqueous extracts possess more storage opportunities.
(f) Manufacturing cost is low as there is no need for special premises to manufacture them. Edible vaccine can be easily produced at mass level in comparison to an animal system.
(g) Edible vaccines are well tolerated, as they do not require administration by injection unlike traditional vaccines. Thus, there is also a reduced need for medical personnel and risk of contamination is low. The feasibility of oral administration compared to injection is also an advantage.
(h) Plant derived vaccines could be the source for new vaccines combining numerous antigens. These multicomponent vaccines are called second generation vaccines as they allow for several antigens to approach M-cells simultaneously.
(i) Edible vaccines are subunit preparations, do not involve attenuated pathogens, and improve the safety of individuals as compared to traditional vaccine since there is no possibility of proteins reforming into infectious organisms.
(j) The separation and purification of vaccines from plant materials is easy and pathogenic contamination from animal cells can be effectively prevented.

Disadvantages of Edible Vaccines

(a) There is a possibility of development of immunotolerance to the vaccine protein or peptide.
(b) Consistency of dosage form differs from plant to plant and generation to generation.
(c) Protein content varies from plant to plant and generation to generation.
(d) Ripeness also affects the proteins that are present in the form of antigens in the fruits.
(e) Limitations of methods for standardization of plant material/product.

(f) Stability of vaccine differs from plant to plant.

(g) Some food cannot be eaten raw (e.g., potato) and needs to be cooked, which will denature or weaken the protein present in it.

(h) Variable conditions for edible vaccine are also a major problem. Potatoes containing vaccine can be stored at 4°C for longer time, while tomato does not last long at this temperature. Thus, these vaccines need to be properly stored to avoid infection through microbial spoilage.

(i) Another concern regarding edible vaccine is the need for proper distinguishing characters to identify between "vaccine fruit" and "normal fruit" to avoid maladministration of vaccine, which could lead to tolerance.

(j) The glycosylation pattern of plants and humans is different, which could affect the functions of vaccines.

Table 3.10 Some patents of edible vaccines

Patent holder	Claim Reference
Ribozyme pharm	Nucleic acid vaccine used to treat or prevent viral infections in plants, animals or bacteria
University Loma Linda	Gene constructs used to produce edible vaccines to treat autoimmune diseases, including diabetes and multiple sclerosis
Rubicon Lab	Retrovirus expressed in animal or plant cells is useful as virus and cancer vaccines
Biosource	Plant viral vector with potential as antiHIV vaccine; recombinant proteins for use in vaccine to protect against parasitic infection
University of Texas	Hepatitis B core antigen recombinant vaccine
University of Yale	Vaccine against invertebrates
Institute of Pasteur	Attenuated *E. colivaccine* for use in gene therapy

EXERCISE

1. Define plant tissue culture. Explain the basic concepts of plant tissue culture.
2. Describe the general steps involved in plant tissue culture.
3. Explain briefly the various types of plant tissue culture with their advantages.
4. Write the applications of plant tissue culture.
5. Explain briefly the nutritional requirements of culture media in plant tissue culture.
6. Explain the growth and maintenance of plant tissue culture.
7. Describe the advantages and disadvantages of plant tissue culture.
8. What is edible vaccine? Explain the basic concept behind edible vaccine.
9. Explain the mechanism of edible vaccine.
10. Describe various methods for production of edible vaccines.

11. Elaborate various applications of edible vaccines.
12. Write a note on the growth curve of plant cell culture.
13. Explain the role of growth regulators in plant tissue culture development.
14. What is cell suspension culture? Explain its types and applications.
15. Describe briefly the protoplast culture.

UNIT IV

Pharmacognosy in Various Systems of Medicine

Objectives

- To recognized the contribution of traditional system of medicine towards development of modern medicine.
- To illustrate the nature, class and therapeutic role of plant secondary metabolites.

4.1 INTRODUCTION

In depth knowledge skills, and practices based on the theories, beliefs, and experience indigenous to different cultures that are used to maintain health as well as to prevent, diagnose, improve, or treat physical and mental illnesses generally termed traditional medicine (TM). Many countries in this world refer to traditional medicine as supplemental or alternative medicine. A majority of people in the region (70-80%) have employed herbal therapies as their primary source of healthcare, making them the most often used traditional medicine. Traditional methods of treating disease inherited from ancient cultures. Many of the ancient medical systems have been around for centuries and have been built around solid foundational concepts and healing techniques. In this context traditional Chinese medicine (TCM) from China and Ayurveda from India are still widely practised systems, whereas Greek medicine and Egyptian medicine are now just of historical significance. A holistic approach to a person's physical, mental, and spiritual well-being has been observed in many ancient systems as whole.

4.1.1 Traditional System of Medicine and Modern Medicine

Pharmacognosy has evolved as an applied science pertaining to the study of all types of drugs of natural origin. However, its subject matter is directed towards the modern allopathic medicine. So the role of pharmacognosy in traditional medicinal systems is undeniable

Plants were being used before 500 BC on belief of their ritual and medicinal power. In successive times of human history, the plants were identified for their curative or healing properties which were being used and conveyed the same knowledge to next generation. The accumulation of such knowledge and transformation to next generations gave birth to traditional system of medicine. This continuous interest towards exploration of medicinal plants by human beings has brought about today's modern and sophisticated stage of herbalism. The developing stages of human civilization undergoes various transitions of raising and perishing but despite of all, the systems of medicine which was developed in various parts and regions in the world still have their immortal print residing towards serving humanity and also popularly known as traditional medicine. The root, principle and philosophical differences of such systems might exist but the purpose for serving the humanity for the treatment, management of diseases and also for maintenance of good health was the prime intention. For example, traditional Chinese medicine (TCM) in China, *Unani* system in Greece, *Ayurvedic* and *Siddha* systems in India, *Amachi* in Tibet, etc., are known as traditional systems of medicine. In this context, *Homoeopathy* system of medicine in Germany is now popularly practised all over the world.

The development of modern allopathic system of medicine, which is also known as modern system of medicine also gradually developed over time on the basis of efforts made by people over the method of scientific and observational even though, the base is still laid on depth of traditional medicinal knowledge and its therapeutic applications. Herbal medicine has a wide range of bioactive chemicals, produced after the cellular metabolisms which are responsible for various therapeutic or pharmacological functions in the living body. Development of many sophisticated and costlier diagnostic methodologies are the part of modern system of medicine (allopathy).

Many modern synthetic drugs may harm more than they help in curing the disease by their serious toxic effects. On the contrary, traditional medicines are much more preferred for being safe and comparatively low or nil harmful effects and cheaper than allopathic medicines. However, one fact must be accepted here that the modern allopathic treatment has developed wonderful techniques of diagnosis and highly effective drugs to provide the best and effective treatment than any other system of medicine till date.

4.1.2 Role of Pharmacognosy in Modern System of Medicine

Era of "modern medicine" starts in the beginning of the nineteenth century with the discovery of morphine, a pharmacologically active compound in 1805. This was the first reported active phytochemical isolated from a medicinal plant by a young German pharmacist, Friedrich Sertürner. Subsequently, countless pharmaceutically active substances have been isolated from natural products. The fundamental difference between the traditional medicine and modern medicine is drug target. Modern medicines basically working on one time one target role where traditional medicine may act on multiple targets in one time, i.e., synergistic action. The isolated compounds as a single chemical entity may act on the basic role of modern medicine but some may follow their traditional uses. However, natural products are important for the development of new drugs, and these products have been in constant use. Some medicines, such as anticancer, antihypertensive, and antimigraine medication, have benefited greatly from natural products. Despite of this western medicine or modern medicine continues to show the influence of ancient practices. For example, cardiac glycosides from *Digitalis purpurea,* morphine from *Papaver somniferum,* reserpine from *Rauwolfia* species, and quinine from *Cinchona* species and artemisinin, an active antimalarial compound from *Artemisia annua,* etc., show the influence of traditional medicine in Western medicine.

4.1.3 Indian Systems of Medicine

India has a golden heritage of traditional system of medicine. Such system is not only comprised of one system moreover it includes different systems, i.e., *Ayurveda*, *Siddha* and *Unani* systems of medicine, etc. Such systems of traditional medicine and the traditional healthcare system have been flourishing since many centuries.

Ayurvedic system of medicine was developed by an extensive use of plant medicines dating back from 1000 BC.

4.1.4 Ayurvedic System of Medicine

Ayurvedic system of medicine is conferred as the oldest written medical system in the world. Despite of losing the actual origin of Ayurveda in prehistoric antiquity, but their concepts were nurtured in ancient times (between 2500 and 500 BC) in India.

The word Ayurveda means: *Ayur* meaning life and '*Veda*' meaning science. Thus, Ayurveda literally means 'science of life'.

The Ayurveda is said to be an *Upaveda* (part) of *Atharva Veda* as per Hindu mythology. *Charaka Samhita* (1900 BC) is the first book with the concept of practice of Ayurveda. This describes 341 plants and plant products used in medicine. *Sushruta Samhit*a (600 BC) was the next ayurvedic literature that has special emphasis on surgery. It described 395 medicinal plants, 57 drugs of animal origin, 4 minerals and metals as therapeutic agents.

Basic Principles of Ayurveda

The basic principle of Ayurveda lies on ancient Indian philosophy, which states that, the whole universe is composed of five basic elements or *pancha maha bhutas.* It includes *prithvi* (earth), *jal* (water), *teja* (fire), *vayu* (air) and *akash* (space). So, a fundamental harmony therefore exists between the macrocosm (the universe) and the microcosm (the individual).

(i) Pancha Mahabhuta theory and the human body

The human body is in a state of continuous flux or dynamic equilibrium. The *pancha bhutas* are represented in the human body as the *doshas*, *dhatus* and *malas*.

(ii) Tridoshas theory

There are three *doshas* in the body, i.e., *vata, pitta* and *kapha.* There are direct equivalents for these three *doshas*, known as *tridoshas*.

- **(a)** ***Vata:*** The factors responsible for movement and sensation in a single cell/whole bodies biological phenomena that are controlled by the functions of central and autonomous nervous system.It is the equilibrium of air and ether.
- **(b)** ***Pitta:*** The factors responsible for digestion, metabolism, tissue building, heat production, blood pigmentation, activities of the endocrine glands and energy. It is the equilibrium state of fire and water.
- **(c)** ***Kapha:*** The factors responsible for strengthening the stomach and the joints, providing firmness to the limbs, and refreshing the sense organs. This is the stage of equilibrium of water and the earth.

There are some special areas in the body in which each *dosha* predominates, namely, the chest for *kapha,* digestive organs for *pitta* and the large intestine for *vata.*

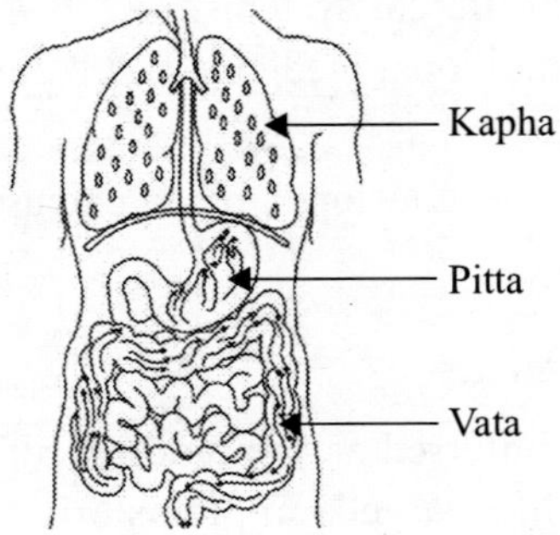

Fig. 4.1 *Dosha* predominated areas in human body

(iii) Dhatus

They are body constituents and play a major role in formation of the basic structure of the body and each one having its own functions to perform.

They are seven in number, known as *sapta dhatus*. These include:

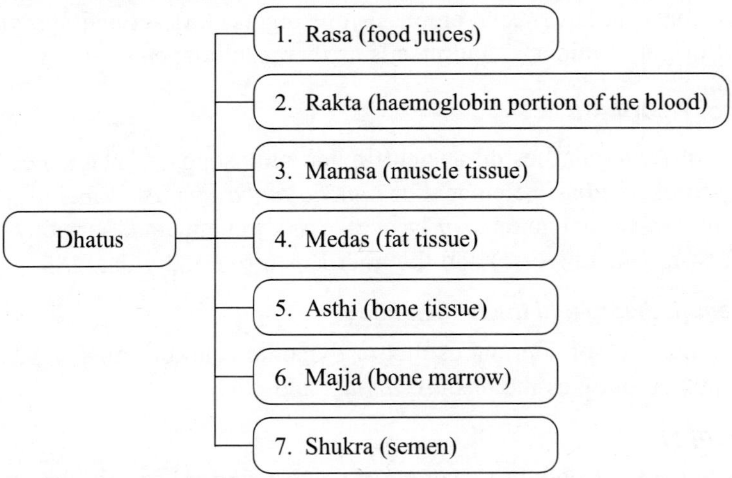

Fig. 4.2 Various *dhatus* in body

Malas

Byproducts of the *dhatus*, partly used by the body and moderately excreted as waste after the digestion process. The useful elements absorbed by the body are retained in the body as *prasad* (useful matter) while those excreted are known as *malas* (waste matter). The *malas include mutra* (urine), *shakrit* (faece) and *sweda* (perspiration).

The *doshas, dhatus* and *malas* should be in a state of perfect equilibrium for the body to remain healthy. Any imbalance among these constituents results in ill health and disease.

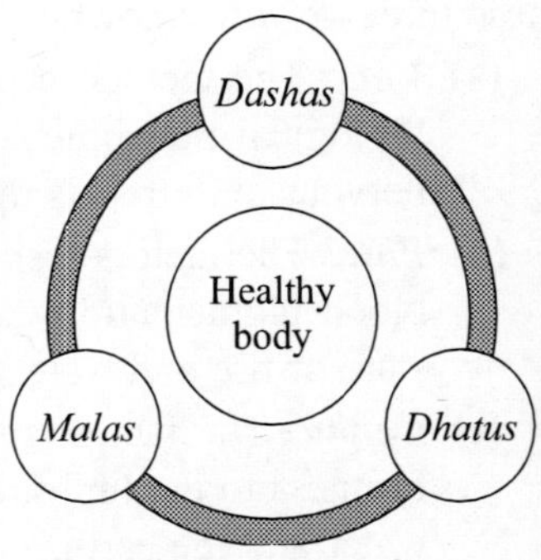

Fig. 4.3 Wheel of equilibrium

Diagnosis

Diagnosis in Ayurveda implies a moment-to-moment monitoring of the interaction between order (health) and disorder (disease). The classical clinical examination in Ayurveda is called *ashta sthana pariksha* (eight-point diagnosis) and includes an assessment of the state of the *doshas* as well as various physical signs. The eight-point diagnose incudes:

1. *Nadi pariksha* (pulse diagnosis)
2. *Mutra pariksha* (urine examination)
3. *Vata/ sparsha* (nervous system assessment)
4. *Pitta/drik* (assessment of digestive fire and metabolic secretions)
5. *Kapha/akriti* (mucous and mucoid secretions assessment)
6. *Mala pariksha* (stool examination)
7. *Jihva pariksha* (tongue examination)
8. *Shabda pariksha* (examination of body sounds).

Treatment

In the treatment of Ayuveda, patients are looked at as individuals as well as in relation to their environment. Ayurvedic treatment attempts to establish a balance among the bodily humours of *vata, pitta* and *kapha,* as well as to improve digestion and elimination of *ama* (undigested food). After determination of a person's constitutional type, drugs are prescribed on the basis of the patient's body type as well as kind of disease or disturbance of the *doshas* they are suffering.

Ayurvedic therapy often begins with *shodhana* (cleansing) in which toxins, emotional or physical, are eliminated or neutralized and then followed by *shamana* (palliative treatment) is used to reduce the intensity of a disease and balance the disordered *doshas*. Finally, *rasayana* (rejuvenation therapy) is used to maintain health and reduce the negative effects of disease.

Properties of herbs

Ayurvedic herbs are described and classified according to five major properties:

1. *Rasa* (taste)
2. *Guna* (physicochemical properties)
3. *Veerya* (potency)
4. *Vipaka* (postdigestive effect)
5. *Prabhava* (unique effect of the drug).

The principle, treatment and philosophy of Ayurveda are one of the best systems that fulfill the needs of human beings. Thus, Ayurveda provides holistic approach of treatment by subjecting the body as a whole giving least importance to *rogabalam*. This may be the reason for time consuming treatment in Ayurveda, but the results last long.

4.1.5 Siddha System of Medicine

The Siddha system of medicine originated from southern part of Indian subcontinent, even before the Aryan occupation of the Sind region and the Gangetic plains. The actual timeline is unknown. As per mythological beliefs the credit of the Siddha medicine goes to Lord Shiva and to Shakti (Parvati) to Nandi. Later on that knowledge was conveyed to seven *siddhas*. All the literature in

Siddha system was written in Tamil language. It was believed that, the Tamil language is attributed to the sage *Agasthya*, and the origin of Siddha medicine is also attributed to him because he was also one of *siddhas* among seven. Siddha medicine was practised basically in the banks of the river Cauvery and Tamirapani, a highly organized civilization of south India.

The therapeutics of Siddha medicine mainly consists of the use of metals and minerals. There is mention of mercury, sulphur, copper, arsenic and gold used as therapeutic agents.

Principle of Siddha system of medicine

As per Siddha philosophy, the whole universe consists of two essential entities, i.e., Siva (matter) and Shakti (energy). Matter cannot exist without energy inherent in it and vice versa. The two coexist and are inseparable. They are the primordial elements (*bhutas*). It includes:

1. *Munn* (solid),
2. *Neer* (fluid),
3. *Thee* (radiance),
4. *Vayu* (gas)
5. *Aakasam* (ether).

These five elements (*bhutas*) are present in every substance, but in different proportions.

The human being is made up of these five elements, in different combinations. The physiological function in the body is mediated by three *doshas* (substances) collaboratively known as *dravyas* (which are made up of the five elements). They are:

1. *Vatham*
2. *Pitham*
3. *Karpam*

Table 4.1 Functions of tridoshas

Dosha	Formation	Function
Vatham	*Aakasam + Vayu*	Controls the nervous actions such as movement, sensation, etc.
Pitham	*Thee*	Controls the metabolic activity of the body, digestion, assimilation, warmth, etc.
Karpam	*Munn + Neer*	Controls stability such as strength, potency, smooths working of joints.

Misbalance of this three *doshas* or disturbances of their equilibrium leads to disease.

Table 4.2 Tridoshas according to Siddha medicine

Doshas	Characteristics	Predominance
Vatham	Dryness, lightness, coldness and motility	Predominates in the bone and first one-third of life when activities, growth, sharpness of function of sense are greater.
Pitham	Heat—mover of the nervous force of the body.	Predominates in the tissue blood and also in the second one-third of life.
Karpam	Smoothness, firmness, viscidity, heaviness	Predominates in other tissues and last one-third of life. Diminishing activity of various organs and limbs.

The *tridoshas* are involved in all functions of the body, physical, mental and emotional.

In each and every cell of the body these three *doshas* coexist and function harmoniously. The tissues are called *dhatus*. There are seven *dhatus* as follows:

1. *Rasa* (lymph).
2. *Kurudhi* (blood).
3. *Tasai* (muscle).
4. *Kozhuppu* (adipose tissue).
5. *Elumbu* (bone).
6. *Majjai* (marrow).
7. *Sukkilam* and *artavam* (male and female hormones).

Method of treatment

The treatments in Siddha system basically focus on to balancing or restoration of equilibrium of the *tridoshas.* By substituting a drug (which is predominantly of the opposite nature) of the same constituents (*guna*), the equilibrium is restored. For example:

1. *Vatham* imbalance is cold, dry; thus the treatment will be oily and warmth.
2. *Pitham* imbalance (increased), produce warmth; to decrease *pitham*, sandalwood is administered, internally or externally because of its cold nature.

Drugs used in *Siddha system*

Classifications of Siddha medicine tabulated below.

Table 4.3 Classes of Siddha medicine

Name	Characteristics
Uppu (Lavanam)	Water-soluble drugs are decrepitated when put into fire giving off vapours (water-soluble inorganic compounds). Example: *kara-charam* (25 varieties), salts and alkalis.
Pashanam	Water-insoluble drugs but give off vapour when put into fire (water- insoluble inorganic compounds).
Uparasam	Water-insoluble chemicals similar to *Pashanam* but differing in their actions. Example: mica, magnetic iron, antimony, zinc sulphate, iron pyrites, and ferrous sulphate.
Loham	Metals and mineral alloys such as gold, silver copper, iron, tin, lead, etc.
Rasam	Drugs that are soluble (sublime when put in fire, and change into small crystals). Example: mercury amalgams, mercury compounds, arsenic, etc.
Gandhakam	Water-insoluble sulphur, burns off when put into fire.
Ratnas and *uparatnas*	Thirteen varieties are described, such as coral, lapis-lazuli, pearls, diamonds, jade, emerald, ruby, sapphire, opal and vaikrantham, rajavantham, spatikam harin mani, etc.

Various metals are used prominently in Siddha system. These include:

1. Mercury

It is used as a catalytic agent in many of its medicines and also used in combination with sulphur which controls the fluidity of mercury. Addition of sulphur converts mercury to mineral acid insoluble mercuric sulphite.

Siddhas used five forms of mercury:

1. *Rasam* (mercury metal)
2. *Lingam* (red sulphide of mercury)
3. *Veeram* (mercury chloride).
4. *Pooram* (mercury chloride).
5. *Rasa chenduram* (red oxide of mercury) lost its poisonous effect once processed as *poorna chandrodayam,* etc.

2. Sulphur

Calcined sulphur or red oxide of sulphur can be obtained by solidifying after purification. It conserves the body, and it is diaphoretic and alterative. Therapeutic ally is used against skin diseases, rheumatic arthritis, asthma, jaundice and blood poisoning.

3. Arsenic

Purified and consolidated arsenic is effective against all fevers, asthma and anaemia.

4. Gold

The absorbance of gold in body is very minute and therapeutically it acts as nervine tonic, antidote and sexual stimulant. Calcinated gold is freed from metallic state and lustre which ensure the safe absorption in human body.

4.1.6 Unani System of Medicine

Unani system of medicine originated in the doctrines of ancient Greece (earlier known as Unan). It is also known as Unani tibb, Arabian medicine or Islamic medicine. The Greek philosopher, physician Hippocrates (460-377 BC), was conferred as the father of Unani medicine. It was believed that, Hippocrates only freed medicine from the realm of superstition and magic of his time. With his efforts, such medicine gains the status of science. The basic theoretical framework of Unani medicine is laid on the teachings of Hippocrates.

After Hippocrates, his successors, i.e., Galen (131-212 AD), Raazes (850-925 AD) and Avicenna (980-1037 AD) followed the system considerably and constructed an imposing edifice of this system with their expertise. Slowly this system of medicine got popularized in Egypt, Syria, Iraq, Persia, India, China, Middle East and Far East countries. In India, Arabs introduced Unani system of medicine with existing systems of medicines.

Popularization of Unani medicine in India was contributed by few well-known Unani physicians, namely, Abu Bakr Bin Ali Usman Kasahani, Sadruddin Damashqui, Bahwabin Khwas Khan, Ali Geelani, Akabl Arzani and Mohammad Hoshim Alvi Khan.

Principles of Unani system

The principle of Unani system based on balance, uniting the physical, mental and spiritual realms of human beings.

Al-Umoor al-tabiyah (basic physiological principles)

According to Unani doctrines, the human body is made up of seven components which have close relationship to the state of individual's health. These include:

1. *Arkan* (elements)
2. *Mizaj* (temperaments)
3. *Aklath* (bodily humours)
4. *Aaza* (organs and system)
5. *Arwah* (vital spirits)
6. *Quo* (faculties)
7. *Afaal* (functions).

Interaction with each other these seven components maintain the balance of the human body. Each individual has a self-regulating capacity or power, called *tabiyat* (or *mudabbira-e-badan*).

According to basic principles of Unani system, the body is made up of the four basic elements, i.e., *Arz* (earth), *hawa* (air), *maa* (water) and *nar* (fire), which have different *mizaj* or temperaments, i.e., cold, hot, wet and dry. After mixing and interaction of four elements, a new compound having new temperament comes into existence, i.e., hot-wet, hot-dry, cold-wet and cold-dry.

The body has simple and compound organs, which get their nourishment through four humours, i.e., *dam* (blood), *balgham* (phlegm), *safra* (yellow bile) and *sauda* (black bile).

Table 4.4 Homours of Unani system

Blood	Hot and wet
Phlegm	Cold and hot
Yellow bile	Hot and dry
Black bile	Cold and dry

Health is a state of body in which there is equilibrium in the humours and functions of the body are normal in accordance to its own temperament and the environment.

Diagnosis

Diseases are mainly diagnosed with the help of pulse (*nabz*), physical examination of the urine and stool.

Treatment

Diseases are treated in the following ways:

1. ***Ilajbil Tadbeer* (regimental therapy):** Some drugless regimens are advised for the treatment of certain ailments, i.e., exercise, massage, *hamam* (Turkish bath), douches (cold and hot) and the regimen for geriatrics.
2. ***Ilajbil Ghiza* (diettherapy):** Different diets are recommended for the patients of different diseases.
3. ***Ilajbil Dava* (pharmacotherapy):** The basic concept of treatment is to correct the cause of the disease that may be abnormal temperament due to envirnmental factors or abnormal humours.

In Unani system of medicine most of the drugs are from plant origin. Some drugs of animal and mineral origins are also used. Patients are treated either by single drug (crude drugs) or by compound drugs (formulations of single drugs).

4.1.7 Traditional Chinese Medicine (TCM) System

This tradictional system of medicine was developed in China but the actual time perioid of its origin is unknown. The agriculture emperors *Materia Medica* published in the Qin dynasty (221–206 B.C.) is considered the the first herbal classic written in China.

Principles of TCM

Traditional Chinese medicine is based on the principle of *Yin* and *Yang* theory. *Yang* represents the forces of light and *Yin* represents the forces of darkness.

Yin and *Yang* is the foundation of the entire universe as per philosophy of the yellow emperor. Every creation in universe underlies therein. As per this theory, these two are the root and source of life and death. It is a must to find the origin of diseases, for treatment and cure.According to this theory, heaven was created by the concentration of *Yang* and the earth by the concentration of *Yin* where *Yang* stands for peace and serenity and *Yin* stands for confusion and turmoil. More elaborately, destruction, disintegration is cused by *Yang* and conservation, shape to things is caused by *Yin.* Similarly,water is an embodiment of *Yin* and fire is an embodiment of *Yang*. In case of natural things like air, created by *Yang* while *Yin* creates the senses or physical body.The physical body dies and the spirit is restored to the air. The spirit receives its nourishment through the air, and the body receives its nourishment through the senses.

The philosophy of TCM states that the nature has four seasons and five elements. To grant long life, these seasons and elements must store up the power of creation in cold, heat, dryness, moisture and wind. Human body composed of five viscera in which those five climates are transformed into joy, anger, sympathy, grief and fear. As like cold and heat are injurious to the body similarly emotions of joy and anger are injurious to the spirit. Violent anger depletes *Yin*; violent joy depletes *Yang*. When disobedient emotions rise to heaven, the pulse expires and leaves the body eventhrough when joy and anger are without moderation, then cold and heat exceed all measures, and life is no longer secure. *Yin* and *Yang* should be respected to an equal extent.

When *Yang* is the stronger, the body is hot, the pores are closed, and people begin to pant; they become boisterous and coarse and do not perspire. They become feverish, their mouths are dry and sore, their stomachs feel tight, and they die of constipation.

When *Yang* is stronger, people can endure winter but not summer. When *Yin* is stronger, the body is cold and covered with perspiration. People realize they are ill; they tremble and feel chilly. When they feel chilled, their spirits become rebellious. Their stomachs can no longer digest food and they die. When *Yin* is stronger, people can endure summer but not winter. Thus, *Yin* and *Yang* are alternate. Their ebbs and surges vary, and so does the character of the diseases.

The treatment is to harmonize both. When one is filled with vigour and strength, *Yin* and *Yang* are in proper harmony.

Treatment

The four types of energies are cold, cool, warm and hot. Usually, cold or cool herbs treat fever, thirst, sore throat and general heat diseases. Hot or warm herbs treat cold sensation in the limbs, cold pain and general cold diseases. The five flavours of herbs are pungent, sour, sweet, salty and bitter.

Table 4.5 Five flavours of herbs

Flavours	Functions
Pungent herbs	Induce perspiration and promote circulation.
Sour herbs	Stop perspiration, diarrhoea, seminal emission and leucorrhoea.
Sweet herbs	Reduce toxicity, relieve pain and slow the progression of acute diseases.
Salty herbs	Soften hardness, lubricate intestines and drain downwards. Used in constipation and goitre.
Bitter herbs	Induce bowel movements; reduce fevers and hot sensations, dry dampness and clear heat. It also nourishes the kidneys too.

After absorption, herbs can move in four different directions: upward towards the head, downward towards the lower extremities, inward towards the digestive organs or outward towards the superficial regions of the body.

Table 4.6 Herbs perform different functions after absorption

Upward-moving herbs	Falling symptoms like prolapsed organs, induce perspiration and treat superficial symptoms that are moving towards the interior of the body.
Downward-moving herbs	Surging symptoms like coughing and vomiting even they can induce bowel movements and promote digestion.

For example, the herbs that are lively alongside respiratory tract disorders travel to the lungs and can be used for asthma or cough.

4.1.8 Homeopathic System of Medicine

It is a specialized medicinal system for therapeutics based on natural law of healing '*Similia Similibus Curantur*, means 'likes are cured by likes'. This system of medicine was developed in 1810 by a German physician, chemist and a pharmacist named Dr Samuel Christian Friedrich Hahnemann (1755–1843).

The word homeopathy stands on two different words, i.e., *homois* means like (similar) and *pathos* means treatment. For this context, administration of any drug possesses same power of producing similar suffering (diseases) in healthy humans.

According to Dr Hahnemenn, the symptoms of any suffering are only the outward reflection of body's inner fight to counter the illness but no longer manifestation of illness.

Principles of Homoeopathy

The whole system of homeopathy treatment is based on certain fundamental principles and they are quite distinct and different from those of other systems of medicine. Dr. Hahnemann had briefly discussed such principles in different sections. They include:

1. **Law of similia:** The entire system is based on this law which states that '*Simillia Similibus Curentur*', which means 'let likes be cured by likes'. According to this law, if the same medicine is administered to a healthy person instead of diseased individual, it would

produce same sufferings (diseases) as like diseased individual. Hence, the developed symptoms of disease are to be matched with the pathogenesis of the medicine.

2. **Law of simplex:** Law of simplex states that the prescription drugs should be simple and single at unit time without admixture of other substance.
3. **Law of minimum:** Lowest concentration of drug must be used as per this law of minimum that is due to hypersensitivity and altered receptivity of tissue to stimuli in disease. The minimum concentration is required to just arouse the body's immunogenic reaction. But in large dose would cause unwanted side effects and damage. The minutest quantity of medicine helps in curative action of drug and expected deprived of unwanted aggravation.
4. **Drug proving:** The drugs which are administered to individuals, should have assured curative power and such potentials must be preknown. Such curative power of the drug includes the ability to produce disease sysmptoms when administered to a healthy individuals.

   Proving the drug singly on healthy human being would serve the only true record of the curative properties of drug.
5. **Drug dynamization or potentization:** Drug dynamization is done by the process such as trituration for insoluble substances and succession for soluble substances. It is required because of the medicine which is used to encounter disease should also have dynamic action to act on the dynamic disturbance or deviations of normal harmonious life force which is belived to be disturbed during disease.
6. **Preparation of potencies:** Three different scales are used to prepare potency, i.e., decimal scale, centesimal scale and millesimal scale.

   According to decimal scale, first potency should contain 1/10 part of original drug where second potency will contain 1/10 part of the first potency, and so on.

   As per centesimal scale, first potency should contain 1/100 of original drug and the second potency will contain 1/100 of the first potency, and so on.

   At last, according to millesimal scale, the first potency should contain 1/50,000 part of the original drug and second potency will contain 1/50,000 of the first potency, and so on.
7. **Vital force:** Vital force is charecterised by spiritual, autocratic, automatic, dynamic, unintelligent and instinctive, etc., while disease and health are quantitative states of this vital force. Disharmonious flow of the vital force causes diseases in human beings and this vital force is to be brought back to normal for health state of body.
8. **Acute and chronic diseases:** The intencity, onset, nature of progress and termination of diseases are basic steps to classify diseases into these categories, i.e., acute or chronic.
9. **Individualization:** Homeopathy philosophy believes that two individuals are never *be are* alike. Therefore, medication can never be administered only basis of the disease without individualizing each case of disease.
10. **Direction of cure:** Cure takes place within outward from above to downward and the symptoms disappears in the reverse of their appearance. If the direction is reverse of that stated then it is not cure but suppression which has occurred.

4.2 SECONDARY METABOLITES

4.2.1 Alkaloids

Alkaloids are the largest group of phytochemicals found in plants. They are basically plant secondary metabolites or byproducts originated from amino acids having bitter taste and also act as a poison in high dose. Due to the a mine characteristics alkaloids produce an alkaline solution in water and hence the origin of their name is alkaloids or alkali-like substances.

A large number of different alkaloids have been isolated and identified by the pharmacists around the world. In this context, there are more than 10,000 alkaloids isolated from around 300 different plant families till date.

Chemically, alkaloids contain heterocyclic ring system with nitrogen atom in outer ring (some alkaloids have exceptions, such as mescaline, the nitrogen atom is not within a carbon ring). Such position of nitrogen atom may vary with different alkaloids from different plant families. In fact, the precise position of nitrogen atom plays the detrimental role of its properties. Alkaloids possess a large number of pharmacological actions, i.e., analgesics, antimalarial, antispasmodics, mydritic (pupil dilation), antihypertensive, antipsychotics (mental disorders), anticarcinogenic, etc.

Alkaloids mainly occur as salt of carboxylic acids in plants such as citric, lactic, oxalic, acetic, maleic acid, tartaric acids, fumaric, benzoic, aconitic, veratric acids, etc. Even some alkaloids have remarkable structural similarities with neurotransmitters in the human central nervous system (CNS) including dopamine, serotonin and acetylcholine. Some well-known alkaloids include morphine, strychnine, quinine, ephedrine, nicotine, etc.

Definition and Occurrence

An alkaloid is defined as 'a bitter nitrogenous basic cyclic organic molecule with nitrogen atom which possesses a specific pharmacological effect on humans and animals in lower dose.

They are a class of compounds which typically contain nitrogen and have complex ring structures.

It is most abundantly found in higher plants. Nearly 25% of higher plants contain these molecules. They are found in any part of the plant like, roots (reserpine from Rauwolfia), aerial parts like (ephedrine from ephedra), barks (quinine from cinchona), leaves (cocaine from coca), seeds (caffeine from coca seeds) or even in entire plant (vinblastin from vinca). In fact, from animal origin nearly 300 alkaloids are reported in the skins of amphibians belongs to over 24 different classes. It occurs in plant as secondary metabolite like vinca and *dhatura* alkaloids, in animals, i.e., in shellfish and fungi. Usually, alkaloids are derived from amino acids. Many alkaloids are poisonous, e.g., strychnine or coniine, etc.

Properties

- Colourless, crystalline solids, have a ring structure, and have definite melting points.
- Derived from plants and have a bitter taste.
- Some alkaloids are not basic and others are brightly coloured like betanidine, beriberine, sanguinarine or nicotine (liquid), etc., are some exceptions.

- They have chiral molecules due to that they have no superimposable mirror images.
- Free bases of alkaloids are freely soluble in organic solvents and insoluble in water.
- Alkaloidal salts are soluble in water and partially soluble in organic solvents. For example, strychnine hydrochloride is much more soluble in water than strychnine as a base.
- Most alkaloids have a very bitter taste.
- Basic in nature because of nitrogen atom in cyclic system.

Classification

Alkaloids are generally classified by their common molecular precursors, based on the biological pathway used to construct the molecule. From a structural point of view, alkaloids are divided according to their shape and origin.

There are three main types of alkaloids:

(1) True alkaloids (2) Protoalkaloids

(3) Pseudoalkaloids

True alkaloids and protoalkaloids are derived from amino acids, whereas pseudoalkaloids are not derived from these compounds.

(1) True Alkaloids: These types of alkaloids are derived from the amino acid precursor and possess a heterocyclic ring with nitrogen atom. The primary precursors of true alkaloids are amino acids, i.e., L-ornithine, L-lysine, L-phenylalanine/L-tyrosine, L-tryptophan and L-histidine. They are highly reactive and show potent biological activity in small doses. Characteristically, true alkaloids have bitter taste and appear as a white crystalline (exception of nicotine which has a brown liquid) water-soluble salt. These alkaloids occur in a limited number of species and families. Examples of true alkaloids include cocaine, quinine, dopamine and morphine, etc.

(2) Protoalkaloids: This category of alkaloids is also derived from amino acid but the free N atom is not a part of the heterocyclic ring system. They are basically derived from the precursor amino acids such as L-tyrosine and L-tryptophan. Protoalkaloids structurally consists of closed ring system as simple alkaloids. Hordenine, mesca-line and yohimbine are good examples of such alkaloids.

(3) Pseudoalkaloids: The pseudoalkaloids are not directly derived from amino acid precursors. In fact, they are connected with amino acid pathways and derived from the precursors or post-cursors of amino acids. Even though pseudoalkaloids may produce by the amination and transamination reactions from amino acids (precursors or post-cursors) connected with different pathways. Sometimes they can also be derived from non-aminoacid precursors too.

Examples of pseudoalkaloids include coniine, capsaicin, ephedrine, solanidine, caffeine, theobromine, etc.

On the basis of their chemical structure or heterocyclic rings, alkaloids are further divided into two categories. These include:

(a) ***Atypical alkaloids:*** These are also known as non-heterocyclic alkaloids and contain nitrogen in aliphatic chain.

Table 4.7 Examples of alkaloids with their chemical structure

Alkaloids	Chemical structure	Examples	Source	Use
Phenyl ethyl amine	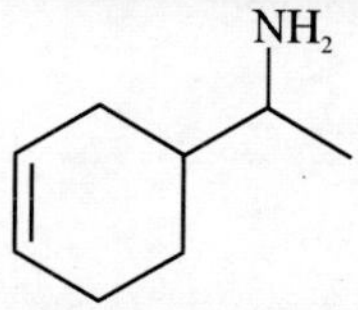	Ephedrine, Mescaline, Hordanine	Ephedra	Asthma
Tropolone alkaloids	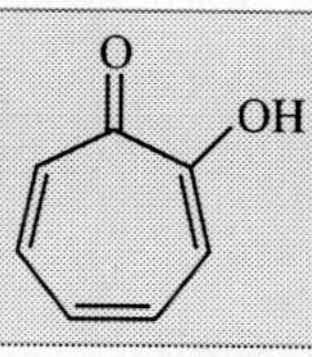	Colchicine	Colchicum	Gout
Modified diterpene	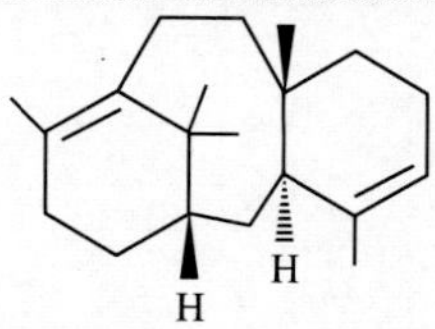	Taxol	Taxus	Anticancer

(b) ***Typical alkaloids:*** These are also known as heterocyclic alkaloids and contain nitrogen in heterocyclic ring system.

(a) Mono-nuclear heterocyclic alkaloids

Table 4.8 Examples of mono-nuclear heterocylic alkaloids

Alkaloids	Chemical structure	Examples	Source	Use
Pyridine	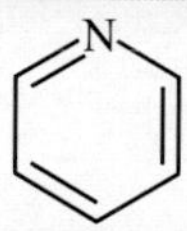	Lobeline	Lobelia	Asthma
Piperidine	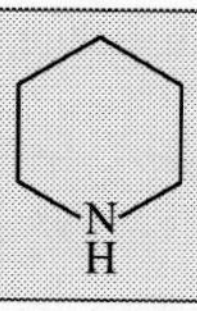	Piperine	Piper	Gonorrhoea, Antioxidant
Pyrrole	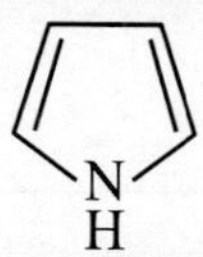	Hygrine	Coca	CNS stimulant
Pyrrolidine	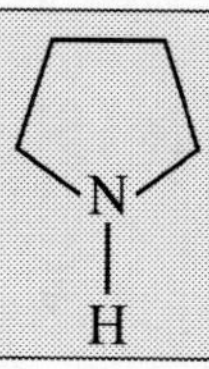	Nicotine	Tobacco	CNS stimulant

Contd.

Imidazole	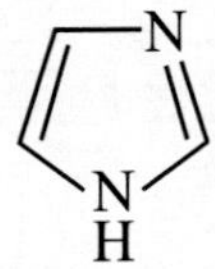	Pilocarpine	Pilocarpus	Contraction of pupil

(b) Poly-nuclear heterocyclic alkaloids

Table 4.9 Examples of poly-nuclear heterocylic alkaloids

Alkaloids	Chemical structure	Examples	Source	Use
Quinoline	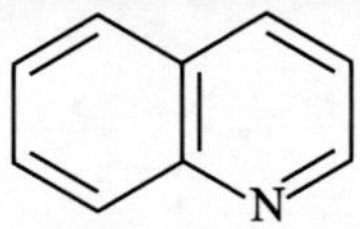	Quinine, quinidine	Cinchona	Antimalarial
Isoquinoline	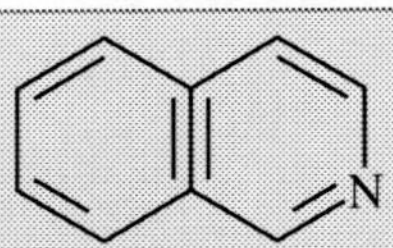	Morphine, papaverine	Opium	Narcotic analgesic
Indole	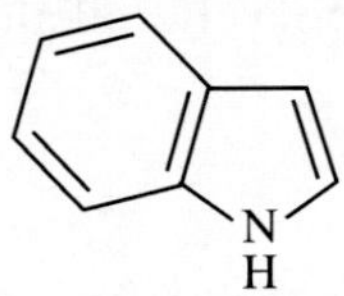	Ergotamine, reserpine, vincristine, strychnine	Ergot, Rauwolfia, Vinca, Nux-vomica	Oxytocic, antihypertensive, anticancer, CNS stimulant
Quinazoline	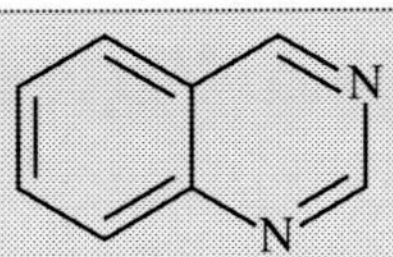	Vasicine	Vasaka	Antitussive
Tropane	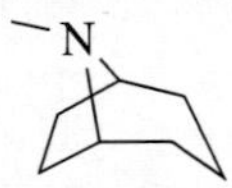	Atropine, hyoscine	Datura, Belladonna	Parasympatholytic
Purine	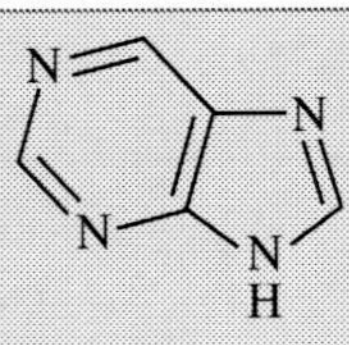	Caffeine	Coffee, Tea	CNS stimulant
Steroids	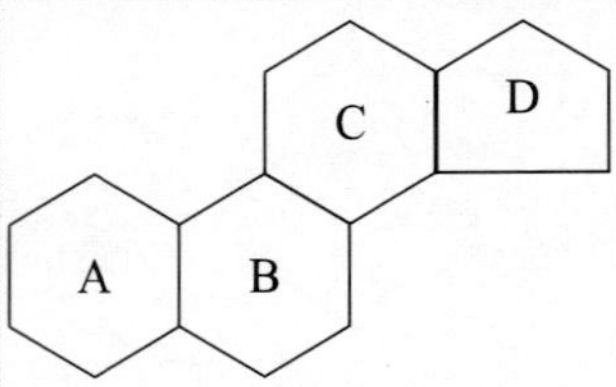	Solasodine	Solanum	Steroidal precursor

Terpenoids	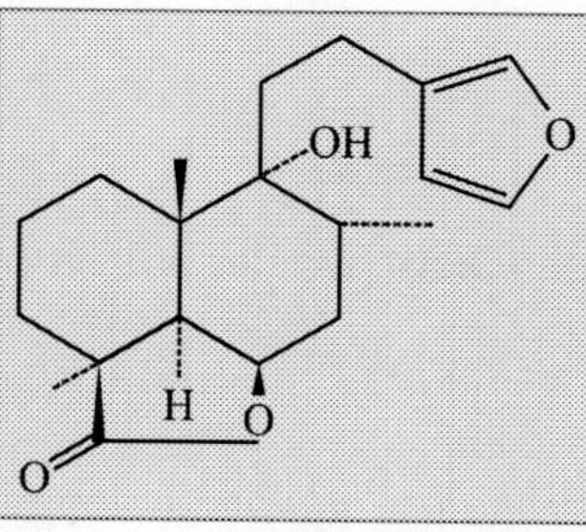	Aconitine	Aconite	Neuralgia

General Chemical Tests

The qualitative chemical tests are performed for alkaloids with neutral or slightly acidic solution of drug sample.

1. **Dragendorff's test:** Drug solution added with Dragendroff's reagent (potassium bismuth iodide), formation of orange or orange-red colour precipitate.
2. **Mayer's test:** Drug solution added with a few drops of Mayer's reagent (potassium mercuric iodide), formation of creamy-white precipitant.
3. **Hager's test:** Drug solution added with a few drops of Hager's reagent (saturated aqueous solution of picric acid), formation of crystalline yellow precipitate.
4. **Wagner's test:** Drug solution added with a few drops of Wagner's reagent (dilute iodine solution), formulation of reddish-brown precipitate.
5. **Tannic acid test:** Drug solution added with a few drops of tannic acid solution, formation of buff coloured precipitate.
6. **Ammonia reineckate test:** Drug solution added with slightly acidified (HCl) saturated solution of ammonia reineckate, formation of pink flocculent precipitate.

Drugs Containing Alkaloids

Tropane Alkaloids

They are frequently found in solanaceae, erythroxylaceae and convolvulaceae families. Chemical structure of tropane alkaloids consists of 8-azabicyclo octane nucleus and basically tropene derivatives. The pyrrolidine and piperidine rings are the basic structural units of tropane ring system or 3-hydroxy tropene.

Tropine and pseudotropine are the stereoisomers of tropene structures made up with combination of esters and acids. Tropane alkaloid can be identified by Vitali-Morin reaction where the esters of tropic acid have been detected.

The acids present are tropic acid in atropine and atropic acid formed by the loss of water from tropic acid in apoatropine. Other organic acids like tiglic acid, acetic acid, isobutyric acid and isovaleric acid are also present.

Tropane alkaloids having several legitimate medicinal uses are probably best known for their toxic properties. For example, three berries of *Hyoscyamus niger* (henbane) and *Atropa belladonna* (deadly nightshade) found lithel for infants.

Belladonna

Synonyms

Belladonna leaf, deadly night shade leaves, banewort, death's herb, dwale, poison black cherry, folia belladonnae.

Biological Source

Belladonna consists of dried leaves and flowering tops of *Atropa belladonna*, belonging to family Solanaceae. It contains about 0.35% of total alkaloids calculated as hyoscyamine.

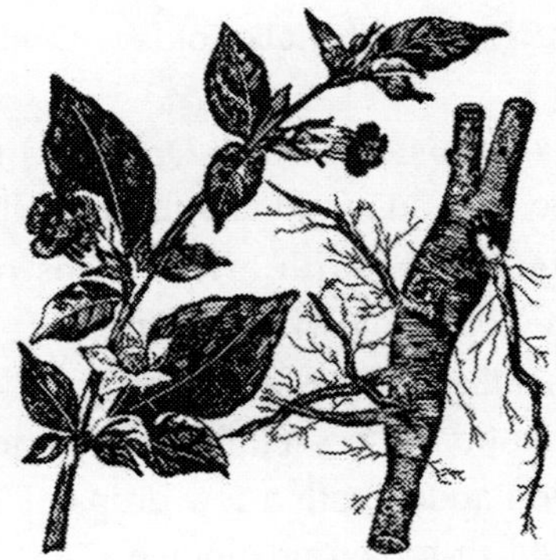

Fig. 4.4 Belladonna herb

Geographical Source

Atropa belladonna is cultivated in United States, Canada, UK, Germany and India.

Chemical Constituents

Belladonna leaves contain 0.3-1.0% total alkaloids, the prominent base is l-hyoscyamine and atropine, apoatropine, belladonnine, cuscohygrine, chrysa tropic acid. The volatile bases, such as atroscine, leucatropic acid; phytosterol, N-methylpyrroline, homatropine, hyoscyamine N-oxide, rutin, kaempferol-3-rhamnogalactoside and 7-glucoside, quercetin-7-glucoside, scopoletin, etc.

Uses

It is used as adjunctive therapy in the treatment of peptic ulcer, digestive disorders, including spastic, mucous and ulcerative colitis, diarrhoea, diverticulitis and pancreatitis. It is also used to control excess motor activity of the gastrointestinal tract and spasm of the urinary tract.

Belladonna is also used as narcotic, antispasmodic (gut or respiratory tract), sedative, diuretic mydriatic and to check secretion. Belladonna acts as a parasympathetic depressant.

Marketed Products

Belladona plaster (Surgi Pharma) for backache, stiffness of muscles and boil, swollen joints.

Indole Alkaloids

Chemically indole (1-H-indole) has the structure of benzopyrrole in which the benzene and pyrrole rings found in 2, 3-positions of the pyrrole ring structure. A large number of plant families have indole nucleus in their naturally occurring compounds. The best commercial importance of indole found as the component of perfumery industry.

The isomar of indole, known as isoindole (I-H-isoindole), made up of benzene and pyrrole rings fused through the 3- and 4-positions of the pyrrole ring system. But such molecules are charecteristically unstable and more exploration yet to be done. N-methylisoindole is one of the simplest examples of such isomaric derivative.

Isolated purified indole compounds are characteristically colourless crystalline solid in nature. It has meling point 52-54°C, where boiling point is 254°C.

Indole has moderate polarity with good solubility in petroleum ether, benzene, chloroform and hot water.

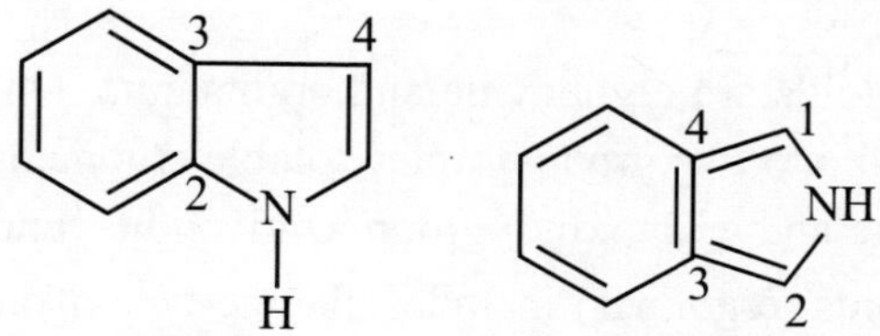

Fig. 4.5 Strecture of indole nucleus

The various plants containing indole alkaloids are vinca, ergot, rauwolfia, nux-vomica, physostigma, etc.

Ergot

Synonyms

Ergot, rye ergot, secale cornutum, spurred rye, ergot of rye, ergota.

Biological Source

Ergot is the dried sclerotium of a fungus, *Claviceps purpurea,* Tulasne, belonging to family Clavicipitaceae, developing in the ovary of rye plant, *Secale cereale* (Family Poaceae).

Ergot should yield about 0.15% of the total alkaloids (ergotoxine) and water-soluble alkaloids equivalent to about 0.01% (ergonovine).

Geographical Source

It is mainly found in Czechoslovakia, Hungary, Switzerland, Germany, France, Yugoslavia, Spain, Russia and India. In India ergot is cultivated at Kodaikanal (Tamil Nadu).

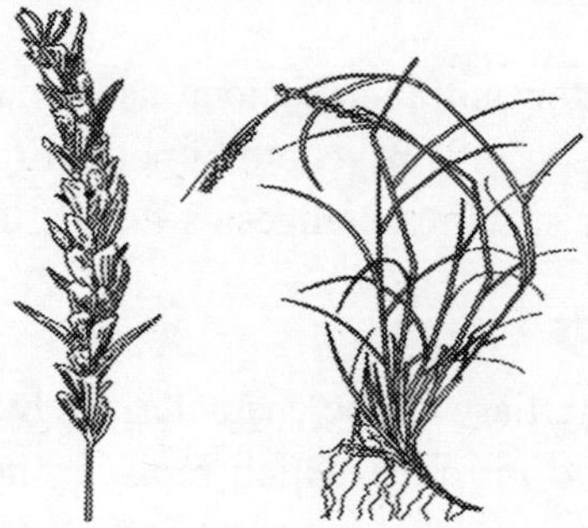

Fig. 4.6 Ergot of rye plant (*Claviceps purpurea*)

Chemical Constituents

Table 4.10 Water-soluble and water-insoluble constituents

Water-soluble Ergometrine	Water-insoluble	
	Ergotamine	Ergotoxine
Ergometrine, Ergometrinine	Ergotamine, Ergotaminine, Ergosine	Ergocristine Ergocristinine Ergocryptine Ergocryptinine Ergocornine Ergocorninine

The most important alkaloids are ergonovine and ergotamine. On the basis of solubility in water the alkaloids are divided into two groups: water-soluble ergometrine (or ergonovine) group or water-insoluble (ergotamine and ergotoxine) group as given hereunder:

The class of ergot alkaloids (ergolines) includes clavine-type alkaloids (e.g., 6, 8-dimethyl-ergoline) and the lysergic acid derivatives (e.g., lysergic acid).

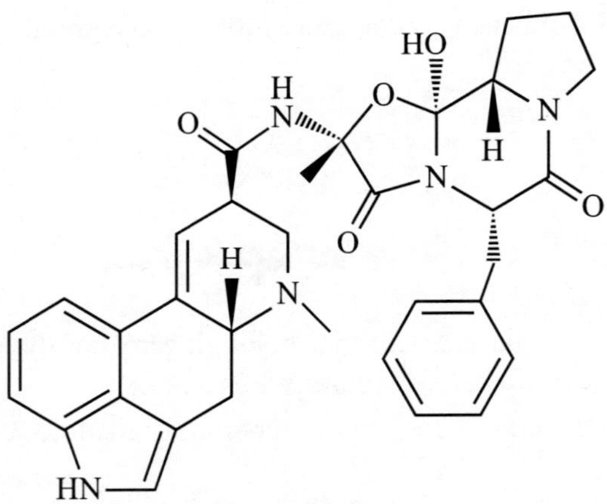
Ergotamine

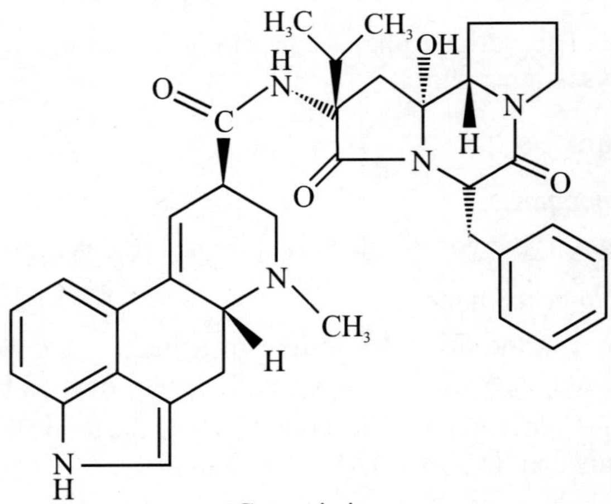
Crgocristine

Fig. 4.7 Structure of Ergotamine and ergocristine

Uses

It is used as oxytocic, vasoconstrictor and abortifacient also reduces post-partum haemorrhage. Lysergic acid (LSD-25) is a potent speczific psychotomimetic. Ergotamine and the semisynthetic dihydroergotamine salts are used as specific analhgesics for the treatment of migraine.

Pyridine and Piperidine Alkaloids

Pyridine is a heterocyclic aromatic tertiary amine characterized by a six-membered ring structure composed of five carbon atoms and nitrogen which replace one carbon-hydrogen unit in the benzene ring (C_5H_5N).

It is a colourless, flammable, toxic liquid with unpleasant odour, miscible with water and with most organic solvents, boils at 115°C. Its aqueous solution is slightly alkaline. Pyridine compounds are found in nature. For example, nicotine from tobacco, ricinine from castor bean, pyridoxine or vitamin B and P products, etc.

Piperidineis a hexa-hydropyridine, belongs to the family of heterocyclic organic compound derived from pyridine through hydrogenation. It has one nitrogen atom in the cycle and hasa clear liquid with pepper-like aroma. It boils at 106°C, soluble in water, alcohol and ether. Piperidine derivative compounds are used as intermediate to make crystal derivative of aromatic nitrogen compounds containing nuclear atoms.

Tobacco

Synonyms

Tobacco, Tabaci Folia.

Biological source

It consists of dried leaves of *Nicotiana tobacum*, belonging to family Solanaceae.

Geographical source

It is mainly found in India, United States, China, Brazil, Russia, Turkey and Italy.

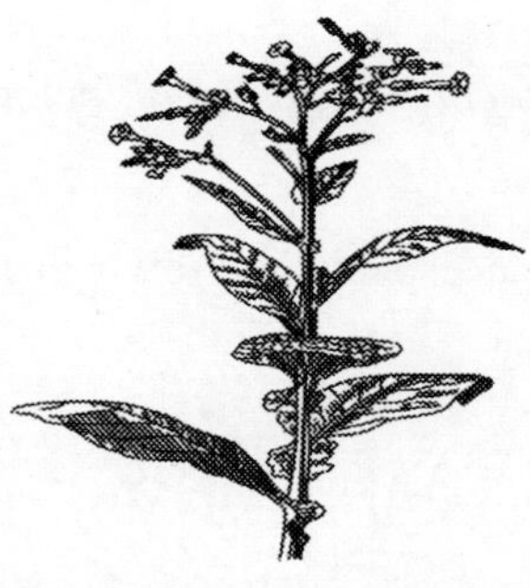

Fig. 4.8 *Nicotiana tobacum*

Chemical Constituents

The most important constituent is nicotine, nicotianin, nicotinine, nicoteine, and nicoteline. After leaves are smoked the nicotine decomposes into pyridine, furfurol, collidine, hydrocyanic acid, carbon monoxide, etc.

The poisonous effects of tobacco smoke are due to these substances of decomposed nicotine.

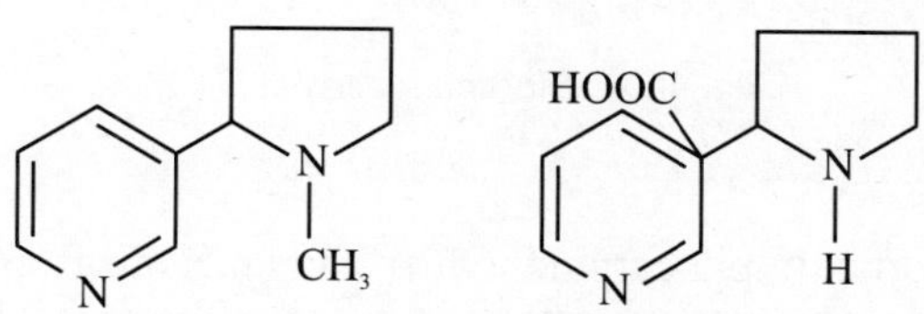

Fig. 4.9 Strucutre of niotine and nicotine acid

Uses

Nicotine is used as a sedative, diuretic, expectorant, discutient and sialagogue. Externally nicotine is an antiseptic and also exerts stimulant effects on heart and nervous system.

The leaves in combination with the leaves of belladonna can be applied for obstinate ulcers, painful tremors and spasmodic affections. Tobacco leaves are made wet and applied for piles.

Imidazole Alkaloids

Imidazole alkaloids are structurally a heterocyclic aromatic organic compound. The ring systems of imidazole act as an important biological building block such as histidine and histamine. It also acts as bases (pKa = 7.0) and as a weak acid (pKa = 14.5). Imidazole exists in two tautomeric forms with a hydrogen atom moving between the two nitrogens. It is a highly polar compound with higher solubility in water. The most important plant of this group is *Pilocarpus jaborandi.*

Pilocarpus

Synonyms

Jaborandi, Arruda do Mato, Arruda brava, Jamguarandi, Juarandi.

Biological source

The drug consists of the leaves of *Pilocarpus jaborandi,* belonging to family Rutaceae

Geographical Source

It is indigenous to South America and especially grown in Brazil. It is found in Venenzuela, Caribbean islands and Central America.

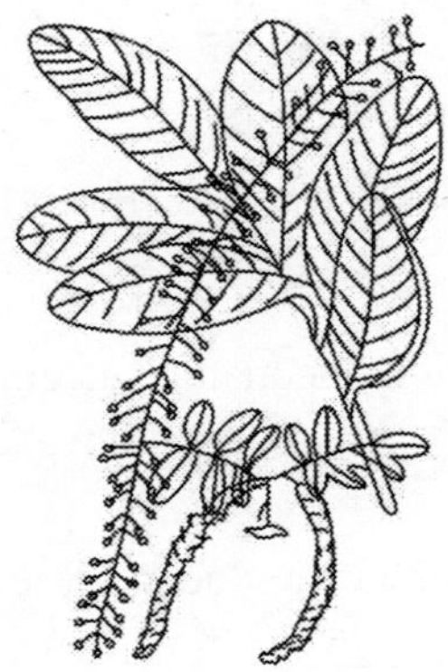

Fig. 4.10 *Pilocarpus jaborandi*

Chemical Constituents

The drug contains most importantly pilocarpine. Other alkaloids are isopilocarpine, pilocarpidine, pilosine, pseudopilocarpine and isopilosine. The range of total alkaloids in different species is between 0.5% and 1%.

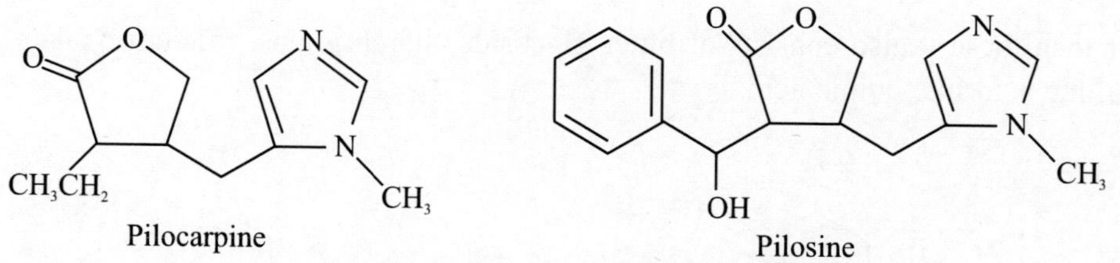

Fig. 4.11 Strucutre of polocarpine and pilosine

Uses

Pilocarpineis a powerful and rapid diaphoretic. Pilocarpine is also used as antagonistic to atropine action (stimulating the nerve endings paralysed by that drug), and contracting the pupil of the eye. It also induces free salivation and excites most gland secretions. It is also used in the treatment of glaucoma.

Quinoline Alkaloids

It is a heterocyclic aromatic organic compound. It consists of double carbon ring containing one nitrogen atom.

It is a colourles hygroscopic liquid with strong order. It is highly soluble in hot water and most organic solvents. Over 200 biologically active quinoline quinozoline alkaloids are identified. The Thalleioquin test basically indentifies quinoline alkaloids.

The most important plant on this catergory is cinchona.

Cinchona

Synonyms

Cortex Cinchonae, Countess, Peruvian or Jesuit's bark, Cinchona.

Biological Source

Cinchona is the dried bark of the stem or of the root of *Cinchona calisaya*, *Cinchona ledgeriana*, *Cinchona officinalis*, and *Cinchona succirubra*, or hybrids of any of the first two species with any of the last two species, belonging to family Rubiaceae.

Geographical Source

Cinchona is a native of South America. At present, it is mainly cultivated Indonesia (Java), Zaire, India, Guatemala, Bolivia, Ceylon, etc. Tropical valleys of the Andes, Bolivia and southern Peru are also a good habitat of this plant.

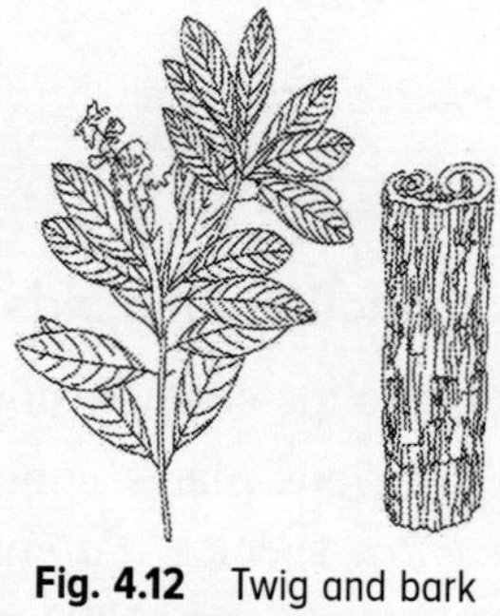

Fig. 4.12 Twig and bark of *Cinchona ledgeriana*

Chemical Constituents

The chiefly identified alkaloids are quinidine, quinine, cinchonine and cinchonidine. These constituents are the stereoisomers of each other.

The other constituents are quiniarnine, cinchotine, hydroquinine, hydrocinchonidine, cinchotannic acid, etc. Quinine and quinidine has a methoxy group in it but cinchonine and cinchonidine do not have a methoxy group.

Other than these it also consists of bitter glycoside, starch grains, calcium oxalate crystals and crystalline acid like quinic acid.

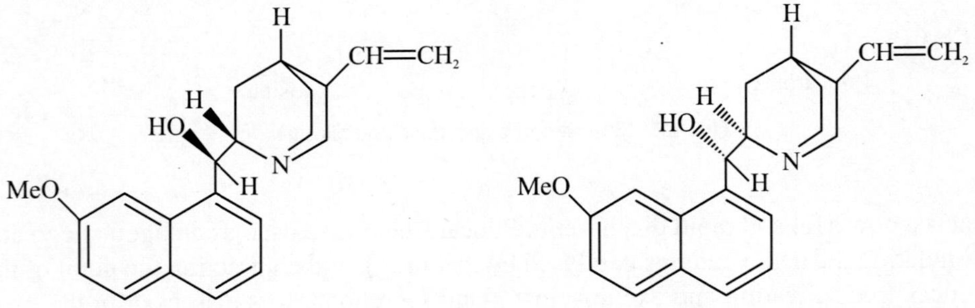

Quinine Quinidine

Fig. 4.13 Strucutre of qunine and quinidine

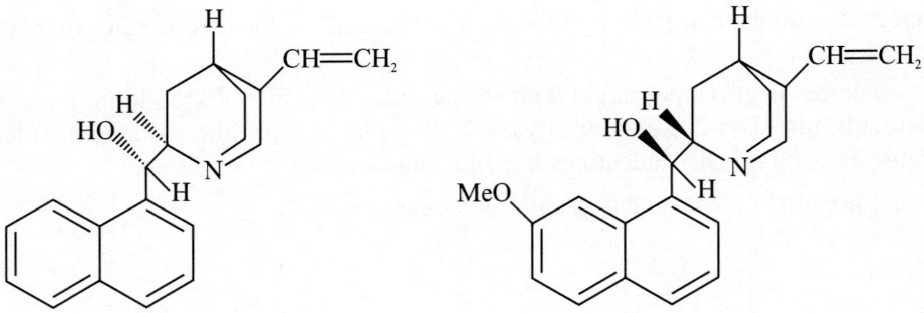

Cinchonine Cinchonidine

Fig. 4.14 Strucutre of cinchonine and cinchonidine

Uses

It is mainly employed as antimalarial drug, but it is also used as analgesic, antipyretic, protoplasmic, bitter stomachic and tonic. Quinidine is cardiac depressant and cinchonidine is used in rheumatism and neuralgia.

Marketed Products

Herbipyrin tablet MP (Vasu Healthcare).

Isoquinoline Alkaloids

Isoquinoline contains double carbon ring system with one nitrogen atom.

Various plants contains isoquinoline alkaloids such as *Prickly poppy*, *Celandine poppy*, *Dicentra* species, *Papaver* species, etc. The isoquinoline alkaloids: papaverine, sangumarine, protoverine, and chelidonine are GI tract irritants and CNS stimulants.

Most of the isoquinolines are noxious in smell and taste and discourage ingestion, thus human toxicity is rare.

Opium

Synonyms

Crude Opium, Raw Opium, Gum Opium, Afim

Biological source

Opium is the air dried milky latex obtained by incision from the unripe capsules of *Papaver somniferum* or *P. album*, belonging to family Papaveraceae. Opium is required to contain not less than 10% of morphine and not less than 2.0% of codeine. The the baine content is limited to 3%.

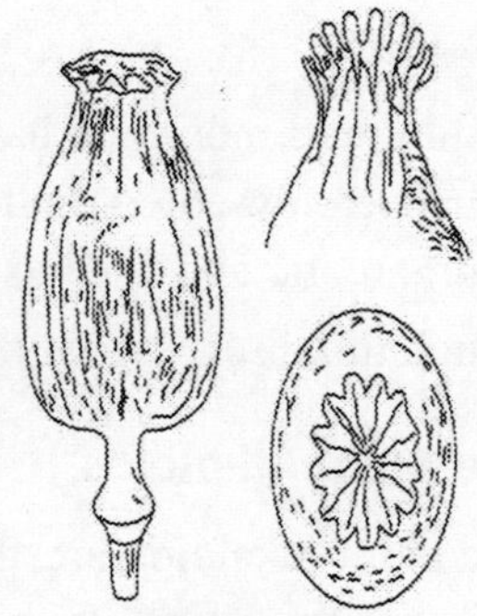

Fig. 4.15 *Papaver somniferum* capsules

Geographical source

It is mainly found in Turkey, Russia, Yugoslavia, Tasmania, India, Pakistan, Iran, Afghanistan, China, Burma, Thailand and Laos. In India, opium is cultivated in M.P. (Neemuch).

Chemical constituents

Opium contains about 35 alkaloids among which morphine (10-16%) is the most important base. The other alkaloids isolated from the drug are codeine (0.8–2.5%), narcotine, thebaine (0.5-2%). noscapine (4-8%), narceine and papaverine (0.5-2.5%).

The different types of alkaloids isolated are: Morphine, codeine, neopine, pseudo or oxymorphine, thebaine and porphyroxine, Hydrocotarnme, narcotoline, 1-narcotine, noscapine, oxynarcotine, narceine, and 5’-O-demethyl-narcotine.

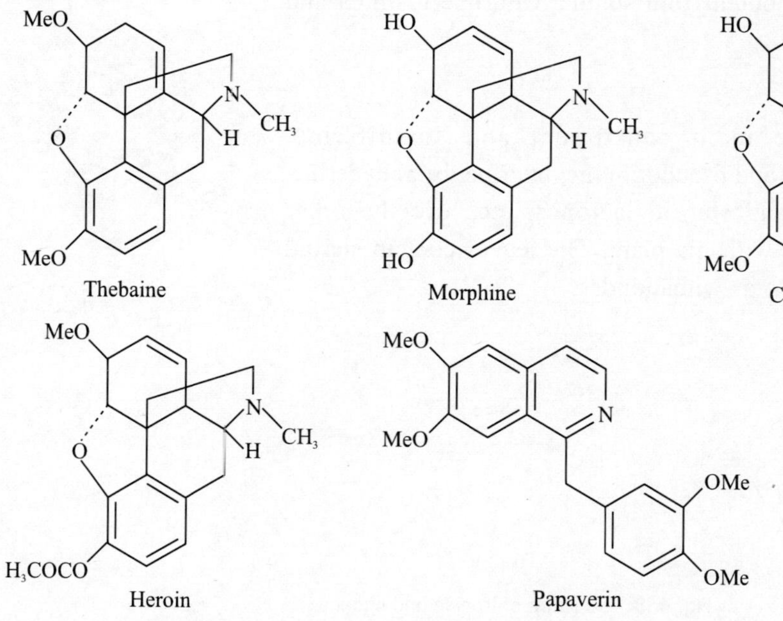

Fig. 4.16 Strucutre of the baine, morphine, codeine, heroin and papaverine

Uses

Opium and morphine have narcotic, analgesic and sedative action and are used to relieve pain, diarrhoea, dysentery and cough. Poppy capsules are astringent, somniferous, soporific, sedative and narcotic and used as anodyne and emollient. Codeine is a mild sedative and is employed in cough mixtures. Papaverine has smooth muscle relaxant action and is used to cure muscle spasms.

Steroidal Alkaloids

Steroidal alkaloids are the steroidal structure molecules, added with nitrogen atom in specific structural position. It contains mainly steroidal (cyclopentenophenanthrene) entity, along with basic nitrogen. They belong to C_{21} or C_{27} group of steroids. Steroidal alkaloids contain a tetracyclic (4-ring) triterpene ring structure called the steroid nucleus or steroidal backbone.

Ashwagandha

Synonyms

Withania root, Ashwagandha, Clustered Wintercherry.

Biological source

It consists of the dried roots and stem bases of *Withania somnifera*, belonging to family Solanaceae.

Geographical source

Withania is widely distributed from southern Europe to India and Africa.

Chemical Constituents

The withanine as the main constituent and somniferine, pseudowithanine, tropine and pseudotropine, hygrine, isopellederine, anaferine, anahygrine and steroid lactones, etc., are the other phytochemicals found in withania plant. The leaves contain steroid lactone, commonly known as withanolides.

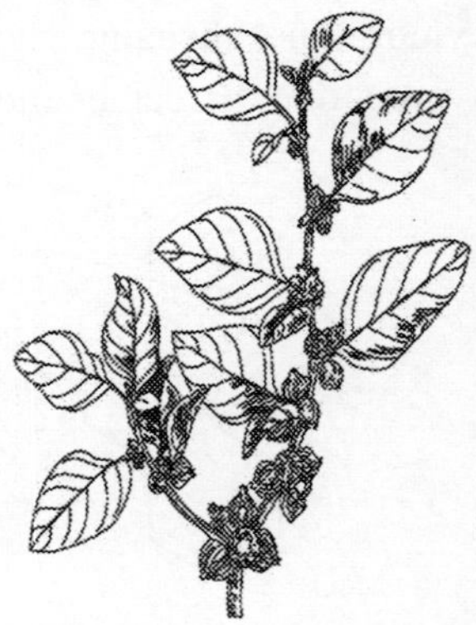

Fig. 4.17 *Withania somnifera*

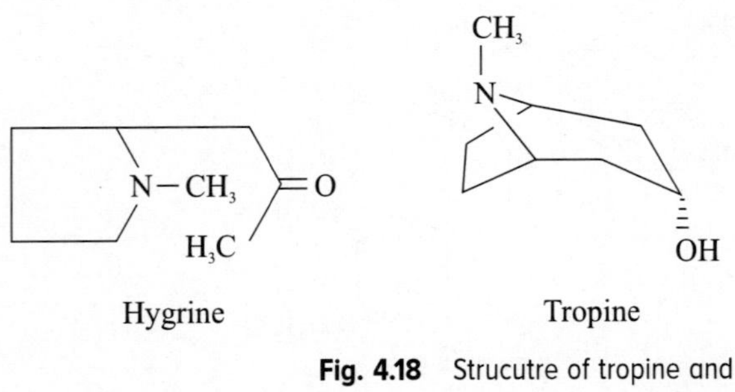

Fig. 4.18 Strucutre of tropine and hygrine

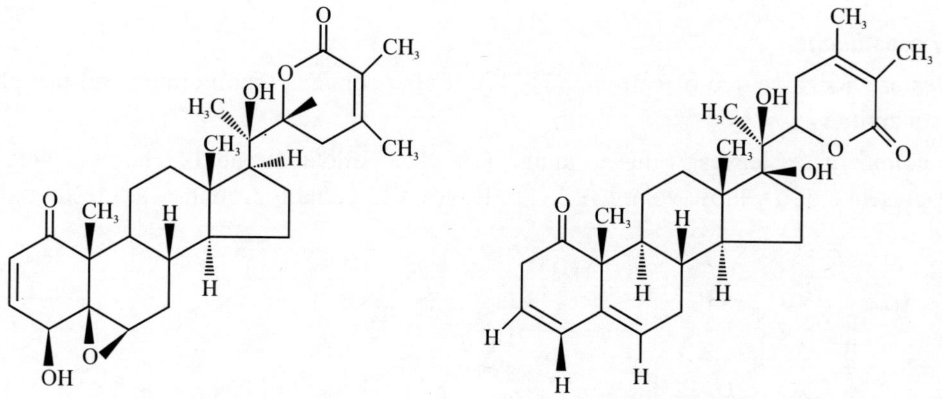

Withanolide D   Withanolide F

Fig. 4.19 Strucutre of withanolides

Uses

The roots, bark, leaves, fruit and seed of ashwagandha are used in nervous disorders, intestinal infections and leprosy. It is also used to treat nervous exhaustion, debility, insomnia, wasting diseases, failure to thrive in children, impotence, infertility, multiple sclerosis, etc.

Externally it has been applied as a poultice to boils, swellings and other painful parts.

Marketed Products

Abana, AntiStress Massage Oil, Nourishing Baby Oil, Nourishing Skin Cream, Anxocare, Galactin Vet, Geriforte Aqua, Geriforte Vet, Immunol, Speman forte Vet, Tentex forte Vet, Ashvagandha tablet (Himalaya Drug Company), Balarishta (Baidyanath), Aswagandha tablet (BAPS AMRUT).

Purine Alkaloids

Purine is composed of double carbon ring system with four nitrogen atoms. Its molecular structure is similar to nitrogenous purine base like adenine. Two important precursors, i.e., iriosine and xanthosine monophosphate are derived via purine biosynthetic pathways. The nucleotides adenosine and guanosine are derived from iriosine and xanthosine derivatives. Most of the purine alkaloids are derived from xanthosine. Purine alkaloids have CNS stimulant effect, relax bronchial smooth muscles and have a diuretic effect.

Tea

Synonyms

Chai patti, Tea leaves

Biological Source

It contains leaves and leaf buds of *Thea sinensis*, belonging to family Theaceae.

Geographical Source

It is predominantly cultivated in India (Assam), Ceylon, Japan and Java.

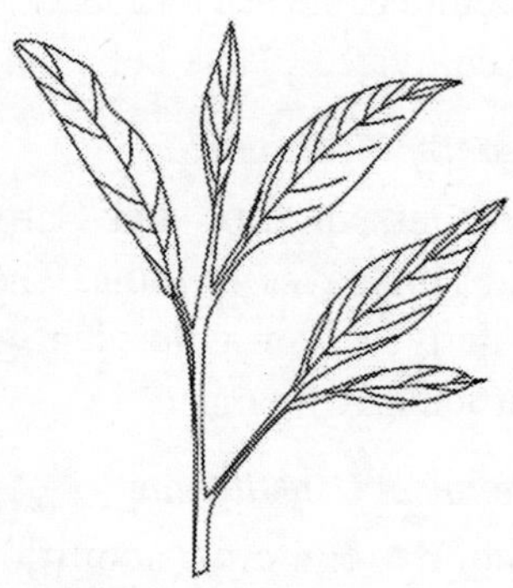

Fig. 4.20 Twig of *Thea sinensis*

Chemical constituents

The leaves are a rich source of caffeine (1–5%). It also contains theobromine and theophylline in minor quantities.

The colour of tea leaves is due to tannin (10–20% gallotannic acid). The agreeable odour is due to presence of a yellow volatile oil. Tea leaves also contain protein, wax, resin and ash.

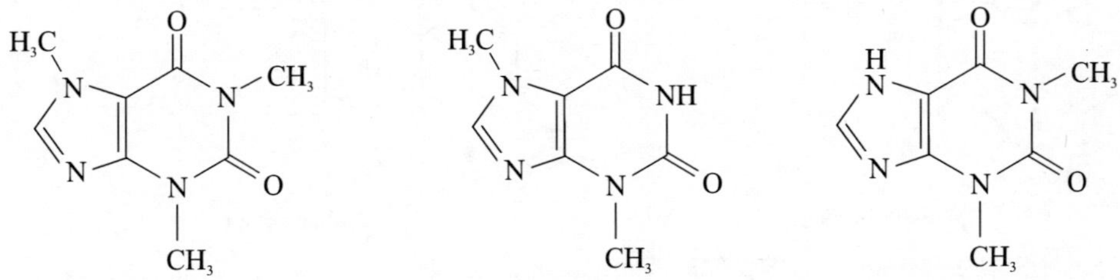

Fig. 4.21 Strucutre of caffeine, theobromine, theophylline

Uses

It is used as stimulant, astringent and also as diuretic.

Diterpene Alkaloids

This type of alokaloid possesses big cyclic ring structure. The bases of diterpenoids are generally classified into two cetegories, i.e., C_{19} skeleton and C_{20} skeleton.

It is accumulated mainly in the plant generas such as Aconitum, Delphinium, Carrya and Thalictrum, etc.

Aconite

Synonyms

Monkshood, Friar's cowl, Mouse-bane, Aconite root, Mitha zahar (Hindi), Radix aconiti.

Biological source

Aconite is the dried roots of *Aconitum napellus*, collected from wild or cultivated plants belonging to family Ranunculaceae.

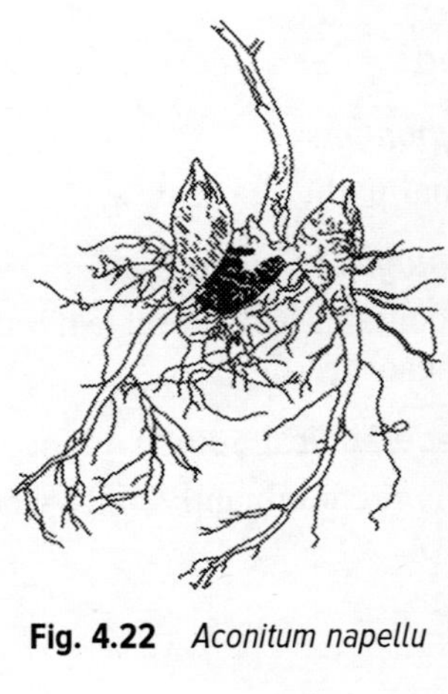

Fig. 4.22 *Aconitum napellu*

Geographical source

It occurs in Alps and Carpathian mountains, hills of Germany and Himalayas in India. The greater part of the commercial drug is derived from wild plant grown in central and southern Europe, particularly Spain.

Chemical Constituents

Aconite contains aconitine (0.4-0.8%), hypaconitine, mesaconitine, aconine, napelline (isoaconitine, pseudoaconitine), neoline, ephedrine, sparteine, picraconitine, acotinic acid, itaconic acid, succinic acid, malonic acid, fat, starch, aconosine, 14-acetyineoline, hokbusine A, senbusines A and C and mesaconitine. The basic skeleton of aconite alkaloid consists of a pentacyclic diterpene.

Uses

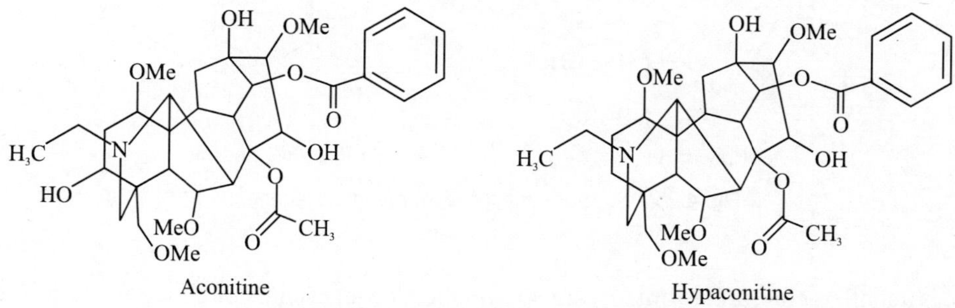

Fig. 4.23 Strucutre of aconiteine, hypaconitine

It is used externally as local analgesic in liniments and to treat neuralgia, rheumatism and inflammation. Tincture aconite is antipyretic in small doses. Aconitine in amount 2–3 mg can lead respiratory failure, heart failure and in the end death. The drug is used for the preparation of an antineuralgic liniment.

Marketed Products

J.P. Painkill oil (Jamuna Pharma).

Amino Alkaloid

It is consist of one or more carbon rings with a nitrogen atom on a carbon side chain. For example, ephedrine has a chemical structure similar to epinephrine (adrenalin) and works like a powerful cardiac stimulant. Pseudoephedrine, an isomer of ephedrine, also occurs in species of Ephedra, and may be produced synthetically. Compared to ephedrine, it causes fewer heart symptoms, such as palpitation, but is equally effective as a bronchodilator.

Ephedra

Synonyms

Ma Huang.

Biological source

Ephedra consists of the dried aerial parts of *Ephedra gerardiana*, *Ephedra sinica*, *Ephedra equisetina*, *Ephedra nebrodensis* and other Ephedra species, belonging to family Ephadreaceae.

Geographical Source

It is mainly found in China, India, Nepal, Turkey, Pakistan and Bhutan.

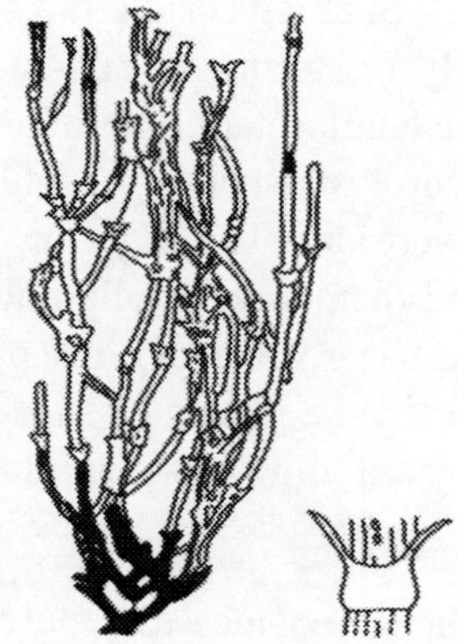

Fig. 4.24 *Ephedra sinica*

Chemical Constituents

Ephedra contains ephedrine (water-soluble salt of an alkaloid), pseudoephedrine (analog of ephedrine), norpseudo ephedrine (an analog of ephedrine).

The leaves and stems of ephedra also contain many potentially active compounds, such as tannins, saponin, flavone and volatile oils.

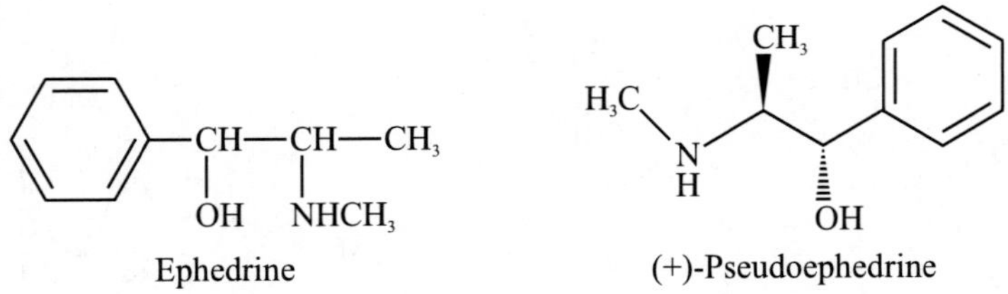

Fig. 4.25 Strucutre of ephedrine, pseudoephedrine

Uses

Ephedrine is antiallergenic, antiasthmatic, antispasmodic, decongestant, cough suppressant, stimulant and vasoconstrictor. Pseudoephedrine is decongestant, cough suppressant and norpseudoephedrine is peripheral vasodilator used to treat angina. As a whole it is decongestant; it opens sinuses, increases sweating, dilates bronchioles (antiasthmatic use), diuretic, CNS stimulant, raises bzlood pressure, alleviates aches and rheumatism, alleviates hay fever/colds, etc.

4.2.2 Glycosides

Glycosides are the group of phytomolecules found in a large number of plant families, comprise with a diverse bioactivities. The term 'glycoside' embraces all and divesed combinations of sugars and nonsugars moieties derived in plants as phyto secondary metabolities. The abundancy of important glycosides found in some plant families includes Scrophulareaceae (*Digitalis purpurea* and *Digitalis lanata, Picrorhiza kurroa*), Apocyanaceae (*Nerium oliander* and *Thevetia peruviana*), Liliacea (*Urgenea indica* and *U. maritima, Aloe vera*), Leguminocae (*Cassia acutefolia* and *C. angustefolia, Glycyrrhiza glabra, Psoralea corylifolia*), Dioscoreaceae (*Dioscorea floribunda*), Rosaceae (*Prunus amygdalus, Carategus oxycantha*), etc. Basically, glycosides are the biomolecules which a sugar group is bonded through its anomeric carbon to another group via glycosidic linkage.

Such glycosidic linkage or bond is a type of chemical bond that conjugates a sugar molecule (glycon) to another non-sugar molecule (aglycon). Specifically, a glycosidic bond is formed between the hemiacetal group of a saccharide and the hydroxyl group of an alcohol. On enzymatic or acid hydrolysis such glycosidic linkage gets seperated into glycon and aglycon or genin moieties of glycosides. The sugar or glycon parts of glycosides mainly consist of monosaccharides (glucose and rhamnose) or oligosaccharides (sucrose, maltose) but rarely deoxysugars (cymarose found in cardiac glycosides). The pharmacological activities of glycosides is due to the aglycon or nonsugar part while glycon or sugar part is be be needed to maintain the overall function of the glycosides since it allows its solubility and absoption.

Definitions

The glycosides are the organic secondary metabolites produced in plant or animals by the condensation of a sugar with non-sugar molecules in which the linkage (alpha and beta) is made with the hemiacetal hydroxyl and easily get hydrolyzed in the presence of enzymes or acid resulted one or more glycon and aglycon moieties.

Properties

In plants, glycosides are crystalline or amorphous substances which have solibility in water or alcohols but insoluble in organic solvents like benzene and ether.

The optically active non-sugar or aglycon part of glycosids is soluble in organic solvents (benzene or ether) and also gets hydrolyzed with water, enzymes and mineral acids.

Classification

The glycosides can be classified into three catergories.

1. On the basis of the nature of glycone or sugar moiety.
2. On the basis of glycosidic linkage.
3. On the basis of aglycone or non-sugar moeity.

1. On the Basis of the nature of Glycone or sugar moiety

(i) **Glucoside:** If the glycone group of a glycoside is glucose, then the molecule is a glucoside.

(ii) **Fructoside:** If the glycon part is fructose, then the molecule is a fructoside.

(iii) **Glucuronide:** If it glucuronic acid, then the molecule is a glucuronide.

(iv) **Rhamnoside:** If it is rhamnose, than the molecule is arhamnoside.

(v) **Pentoside:** If the glycone group of a glycoside is pentose, then the molecule is a pentoside.

(vi) **Arabinoside:** If the glycone group of a glycoside is arabinose, then the molecule is aarabinosid.

2. On the basis of glycosidic linkage

1. **C-glycosides:** Sugar molecule is directly attached with C-atom of aglycon, for example, Anthraquinone glycosides like Aloin, Barbaloin, Cascaroside and Flavan glycosides, etc.

   Glycon – OH + HC – Aglycon – Glycon – C – Aglycon + H_2O

   Such type of glycosides do not hydrolyse by heating with dilute acid or alkali but undergoes oxidative hydrolysis with $FeCl_3$.
2. **N-glycosides:** Sugar molecule is combined with N of the –NH (amino group) of aglycon, for example, nucleosides.

   Glycon – OH + HN – Aglycon — Glycon – N – Aglycon + H_2O
3. **O-glycosides:** Sugar molecule is combined with phenol or –OH group of aglycon, for example, amygd-aline, indesine, arbutin, salicin, cardiac glycosides, anthraxquinone glycosides like sennosides, etc. They are easily hydrolysed by treatment with acid or alkali.

   Glycon – OH + HO – Aglycon — Glycon – O – Aglycon + H_2O
4. **S-glycosides:** Sugar molecule is combined with the S or SH (thiol group) of aglycon, for example, Sinigrin (black mustard).

   Glycon – OH + HS – Aglycon — Glycon – S – Aglycon + H_2O

3. On the basis of aglycone or non-sugar moiety

The various classes according to aglycone moiety are given below.

Table 4.11 Examples of aglycone moiety

Sl no.	Aglycon moiety	Example
1.	Anthraquinone glycoside	Senna, Aloe, Rhubarb
2.	Aldehyde glycosides	Vanilla pods
3.	Cyanogenic and cyanophoric glycosides	Bitter almond, Wild cherry bark
4.	Coumarin glycosides	Celery fruits
5.	Flavonoid glycosides	Citrus bio flavonoids, Ginkgo
6.	Phenol glycosides	Bearberry
7.	Sterol or cardiac glycoside	Digitalis, Squill, Thevetia
8.	Saponin glycosides	Dioscorea, Liquorice, Ginseng
9.	Steroidal glycosides	Solanum
10.	Thiocynate and isothiocynate glycosides	Black mustard
11.	Glucosidal bitter and miscellaneous	Gentian, Picrrohiza, Chirta

4. On the basis of therapeutic nature of glycosides

Table 4.12 Therapeutic actions of glycosides

Therapeutic nature	Examples
Cardiac glycosides	Didgitalis
Laxatives glycosides	Senna
Anti-ulcer glycosides	Liquorice
Bitter glycosides	Quassia

Chemical Tests of Glycosides

Generally, aqueous or alcoholic extracts of crude drugs are tested with specific reagents for the presence of various types of glycosides.

Chemical Tests for Anthraquinone Glycosides

Borntrager's test

To 1 gm of drug add in 5–10 mL of dilute HCl and boil on water bath for 10 min and filter. Filtrate is extracted with chloroform / benzene and add equal amount of ammonia solution to filtrate and shake. The ammonical layer trun into pink or red colour which indicates the presence of anthraquinone moiety.

Modified borntrager's test

To 1 gm of drug, add 5 mL dilute HCl followed by 5 mL ferric chloride (5% w/v). Boil for 10 min on water bath, cool and filter, filtrate further extracted with carbon tetrachloride or benzene and add equal volume of ammonia solution, formation of pink to red colour due to presence of anthraquinone moiety. This is used C-type of anthraquinone glycosides.

Chemical tests for saponin glycosides

Haemolysis test

A drop blood on slide mixed with few drops of aqueous saponin solution, RBCs become ruptured in the presence of saponins.

Foam test

To 1 gm of drug add in 10–20 mL of water; shake for a few minutes, formation frothing which persists for 60–120 seconds indicates the presence of saponins.

Chemical Tests for Steroid and Triterpenoid Glycosides

Libermann burchard test

Alcoholic extract of drug evaporated to dryness and extracted with $CHCl_3$, add a few drops of acetic anhydride followed by conc. H_2SO_4 from side wall of test tube to the $CHCl_3$ extract. Formation of violet to blue coloured ring at the junction of two liquid, indicates the presence of steroid moiety.

Salkowaski test

Alcoholic extract of drug evaporated to dryness and extracted with $CHCl_3$, add conc. H_2SO_4 from sidewall of test tube to the $CHCl_3$ extract. Formation of yellow coloured ring at the junction of two liquids, which turns red after 2 min, indicates the presence of steroid moiety.

Antimony trichloride test

Alcoholic extract of drug evaporated to dryness and extracted with $CHCl_3$, add saturated solution of $SbCl_3$ in $CHCl_3$ containing 20% acetic anhydride. Formation of pink colour on heating indicates presence of steroids and triterpenoids.

Trichloro acetic acid test

Triterpenes on addition of saturated solution of trichloro acetic acid forms coloured precipitate.

Tetranitro methane test

It forms yellow colour with unsaturated steroids and triterpenes.

Zimmermann test

Meta dinitrobenzene solution added to the alcoholic solution of drug containing alkali, on heating it forms violet colour in the presence of keto steroid.

Chemical Tests for Cardiac Glycosides

Keller-kiliani test

To the alcoholic extract of drug equal volume of water and 0.5 mL of strong lead acetate solution added, shaked and filtered. Filtrate further extracted with equal volume of chloroform. Chloroform extract evaporated to dryness and residue dissolved in 3 mL of glacial acetic acid followed by addition of a few drops of $FeCl_3$ solution. The resultant solution is transferred to a test tube containing 2 mL of conc. H_2SO_4. Reddish brown layeris formed, which turns bluish green after standing due to presence of digitoxose.

Legal test

To the alcoholic extract of drug equal volume of water and 0.5 mL of strong lead acetate solution is added, shaked and filtered. The filtrate is further extracted with equal volume of chloroform and the chloroform extract is evaporated to dryness. The residue dissolved in 2 mL of pyridine and 2 mL of sodium nitropruside added and followed by addition of NaOH solution to make alkaline. Formation of pink colour in presence of glycosides or aglycon moiety.

Baljet test

Thick section of leaf of digitalis or the part of drug containing cardiac glycoside, when dipped in sodium picrate solution, it forms yellow to orange colour in presence of aglycones or glycosides.

3,5-dinitro acid test

To the alcoholic solution of drug a few drops of NaOH followed by 2% solution of 3,5-dinitro benzoic acid added. Formation of pink colour indicates presence of cardiac glycosides.

Chemical Tests for Coumarin Glycosides

$FeCl_3$ test

To the concentrated alcoholic extract of drug a few drops of alcoholic $FeCl_3$ solution added. Formation of deep green colour, which turned yellow on addition of conc. HNO_3, indicates presence of coumarins.

Fluorescence test

The alcoholic extract of drug mixed with 1 N NaOH solution (one mL each). Development of blue-green fluorescence indicates presence of coumarins.

Chemical tests for cynophoric glycoside

Sodium picrate test

Powdered drug moistened with water in a conical flask and a few drops of conc. H_2SO_4 is added. Filter paper impregnated with sodium picrate solution followed by sodium carbonate solution trapped on the neck of flask using cork. Formation of brick red colour due to volatile HCN in presence of cynophoric glycosides.

Chemical Tests for Flavonoid Glycosides

Ammonia test

Filter paper dipped in alcoholic solution of drug and exposed to ammonia vapour. Formation of yellow spot on filter paper indicates the presence of flavonoids.

Shinoda test

(i) To the alcoholic extract of drug add with magnesium turning and dil. HCl, formation of red colour indicates the presence of flavonoids.

(ii) To the alcoholic extract of drug add with zinc turning and dil. HCl, formation of deep red to magenta colour indicates the presence of dihdro flavonoids.

Vanillin HCl test

Vanillin HCl added to the alcoholic solution of drug, formation of pink colour due to presence of flavonoids.

Drugs Contain Glycosides

Anthracene Glycosides

It consists of glycosides formed from aglycone moieties like anthraquinones, anthranols, anthrones or dimers of anthrones or their derivatives. Anthrones are insoluble in alkali and do not show strong fluorescence with them, while anthronols which are soluble in alkali show strong fluorescence. The reduced anthraquinones are biologically more active. Anthroquinones that are present in fresh drugs are in reduced form, which on long storage get oxidized and hydrolysed, Glycosides of reduced derivatives are more active than oxidized aglycones. This is due to the fact that sugars take the glycosides to the site of action and thus are more active.

Anthraquinone is an aromatic organic compound and a derivative of anthracene. It has the appearance of yellow or light grey to grey-green solid crystalline powder. Its chemical formula is $C_{14}H_8O_2$. It melts at 286°C, boils at 379.8°C. It is insoluble in water or alcohol, but dissolves in nitrobenzene and aniline. It is chemically fairly stable under normal conditions.

Anthraquinone naturally occurs in some plants (e.g., aloe, senna, rhubarb and cascara), fungi, lichens and insects, where it serves as a basic skeleton for their pigments. Natural anthraquinone derivates tend to have laxative effects.

These glycosides are characterized by a chemical test, known as Borntrager test and show the property of micro-sublimation. Most of the glycosides are O-glycosides and S-glycosides, by their hydrolysis derivatives of 1,8-dihydroxy anthraquinone, anthranol, anthrone, or dianthrone are obtained.

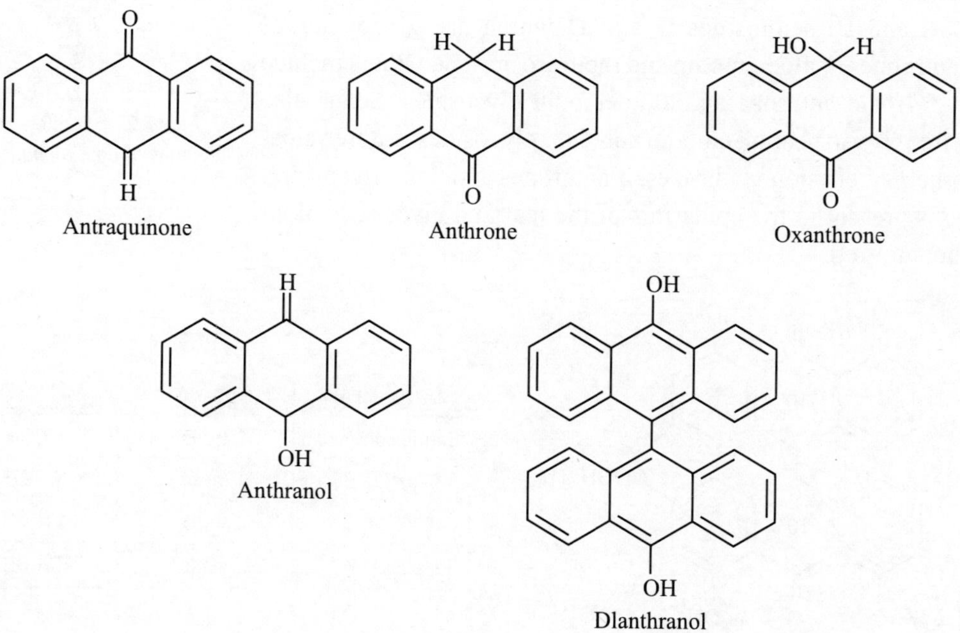

Fig. 4.26 Strucutre of Anthracene glycosides

The common aglycones are aloe-emodin, emodin, rhein, chrysophanol and physcion which may exist as anthraquinones, anthranols or anthrones. The sugars present are usually arabinose, rhamnose and glucose. During drying and storage by hydrolysis and oxidation free anthraquinones are produced.

Senna Leaf

Synonyms

Alexandrian senna, Tinnevelly senna, Folia senna.

Biological source

Senna leaf consists of the dried leaflets of *Cassia acutifolia* (known as Alexandrian senna) or *C. angustifolia* (known as Tinnevelly senna), belong to family Leguminosae.

Geographical source

Alexandrian senna is indigenous to South Africa and widely grows and cultivated in Egypt and in the middle upper territories of Nile River. Indian or Tinnevelly senna is indigenous to southern Arabia and cultivated largely in Tinnevelly and Ramnathpuram districts of Tamilnadu. It also grows in Sindh and Punjab region.

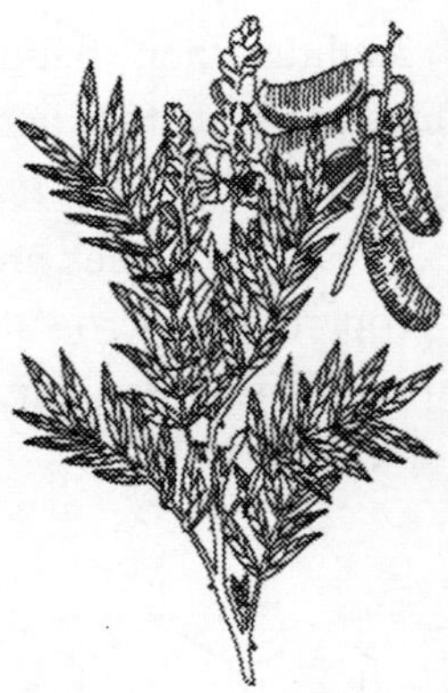

Fig. 4.27 Leaflets and legumes of *Cassia angustifolia*

Chemical constituents

Senna contains sennosides A and B (2.5%) based on the aglycones sennidin A and B, sennosides C and D which are glycosides of heterodianthrones of aloe-emodin and rhein are present. Others include palmidin A, rhein anthrone and aloe-emodin glycosides. Senna also contains free chryso phanol, emodin and their glycosides and free aloe-emodin, rhein, their monoanthrones, dianthrones and their glycosides. Mucilage is present in the epidermis of the leaf and gives red colour with ruthenium red.

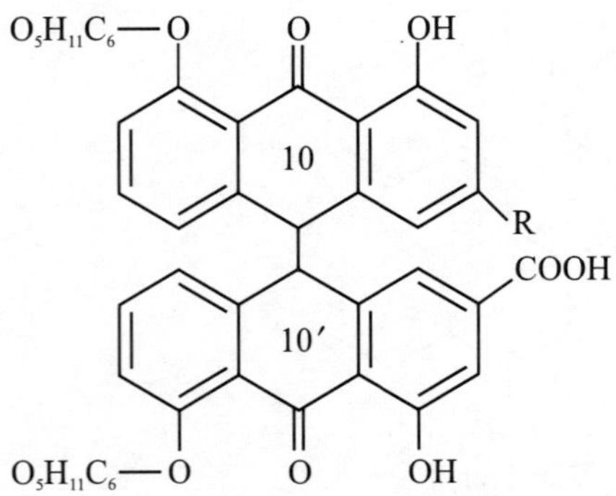

Glycoside	10 - 10′	R
Sennoside A	trans	COOH
Sennoside B	meso	COOH
Sennoside C	trans	CH_2OH
Sennoside D	meso	CH_2OH

Fig. 4.28 Strucutre of sennoside

Uses

Senna leaves are used as laxative. It causes irritation of large intestine and have some griping effect. Thus they are prescribed along with carminatives. Senna is stimulant cathartic and exerts its action by increasing the tone of the smooth muscles in large intestine.

Marketed products

Constivac, Softovac (Lupin Herbal Laboratory) and Isova powder, Kultab tablet (Vasu Healthcare).

Sterol or Cardiac Glycosides

The cardiac glycosides are an important class of naturally occurring drugs whose actions include both beneficial and toxic on the heart. Plants containing cardiac steroids have been used as poison and heart drugs since 1500 BC. These plants or their extracts have been variously used as arrow poisons, emetics, diuretics and heart tonics. Cardiac steroids are widely used in treatment of congestive heart failure and atrial fibrillation and flutter.

Cardiac glycosides are composed of two structural features: the sugar (glycone) and the non-sugar (aglycone-steroid) moieties. The steroid nucleus has a unique set of fused ring system with hydroxyls at 3- and 14-positions. The lactone moiety at C-17 position is an important structural feature. Normally, plant sources provide a five-membered unsaturated lactone while animal sources give a six-membered unsaturated lactone. Two classes have been observed in nature, the cardenolides and the bufadienolides.

Table 4.13 Comparison between caardenolides and bufadienolides

Cardenolides	Bufadienolides
Unsaturated butyrolactone ring.	Pyrone ring.
One double bond and is attached at the C-17 position of steroidal nucleus.	Two double bond which is attached at the 17 α-position of the steroidal nucleus.
Five-membered lactone ring and form a C_{23} steroids (leguminosae, cruciferae, euphorbiaceae, etc.)	Six-memberd lactone ring and form C_{24} steroids (liliaceae, ranunculaceae).

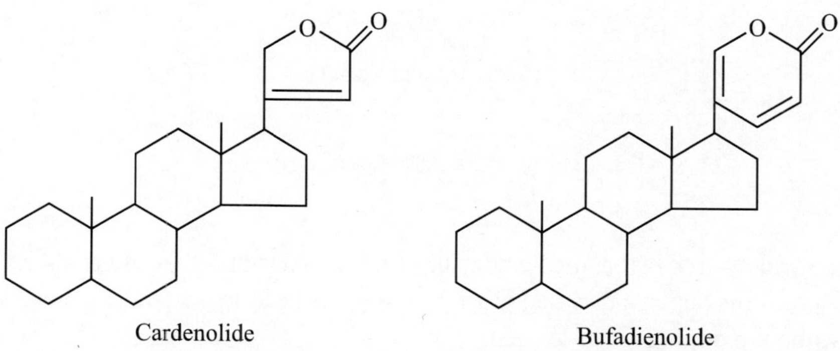

Fig. 4.29 Strucutre of *cardenolides, bufadienolides*

Digitalis Leaves

Synonyms

Digitalis, purple foxglove, finger flower, lady's glove, Fox-glove leaves, *Folia digitalis*.

Biological sources

Digitalis consists of dried leaves of *Digitalis purpurea*, belonging to family Scrophulariaceae.

Geographical sources

It is mainly found in England, Germany, France, North America, India, Iraq, Japan, Kurdistan, Mexico, Nepal, Spain and Turkey.

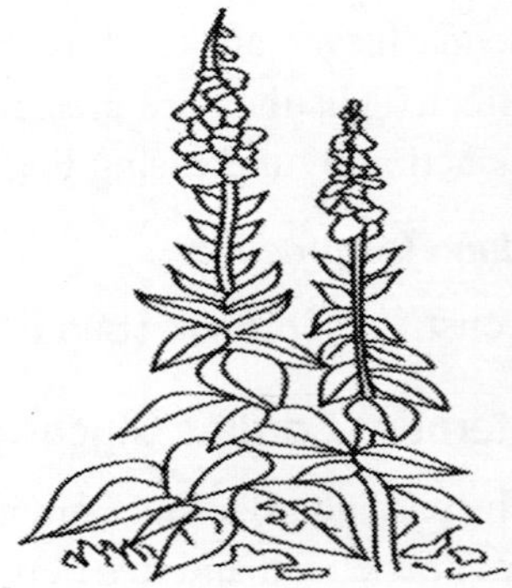

Fig. 4.30 *Digitalis purpurea*

Chemical Constituents

Digitalis leaves contain 0.2–0.45% of both primary and secondary glycosides. Purpurea glycosides A and B and glucogitoloxin are primary glycosides. Purpurea glycosides A and B on hydrolysis produce digitoxin and glucose or gitoxin and glucose. Digitalis leaves also contain glycosides like odoroside-H, gitaloxin, verodoxin and glucoverodoxin.

Digitoxose and digitalose are desoxy sugars found only in cardiac glycosides and show positive in Keller–Killiani test. The important saponins include digitonin, tigonin and gitonin, and luteolin, a flavone responsible for the colour of the drug are also present in the leaves.

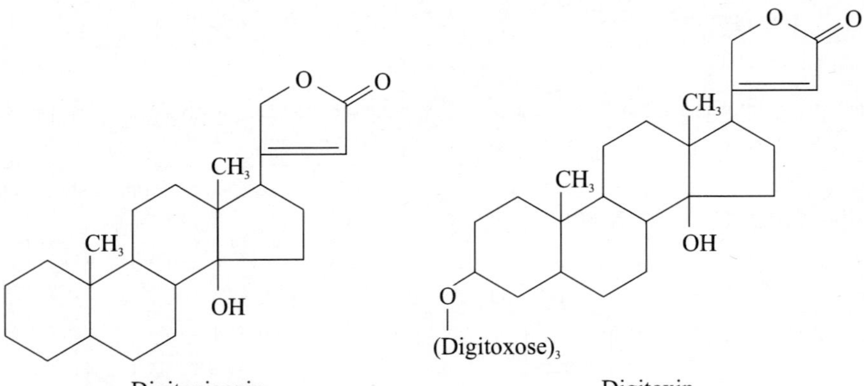

Fig. 4.31 Strucutre ofdiitoxigenin, digtoxin

Uses

The foxglove is a widely used herbal medicine with a recognized stimulatory effect upon the heart. It has a profound tonic effect upon a diseased heart, enabling the heart to beat more slowly, powerfully and regularly without requiring more oxygen.

It has also been employed in the treatment of internal haemorrhage, in inflammatory diseases, in delirium tremens, in epilepsy, in acute mania and various other diseases.

Marketed products

Lanoxin tablets (Glaxo Smith Kline).

Saponin Glycosides

Saponins are glycoside compounds often referred to as a 'natural detergent' because of their foamy texture. Foremost among this is the strong tendency to froth formation when shaken with water. The other properties are hemolytic activity, sneezing effect, toxicity, complex formation with cholesterol and antibiotic properties.

They consist of a polycyclic aglycone that is either a choline steroid or tritetpenoid attached via C_3 and an ether bond to a sugar side chain. The aglycone is referred to as the sapogenin and steroid saponins are called sarsaponins.

1. Steroid saponins

Steroid saponins are similar to the sapogenins and related to the cardiac glycosides distributed in such families like Solanaceae, Apocynaceae, Liliaceae, Leguminosae, etc. They have ability to interact medically and beneficially with the cardiac glycosides, sex hormones, Vitamin D and other factors, render these phytochemicals components of great medical significance. Diosgenin is the important steroid sapogenin. Recently, from these saponins steroid hormones like progesterone, cortisone, etc. have been obtained by partial synthesis and thus their importance has increased considerably.

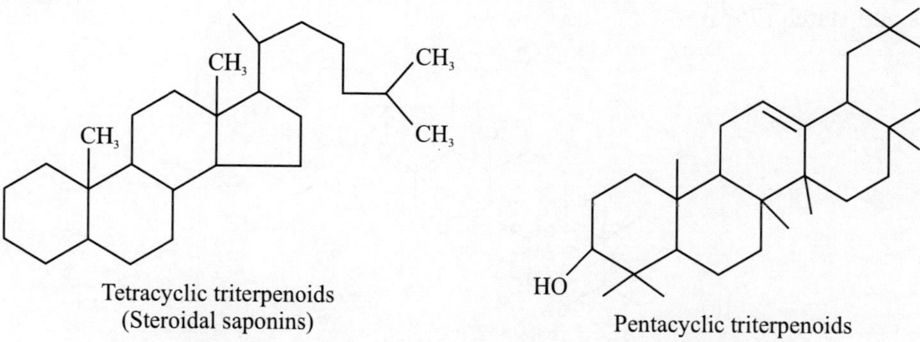

Fig. 4.32 Strucutre of saponin glycosides (steriodal andnon-steroidal)

2. Triterpenenoid saponins

Triterpenoid saponins, or sapogenins, are plant glycosides (belonging to the family Rubiaceae, Compositae, Rutaceae, Umbelliferae, etc.) which lather in water and are used as detergents, or foaming agents, antimicrobial, and adaptogenic properties.

Saponins are rarely crystalline and generally amorphous powder with high molecular weight. They carry many asymmetric centres and are optically active. They are generally soluble in water and form colloidal solutions. These are also soluble in ethyl and methyl alcohol and are usually insoluble in organic solvents like petroleum ether, chloroform and acetone, etc. They are bitter in taste and non-alkaline in nature.

Saponins show fungicidal, bactericidal activity, antiviral activity, antibiotic property, inflammation inhibition activity, spermicidal, antifertility, molluscicidal, etc. Saponins have been reported to possess blood purifying and abortion causing properties, anthelmintic effect, sedative property and antispasmodic effects. Saponins have also been identified in the animal kingdom in snake venom, starfish and sea cucumber, etc.

Dioscorea

Synonym

Yam

Biological source

Dioscorea is the dried rhizome of several species of *Dioscorea* like *D. villosa, D. prazeri, D. composite, D. spiculiflora, D. deltoidea* and *D. floribunda,* belonging to family Dioscoreaceae.

Geographical source

It is mainly found in North America, Mexico, India (Himalayas from Kashmir and Punjab up to an altitude of 3000 m), Nepal and China.

Chemical constituents

The roots contain diosgenin (4-6%) a steroidal sapogenin and its glycoside smilagenin, epismilagenin and beta isomer yammogenin. It also contains sapogenase (enzyme), phenolic compounds and starch (75%).

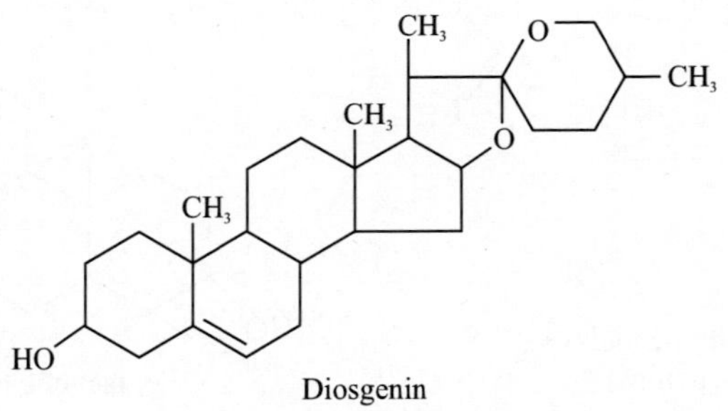

Diosgenin

Fig. 4.33 Strucutre of diosgenin

Uses

It is a main source of diosgenin. This is widely used in modern medicine in order to manufacture progesterone and other steroid drugs. These are used as contraceptives and in the treatment of various disorders of the genitary organs as well as in a host of other diseases such as asthma and arthritis.

Marketed products

Explode (Herbotech Pharmaceuticals).

Cyanogenic Glycosides

These are the glycosides which on hydrolysis yield hydrocynic acid (HCN), benzaldehyde and sugars. The medicinal activity of cyanogenetic glycosides is due to the presence of hydrocyanic acid and these are the characteristics of family Rosaceae. For examples, amygdalin obtained from bitter almond (*Prunus amygdalus*), Prunasin obtained from wild cherry bark.

Almond

Synonyms

Sweet almond

Biological source

Almond oil is a fixed oil obtained by expression from the seeds of *Prunus amygdalus* (sweet almonds), or *P. amygdalus* (bitter almonds) belongs to family Rosaceae.

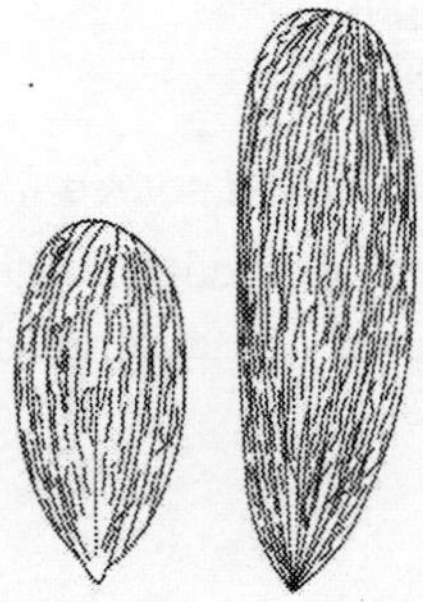

Fig. 4.34 Almond

Geographical source

The oil is mainly produced from almonds grown in the countries like Italy, France, Syria, Spain and North Africa and Iran.

Chemical Constituents

Both varieties of almond contain 40-55% of fixed oil, about 20% of proteins, mucilage and emulsin. The bitter almonds contain in addition 2.5-4.0% of the colourless, crystalline, cyanogenelic glycoside amygdalin.

Almond oil consists of a mixture of glycerides of oleic (62-86%), linoleic (17%), palmitic (5%), myristic (1%), palmitoleic, margaric, stearic, linolenic, arachidic, gadoleic and erucic acid.

Bitter almond oil contains benzaldehyde and 2-4% of hydrocyanic acid. Purified volatile oil of bitter almonds has all its hydrocyanic acid removed and, therefore, consists mainly of benzaldehyde. The unsaponifiable matter contains β-sitosterol, Δ^5-avenasterol, cholesterol, brassicasterol and tocopherols.

Uses

Almond oil is an emollient and an ingredient in cosmetics. It is used as a laxative, emollient, in the preparation of toilet articles and as a vehicle for oily injections. The volatile almond oils are used as flavouring agents.

Marketed Products

Baidyanath Lal Tel (Baidyanath Company), Himcolin gel, Mentat, Tentex Royal (Himalaya Drug Company) and Sage Badam Roghan (Sage Herbals).

Isothiocynate Glycosides

These are sulphur containing compounds rich in family cruciferae, also known as glucosinolates and on hydrolysis yields isothiocyanate (-NCS) group. These glycosides are generally irritant and hence used externally as counter-irritant, for example, sinigrin from black mustard, sinalbin from white mustard and gluconapin from rapeseed.

Mustard

Synonyms

Sarson

Biological source

It is a fixed oil obtained from matured seeds of *Brassica nigra* or *Brassica juncea* belonging to family Cruciferae (Brassicaceae).

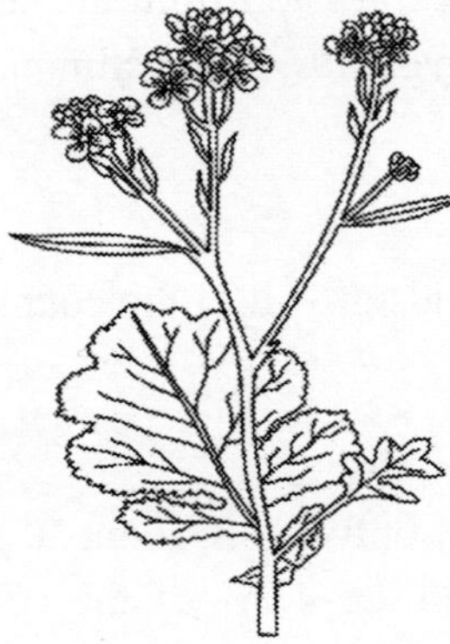

Fig. 4.35 Mustard

Geographical source

It is cultivated in India, China, Canada and England.

Chemical constituents

Mustard oil contains glycerides of arachidic (0.5%), behenic (2-3%), eicosenoic (7-8%), erusic (40–60%), lignoceric (1-2%), linoleic (14-18%), linolenic (6.5-7.0%), oleic (20-22%) and myristic (0.5-10%) acids.

Black mustard seeds contain 35-40% of fixed oil and a glycoside known as sinigrin along with an enzyme myrosin. Allyl isothiocynate is responsible for the strong acrid smell of volatile oil of mustard produced on hydrolysis of glycoside.

Brassica nigra

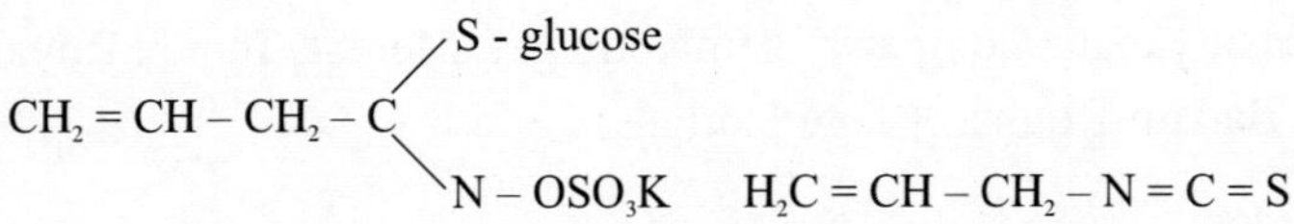

Sinigrin   Allyl isothiocyanate

Uses

Fixed oil is used as edible oil after refining, but medicinal properties are due to allyl isothiocynate, which is a local irritant and emetic. If applied externally, it is rubefacient and vasicant. It is also used as condiment and in manufacture of soap. Refined mustard oil is used in vegetable ghee.

Marketed products

Dabur Mustard Oil, Saaf Organic Eraser Body Oil.

Flavone Glycosides

These are complex organic compounds containing phenyl-benzopyrone ring system. Flavones are present in plants in a free state or in glycosidal state (O-glycoside or C-glycoside) with its different derivatives like flavane, flavonol, flavonone, isoflavone and chalcones, for example, rutin, quercitrin, hyperoside, diosmin (buchu leaf), hesperidin (lemon and orange peel) and vitexin (Carategus).

Ginkgo

Synonym

Biological source

The leaves of Ginkgo are obtained from the dioeceous tree *Ginkgo biloba*, belonging to family Ginkgoaceae.

Geographical source

It is a native of China and Japan and cultivated ornamentally in many temperate regions.

Chemical constituents

The diterpene lactones and flavonoids possess therapeutic activity. Five diterpene lactones (ginkgolides A, B, C, J, M) have been characterized; these have a cage structure involving a tertiary butyl group and six 5-membered rings including a spirononane system; a tetrahydrofuran moiety and three lactonic groups.

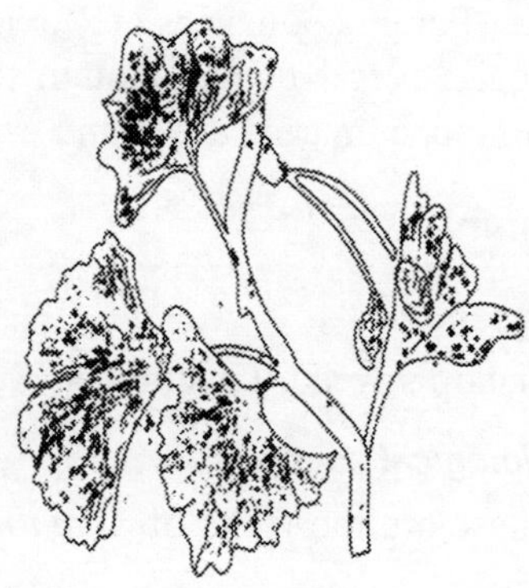

Fig. 4.36 Ginkgo

About 40 flavonoids have now been isolated from the leaves including glycosides of kaempferol, quercetin and isorhamnetin derivatives.

Ginkgo biloba

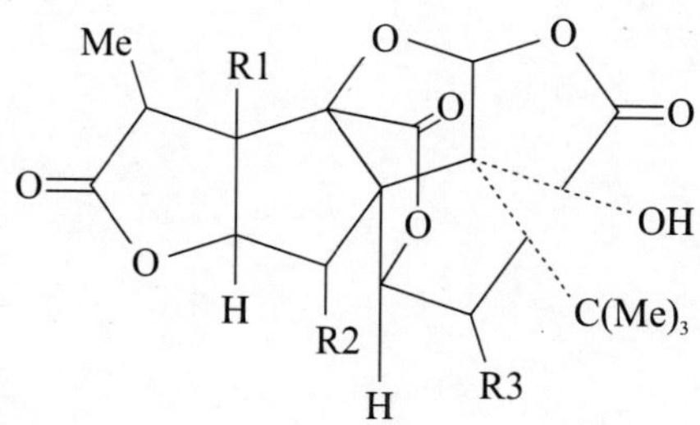

	R1	R2	R1
Ginkgolide A	OH	H	H
Ginkgolide B	OH	OH	H
Ginkgolide C	OH	OH	OH
Ginkgolide J	OH	H	OH
Ginkgolide M	H	OH	OH

Fig. 4.37 Strucutre of ginkgolides

Uses

Ginkgo is used as an antiasthmatic and bronchodilator. Leaf constituents are used for improving peripheral and cerebral circulation in those elderly with symptoms of loss of short-term memory, hearing and concentration; it is also claimed that vertigo, headaches, anxiety and apathy are cured.

Coumarin and Furanocoumarin Glycosides

In these types of glycosides the aglycone is coumarin. Coumarin is a chemical compound found in many plants, notably in high concentration in the tonka bean, woodruff, and sweet grass. They are benzopyrone derivative, have aromatic smell and their alcoholic solutions when made alkaline show blue or green fluorescence. The biosynthesis of coumarin in plants is via hydroxylation, glycolysis and cyclization of cinnamic acid.

It acts as precursor for several anticoagulants, notably warfarin. Some naturally occuring coumarin derivatives include umbelliferone (7-hydroxycoumarin), herniarin (7-methoxy-coumarin), psoralen and imperatorin. Medicinally, coumarin glycosides have been shown to have hemorrhagic, antifungicidal and antitumor activities.

Furanocoumarins are toxic compounds that consist of a coumarin nucleus bonded to a furan ring. Several plants contain the psoralens that are generally the precursors of furocoumarins. Furanoccumarins are found especially in rutaceae, umbelliferae and leguminosae.

Ammi

Synonyms

Bishop's weed, Laceflower, Large Bullwort, Toothpick Arami.

Biological source:

These are the fruits of *Ammi majus*, belonging to family Umbelliferae.

Geographical source

It is mainly found in Europe, Egypt, West Africa and India.

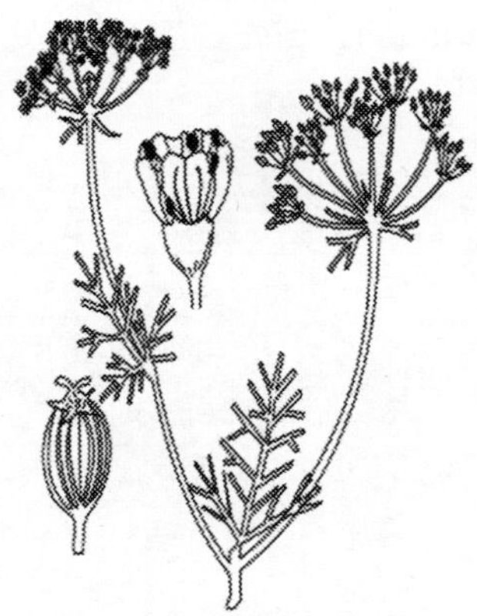

Fig. 4.38 *Ammi majus*

Chemical constituents

The drug contains furanocoumarins, xanthotoxin (0.4–1.9%), imperatorin, bergapten and isopimpilin.

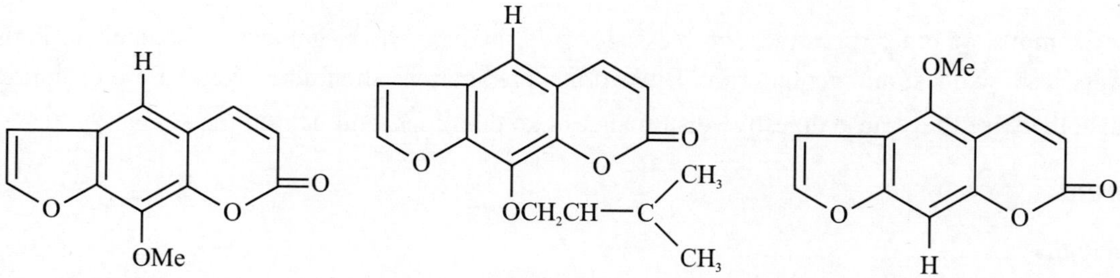

Xanthotoxin Imperatorin Bergapten

Fig. 4.39 Strucutre of xanthotoxin, imperatorin, bergapten

Uses

Furanocoumarins stimulate skin pigmentation when exposed to bright sunlight and are used in the treatment of vitiligo (piebald skin) and psoriasis.

Marketed Products

Lukoskin Ointment (Aimil Pharmaceuticals).

Steroidal Glycosides

It consists of steroidal nucleous.

Solanum

Biological source

It consists of dried berries of *Solanum khasianum*, belonging to family Solanaceae.

Geographical source

The plant is found widely growing at various altitudes in India right from coastal region up to 2000 m. It is found in hilly regions of Assam, Manipur, Sikkim, Nilgiris, Central India and also in Myanmar and China.

Chemical constituents

It contains about 3% of steroidal glycoalkaloid called solasodine. A new glycoalkaloid solakhasianin having rhamnose and galactose as sugar components have been isolated. Mucilage surrounding part of the seeds contain highest amount of alkaloide.

Uses

Solasodine is used as a precursor for steroidal synthesis. Like diosgenin, it is first converted to 16-dehydropregnenelone acetate. The latter is a precursor for steroids, like corticosteroids, pregnane and androstanes. All of these are useful as sex hormones, oral contraceptives, etc.

Bitter and Miscellaneous Glycosides

Bitter glycosides are a class of compounds that plays an important role in the digestive process. Bitter drugs and bitter constituents are used since a very early period as stomachics, febrifuges, and bitter tonics and in digestive disturbances.

Examples of bitter digestives are blessed thistle, barberry bark, goldenseal, dandelion, hops flowers, yellow dock, and gentian root. Bitter drugs preparations should be taken before or during meals otherwise they cause digestive disturbances like diarrhoea, and pain in the stomach.

Chirata

Synonyms

Indian Gentian, Indian Balmony, Chirayta, *Ophelia chirata, Swertia chirayita.*

Biological source

Chirata consists of the entire herb of *Swertia chirata*, belonging to family Gentianaceae. It contains not less than 1.3% bitter constituent.

Geographical source

It is mainly found in India, Nepal and Bhutan.

Chemical constituents

Chirata contains chiritin, gentiopicrin and amarogentin. Amarogentin is phenol carboxylic acid ester of sweroside a substance related to gentiopicrin. Ophelic acid a non-crystalline bitter substance is present. It also contains gentianine and gentiocrucine.

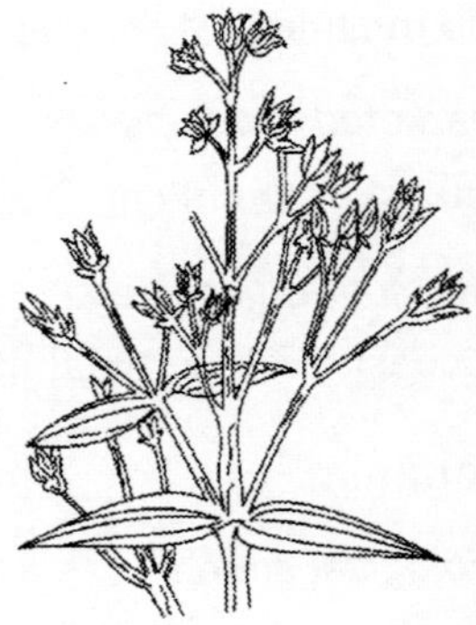

Fig. 4.40 *Swertia chirata*

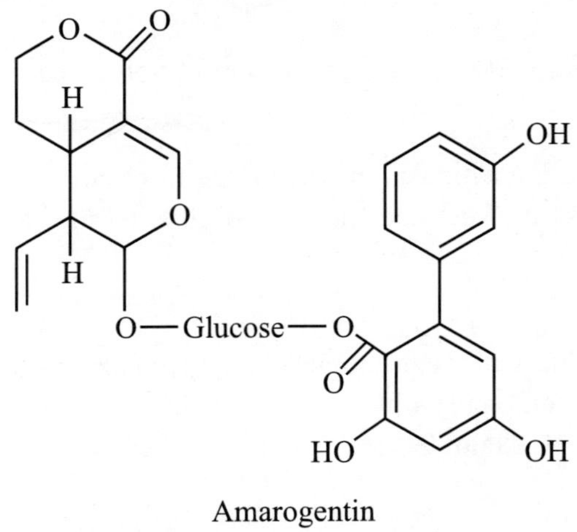

Amarogentin

Fig. 4.41 Strucutre of amerogentin

Uses

It is an important ingredient for ayurvedic preparations Mahasudarshan churna and Sudarshan churna used in chronic fever. The whole plant is an extremely bitter tonic digestive herb that lowers fevers and is stimulant. The herb has a beneficial effect on the liver, promoting the flow of bile; it also cures constipation and is useful for treating dyspepsia.

Marketed products

Diabecon (Himalaya), Mehmudgar Bati (Baidyanath), Sabaigo (Aimil Company), J.P. Liver Syrup (Jaumana Pharma), Fever End Syrup (Chirayu), Sage Chirata (Sage Herbals) and Safi (Hamdard Laboratories).

4.2.3 Flavonoids

Flavonoids are a group of natural compounds with variable phenolic structures and are found in plants. In 1930 a new substance was isolated from oranges and it was believed to be a member of a new class of vitamins and was designated as vitamin P. Later on it became clear that this substance was a flavonoid (rutin) and till now more than 4000 varieties of flavonoids have been identified. The term 'flavonoids (or bioflavonoids)' obtained from the Latin word 'flavus' meaning yellow.

It consists of a large group of polyphenolic compounds having a benzo-γ-pyrone structure. They are synthesized by phenylpropanoid pathway. The chemical nature of flavonoids depends on their structural class, degree of hydroxylation, other substitutions and conjugations, and degree of polymerization. Chemically flavonoids are based upon a fifteen-carbon skeleton consisting of two benzene rings (A and B) linked via a heterocyclic pyrane ring (C). They can be divided into a variety of classes such as flavones (e.g., flavone, apigenin, and luteolin), flavonols (e.g., quercetin, kaempferol, myricetin, and fisetin), flavanones (e.g., flavanone, hesperetin, and naringenin), and others. The various classes of flavonoids differ in the level of oxidation and pattern of substitution of the C ring, while individual compounds within a class differ in the pattern of substitution of the A and B rings.

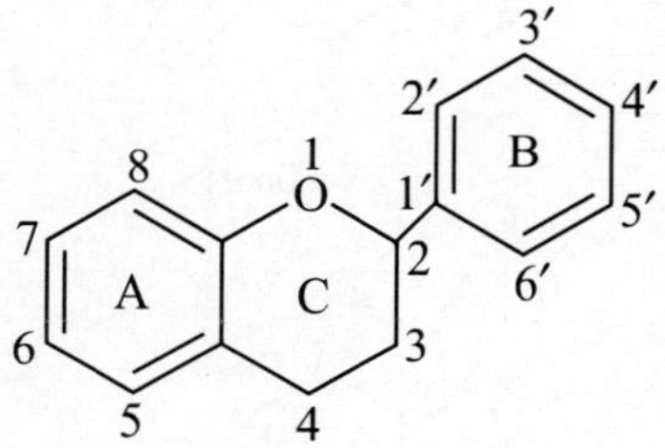

Fig. 4.42 General structures of flavanoids

Definitions and Occurrence

Flavonoids are defined as a group of polyphenolic compounds, diverse in chemical structure and characteristics, found ubiquitously in plants as secondary metabolites.

The major flavonoid classes are flavonols, flavones, flavanones, catechins, anthocyanidins, isoflavones, dihydroflavonols and chalcones, etc.

This polyphenolic compounds are found in fruits, flowers, seeds and vegetables, moreover abundant in higher plant families like Polygonaceae, Rutaceae, Leguminosae, Umbelliferae and Compositae.

Properties of Flavones and Flavonols

These are crystalline compounds, soluble in water, dilute mineral acids, alkalis, alcohol, etc. They are precipitated by means of lead acetate and give a dull green or a red brown colour with ferric chloride solution. Flavonoids show highly coloured in the acidic medium than in the bases from which they are derived. In acidic medium they form oxonium salts colour.

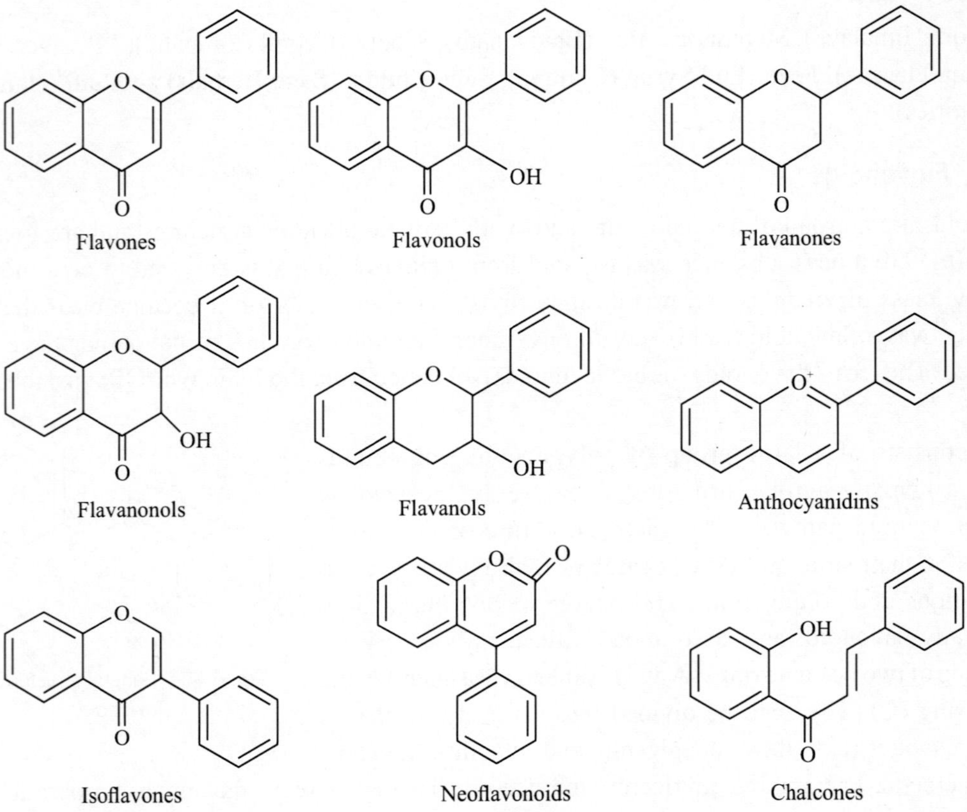

Fig. 4.43 Flavonoid subclasses

Classification

Flavonoids are classified into different subclasses depending on the carbon of the C ring on which B ring is attached, and the degree of unsaturation and oxidation of the C ring.

Flavonoids in which B ring is linked in position 3 of the ring C are called isoflavones; those in which B ring is linked in position 4, neoflavonoids, while those in which the B ring is linked in position 2 can be further subdivided into several subgroups on the basis of the structural features of the C ring.

This subgroup includes flavones, flavonols, flavanones, flavanonols, flavanols or catechins and anthocyanins. Flavonoids with open C ring are called chalcones. (Fig. 4.43)

1. **Flavones:** It has a double bond between positions 2 and 3 and a ketone in position 4 of the C ring. Most flavones of vegetables and fruits has a hydroxyl group in position 5 of the A ring, while the hydroxylation in other positions, for the most part in position 7 of the A ring or 3′ and 4′ of the B ring may vary according to the taxonomic classification of the particular vegetable or fruit. Glycosylation occurs primarily on position 5 and 7, methylation and acylation on the hydroxyl groups of the B ring. Some flavones, such as nobiletin and tangeretin, are polymethoxylated. (Fig. 4.44)

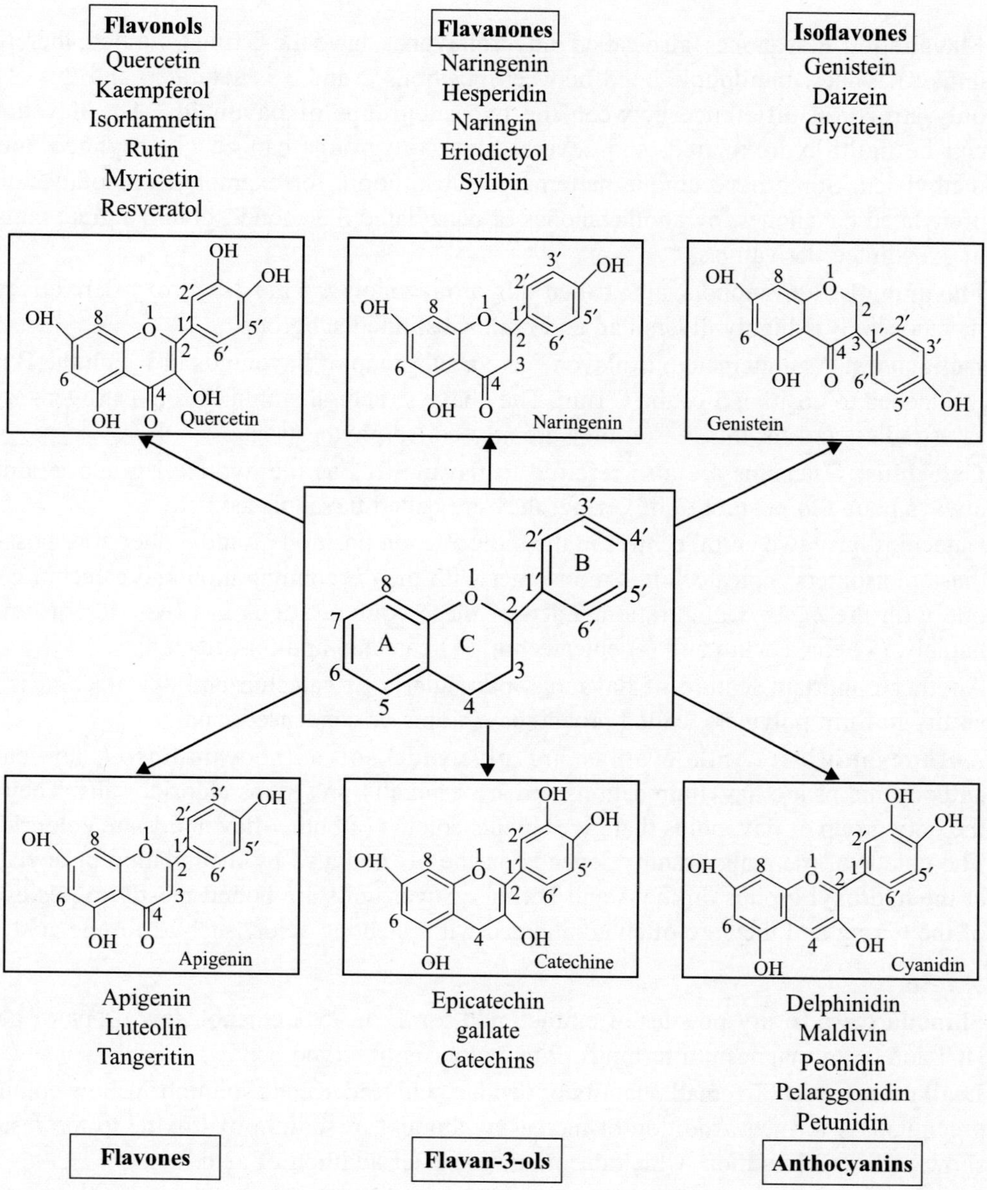

Fig. 4.44 Different structures of flavonoids

2. **Flavonols:** Compared to flavones, they have a hydroxyl group in position 3 of the C ring, which may also be glycosylated. Again, like flavones, flavonols are very diverse in methylation and hydroxylation patterns as well, and considering the different glycosylation patterns, they are perhaps the most common and largest subgroup of flavonoids in fruits and vegetables. For example, quercetin.

3. **Flavanones:** Flavanones, also called dihydroflavones, have the C ring saturated; therefore, unlike flavones, the double bond between positions 2 and 3 is saturated and this is the only structural difference between the two subgroups of flavonoids. The flavanones can be multi-hydroxylated, and several hydroxyl groups can be glycosylated and/or methylated. Some have unique patterns of substitution, for example, furanoflavanones, prenylated flavanones, pyranoflavanones or benzylated flavanones, giving a great number of substituted derivatives.
4. **Flavanonols:** Flavanonols, also called dihydroflavonols are the 3-hydroxy derivatives of flavanones. It is highly diversified and multisubstituted subgroup.
5. **Isoflavones:** As anticipated, isoflavones are a subgroup of flavonoids in which the B ring is attached to position 3 of the C ring. They have structural similarities to estrogens, such as estradiol, and for this reason they are also called phytoestrogens.
6. **Catechins:** Catechins are also referred to flavan-3-ols as the hydroxyl group is almost always bound to position 3 of C ring; they are called flavanols as well.

   Catechins have two chiral centres in the molecule, on positions 2 and 3, then four possible diastereoisomers. Epicatechin is the isomer with the *cis* configuration and catechin is the one with the *trans* configuration. Each of these configurations has two stereoisomers, namely, (+) epicatechin and (-) epicatechin, (+)-catechin and (-)-catechin.

   Another important feature of flavanols, particularly of catechin and epicatechin, is the ability to form polymers, called proanthocyanidins or condensed tannins.
7. **Anthocyanidins:** Anthocyanins are glycosides of anthocyanidins. Chemically, anthocyanidins are flavylium cations and are generally present as chloride salts. They are the only group of flavonoids that gives plants colours (all other flavonoids are colourless). The colour of the anthocyanins depends on the pH and also by methylation or acylation at the hydroxyl groups on the A and B rings. Sugar units are bound mostly to position 3 of the C ring and they are often conjugated with phenolic acids, such as ferulic acid.

Chemical Tests

1. **Shinoda test:** To dry powder or extract, add 5 mL of 95% ethanol, few drops of conc. HCl and 0.5 g magnesium turnings. Pink colour is observed.
2. **Lead acetate test:** To small quantity of residue, add lead acetate solution. Yellow coloured precipitate is formed. Addition of increasing amount of sodium hydroxide to the residue show yellow colouration, which decolouration after addition of acid.
3. **Aluminum chloride test:** Reaction with aluminum chloride, flavonoids give yellow colour.
4. **Antimony pentachloride test for chalcones:** Alcoholic solution added with antimony pentachloride ($SbCl_5$), red or violet colour is produced.
5. **Sodium hydroxide test:** To the aqueous extract added with 10% aqueous sodium hydroxide. This gives a yellow colour. A change in colour from yellow to colourless on addition of dilute HCl is an indication for the presence of flavonoids.
6. ***p*-Dimethylaminocinnamaldehyde test:** A colorimetric assay based upon the reaction of A-rings with the chromogen p-dimethylaminocinnamaldehyde (DMACA) has been developed for flavanoids in beverages that can be compared with the vanillin procedure.

4.2.4 Tannins

Tannins are a large group of phytochemicals widely distribute in plants. The term 'tannin' derives from French word 'tanin' which means tanning substance or have the ability to combine with animal hides to convert them into leather.

These compounds widely distributed in the plant kingdom. The term 'tannin' was first used by Seguin in 1796 to denote substances which have the ability to combine with animal hides to convert them into leather which is known as tanning of the hide. According to this, tannins are substances which are detected by a tanning test due to its absorption on standard hide powder. The test is known as Goldbeater's skin test.

Definitions and occurrence

Tannins are defined as the naturally occurring complex organic compounds possessing nitrogen free polyphenols of high molecular weight which forms colloidal solution with water giving acid reactions and have the capacity to precipitate proteins and alkaloids.

They occur normally in the roots, wood, bark, leaves, and fruit of many plants, particularly in the bark of oak (Quercus) species and in sumac (Rhus) and myrobalan (*Terminalia chebula*). They also occur in galls, pathological growths resulting from insect attacks.

Properties of Tannins

1. Tannins are colloidal solutions with water.
2. Non-crystalline substance.
3. Soluble in water (exception of some high molecular weight structures), alcohol, dilute alkali, and glycerin.
4. Sparingly soluble in ethyl acetate.
5. Insoluble in organic solvents, except acetone.
6. Molecular weight ranging from 500 to >20,000.
7. Oligomeric compounds with multiple structure units with free phenolic groups.
8. Can bind with proteins and form insoluble or soluble tannin-protein complexes.

Classification

The tannin compounds can be divided into two major groups on the basis of Goldbeater's skin test. A group of tannins showing the positive tanning test may be regarded as true tannins, whereas those, which are partly retained by the hide powder and fail to give the test, are called pseudotannins.

Most of the true tannins are high molecular weight compounds. These compounds are complex polyphenolics, which are produced by polymerization of simple polyphenols. They may form complex glycosides or remain as such which may be observed by their typical hydrolytic reaction with the mineral acids and enzymes. Two major chemical classes of tannins are usually recognized based on this hydrolytic reaction and nature of phenolic nuclei involved in the tannins structure. The first class is referred to as hydrolysable tannins, whereas the other class is known as condensed tannins.

1. **Hydrolysable Tannins:** As the name implies, these tannins are hydrolysable by mineral acids or enzymes such as tannase. Their structures involve several molecules of polyphenolic acids such as gallic, hexahydrodiphenic, or ellagic acids, bounded through ester linkages to a central glucose molecule. On the basis of the phenolic acids produced after the hydrolysis, they are further categorized under gallotannins composed of gallic acid or ellagitannins which contains hexahydrodiphenic acid which after intraesterification produces ellagic acid.

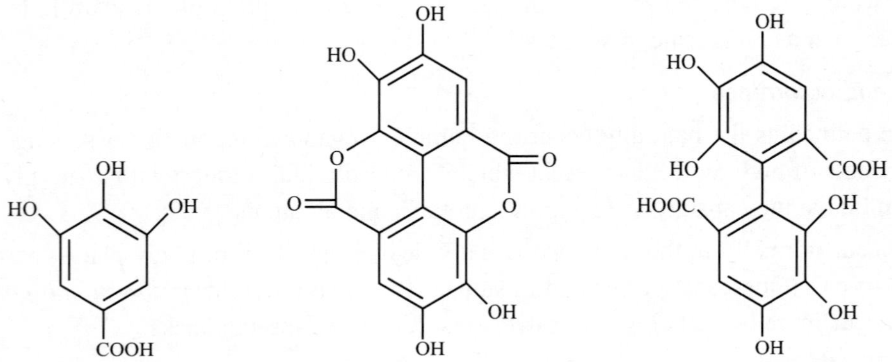

Gallic acid Ellagic acid Hexahydroxydiphenic acid

Fig. 4.45 Different structures of tannins

Hydrolysable tannins are sometimes referred to as pyrogallol tannins as the components of phenolic acids on dry distillation are converted to pyrogallol derivatives. The hydrolysable tannins are soluble in water, and their solution produces blue colour with ferric chloride.

2. **Non-hydrolysable or Condensed Tannins:** Condensed tannins, unlike the previously explained group are not readily hydrolysable to simpler molecules with mineral acids and enzymes, thus they are also referred to as nonhydrolysable tannins. The term proanthocyanidins is sometimes alternatively used for these tannins. The compounds containing condensed tannins contain only phenolic nuclei which are biosynthetically related to flavonoids. Catechin which is found in tannins is flavan-3-ol, whereas leucoanthocyanidins are flavan-3,4-diol structures. These phenolics are frequently linked to carbohydrates or protein molecules to produce more complex tannin compounds. When treated with acids or enzymes, they tend to polymerize yielding insoluble red coloured products known as phlobaphens. The phlobaphens give characteristic red colour to many drugs such as cinchona and wild cherry bark. On dry distillation, they yield catechol derivatives. Condensed tannins are also soluble in water and produces green colour with ferric chloride.

The families of the plants rich in both of the above groups of tannins include Rosaceae, Geraniaceae, Leguminosae, Combretaceae, Rubiaceae, Polygonaceae, Theaceae, etc. The members of families Cruciferae and Papaveraceae on the other hand are totally devoid of tannins. In the plants in which tannins are present, they exert an inhibitory effect on many enzymes due to their nature of protein precipitation and therefore contribute a protective function in barks and heartwood.

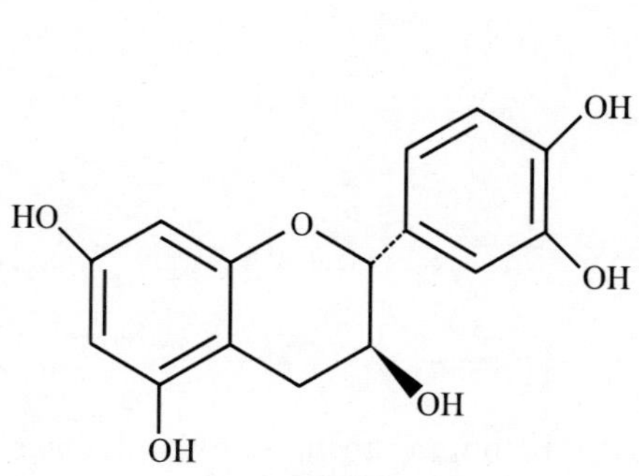

Fig. 4.46 Catechin

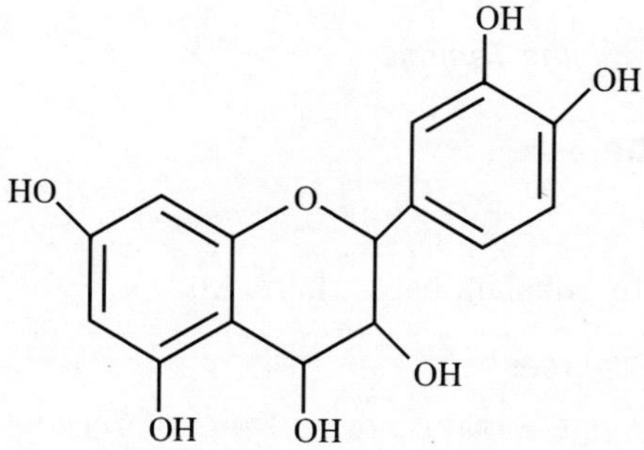

Fig. 4.47 Leucoaanthcyanidin

3. **Pseudotannins:** Pseudotannins are simple phenolic compounds of lower molecular weight. They do not respond to the tanning reaction of Goldbeater's skin test. Gallic acid, chlorogenic acid, or the simple phenolics such as catechin are pseudotannins which are abundantly found in plants, especially in dead tissues and dying cells.

Chemical Tests

1. **Goldbeater's skin test:** Goldbeater's skin is a membrane produced from the intestine of Ox. It behaves just like untanned animal hide. A piece of Goldbeaters skin previously soaked in 2% hydrochloric acid and washed with distilled water is placed in a solution of tannin for 5 minutes. It is then washed with distilled water and transferred to 1% ferrous sulphate solution. A change of the colour of the Goldbeater's skin to brown or black indicates the presence of tannin.
2. Hydrolysable and condensed tannins both give the positive Goldbeater's test, whereas pseudotannins show very little colour or negative test.
3. **Phenazone test:** To 5 mL of aqueous solution of tannin containing drug, add 0.5 g of sodium acid phosphate. Warm the solution, cool, and filter. Add 2% phenazone solution to the filtrate. All tannins are precipitated as bulky, coloured precipitate.
4. **Gelatin test:** To a 1% gelatine solution, add little 10% sodium chloride. If a 1% solution of tannin is added to the gelatine solution, tannins cause precipitation of gelatine from solution.
5. **Test for Catechin (Matchstick test):** Catechin test is the modification of the well-known phloroglucinol test for lignin. Matchstick contains lignin. Dip a matchstick in the dilute extract of the drug, dry, moisten it with concentrated hydrochloric acid, and warm it near a flame. Catechin in the presence of acid produces phloroglucinol which stains the lignified wood pink or red.
6. **Test for chlorogenic acid:** A dilute solution of chlorogenic acid containing extract, if treated with aqueous ammonia and exposed to air, slowly turns green indicating the presence of chlorogenic acid.
7. **Vanillin-hydrochloric acid test:** Drug shows pink or red colour with a mixture of vanillin:alcohol:dilute HCl in the ratio 1:10:10. The reaction produces phloroglucinol which along with vanillin gives pink or red colour.

Drugs Containing Tannins

Myrobalan

Synonyms

Chebulic myrobalan, harde, haritaki.

Biological sources

Myrobalan is the mature dried fruits of *Terminalia chebula,* belonging to family Combretaceae.

Geographical source

Myrobalan trees are found at an elevation of 300 to 900 m in North India, Satpura ranges of Madhya Pradesh, Maharashtra, and Panchamahal district in Gujarat. It is also found in Myanmar and Sri Lanka.

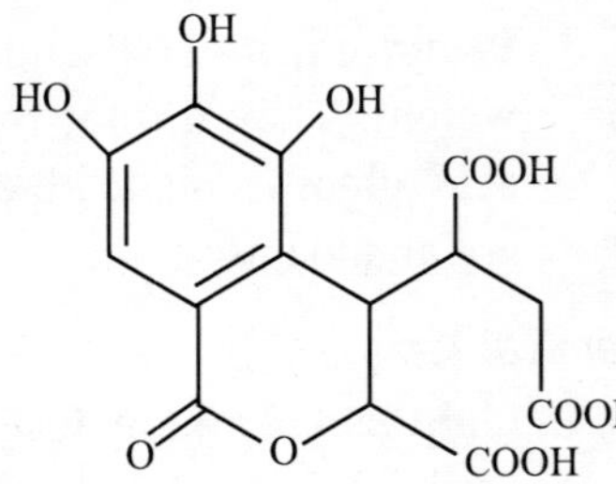

Fig. 4.48 Chebulic acid

Chemical Constituents

Myrobalan contains about 30% of the hydrolysable tannins, which consists of chebulinic acid, chebulagic acid and D-galloyl glucose. It contains free tannic acid, gallic acid, ellagic acid, and resin myrobalanin. Anthraquinone glycosides, sennosides have been reported in myrobalan.

Uses

Myrobalan is reputed in Indian system of medicine as antiseptic and healing properties of tannins, it is used externally in chronic ulcers, wounds, piles, and as stomachic. It is one of the drugs of the well-known preparation, 'Triphala'. It has purgative properties. Fine powder of myrobalan is used in dental preparations. Commercially, it is used in dyeing and tanning industry and also in treatment of water used for locomotives.

Marketed products

Constivac (Lupin Herbal Laboratory), Pilect (Aimil Pharmaceuticals), Abana, Bonnisan, Gariforte, Koflet, Menosan (Himalaya Drug Company), Haritakh churna, Triphala churna, Tentex forte (Baidyanath Company).

4.2.5 Volatile Oils

Volatile oils are odorous volatile principles of plant and animal source, evaporate when exposed to air at ordinary temperature, and hence known as volatile or etheral oils. These represent essence of active constituents of the plant and hence also known as essential oils. In most instances the volatile oil pre-exists in the plant and is usually contained in some special secretory tissues, for example, the oil ducts of umbelliferous fruits, the oil cells, or oil glands occurring in the sub-epidermal tissue of the lemon and orange, mesophyll of eucalyptus leaves, trichomes of several plants, etc.

In few cases the volatile oil does not pre-exist, but is formed by the decomposition of a glycoside. For example, whole black mustard seeds are odourless, but upon crushing the seeds and adding water to it a strong odour is evolved. This is due to allyl isothiocyanate (the main constituent of essential oil of mustard) formed by decomposition of a glycoside, sinigrin, by an enzyme, myrosin. Glycoside and enzyme are contained in different cells of the seed tissue and are unable to react until the seeds are crushed with water present, so that the cell contents can intermingle.

Definition and Properties

Volatile oils are defined as a mixture of hydrocarbon terpenes, sesquiterpenes and polyterpenes and their oxygenated derivatives obtained from various parts of the plant which evaporates on exposure to air at ordinary temperature and are the odorous constituents.

It is chemically derived from terpenes (mainly mono- and sesquiterpenes) and their oxygenated derivatives. These are soluble in alcohol and other organic solvents, practically insoluble in water, lighter than water (clove oil heavier), possess characteristic odour, have high refraction index, and most of them are optically active. The volatile oils dissolve many of the proximate principles of plant and animal tissues, such as the fixed oils and fats, resins, camphor, and many of the alkaloids when in the free state.Volatile oils are colourless liquids, but when exposed to air and direct sunlight these become darker due to oxidation. Unlike fixed oils, volatile oils neither leave permanent grease spot on filter paper nor saponified with alkalis.

Classification of Volatile Oils

Volatile oils are classified on the basis of functional groups present as given in Table 4.14.

Table 4.14 Classification of volatile oils on basis of functional groups

Chemical groups	Examples
Hydrocarbons	Turpentine oil
Alcohol	Peppermint oil, sandalwood oil
Aldehyde	Cymbopogon species, lemongrass oil, cinnamon, cassia
Ketones	Campor, caraway, fennel
Phenol	Clove, ajowan, tulsi
Phenolic ether	Nutmeg, calamus
Oxides	Eucalyptus oil, cardamom, chenopodium oil
Ester	Valerian, rosemary oil, garlic, gaultheria oil

Chemical Tests for Volatile Oils

1. Thin section of drug treated with alcoholic solution of Sudan III develops red colour in the presence of volatile oils.

2. Thin section of drug is treated with tincture of alkana, which produces red colour that indicates the presence of volatile oils in natural drugs.

Drugs Containing Volatile Oils

Volatile Oils Containing Hydrocarbons

Hydrocarbons are present in all volatile oils. Limonene is the most widely distributed of the monocyclic terpenes. It occurs in citrus, mint, myristica, caraway, thyme, cardamom, coriander, and many other oils. Another monocyclic hydrocarbon monoterpene is p-cymene, present in coriander, thyme, cinnamon, and myristica oils. Pinene, a dicyclic monoterpene, is also widely distributed. Acyclic monoterpene myrcene occurs in myricia, lemon, and myristica. Cadinene occurring in juniper tar, is a sesquiterpene hydrocarbon. β-Caryophyllene is a sesquiterpene found in wormwood, peppermint, cinnamon, and clove oils.

A volatile oil drug is composed mainly of hydrocarbons is turpentine oil.

Turpentine Oil

Synonyms

Oleum terbinthae, rectified oil of turpentine.

Botanical source

Turpentine oil is the volatile oil obtained by the distillation of oleoresin from *Pinus longifolia* Roxb and various species of Pinus, belonging to family Pinaceae.

Geographical source

Pinus longifolia is cultivated in India and Pakistan; the other species are cultivated in the United States, France, Europe, and Russia.

Chemical constituents

Oil of turpentine contains more than 40 terpenes; the chief terpenes are α- and β-pinene with small quantity of camphene, limonene, etc.

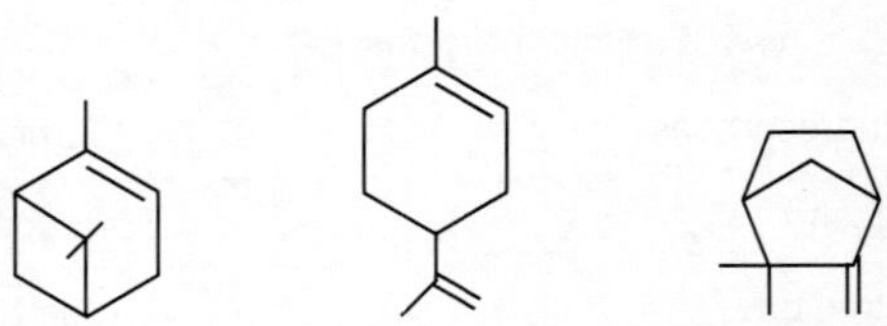

Fig. 4.49 Strucutre of pinene, limonene, camphene

Uses

Turpentine oil is used as counter-irritant, rubefacient, in swelling, neuralgia, as mild antiseptic, as an expectorant in chronic bronchitis, as diuretic, and urinary antiseptic. When taken internally it causes irritation of kidney also. In industries it is used in the preparation of disinfectants, insecticides, paints, varnishes, and pine oil.

Marketed Products

Rumalaya gel and Pain balm (Himalaya Drug Company).

Volatile Oils Containing Alcohols

Methyl, ethyl, isobutyl, isoamyl, hexyl, and the higher aliphatic alcohols occur in volatile oils.

Table 4.15 Volatile oils containing alcohol

Class	Example
Acyclic alcohols	Geraniol, Linalool, Citronellol
Monocyclic alcohols	Menthol, α-terpineol
Dicyclic terpene alcohol	Borneol
Sesquiterpene alcohols	Zingiberol, santalols, Artemisin

Peppermint, cardamom oil, coriander oil, rose oil, orange flower oil, juniper oil, and pine oil are the major alcohol volatile oils containing drugs.

Peppermint

Synonym

Brandy Mint.

Botanical source

It is the oil obtained by the distillation of *Mentha piperita*, belonging to family Labiatae.

Geographical source

It is mainly found in Europe, United States, and also in damp places of England.

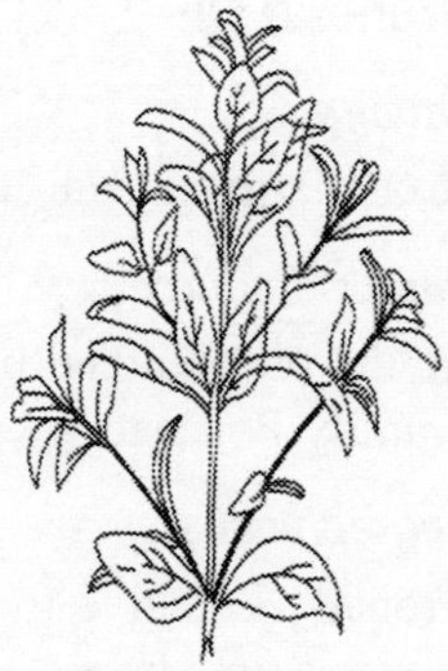

Fig. 4.50 *Mentha piperita*

Chemical constituents

The chief constituent of peppermint oil is menthol, along with other constituents like menthyl acetate, isovalerate, menthone, cineol, inactive pinene, limonene, etc. Menthol separates on cooling it to a low temperature (–22°C). The flavouring properties of the oil are due to both the ester and alcoholic constituents, whereas the medicinal value is attributed only due to the alcoholic components.

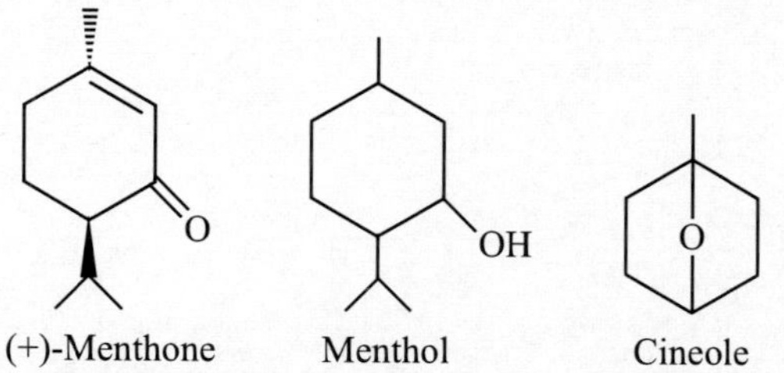

Fig. 4.51 Structure of menthone, menthol, cineole

Uses

It is used as stimulant, stomachic, carminative, flatulence, colic, dyspepsia, sudden pains, and also in cholera and diarrhoea. Peppermint is good to aid in raising internal heat and inducing perspiration. It is also used in cases of hysteria and nervous disorders.

Marketed products

Dabur Lal Tooth Powder (Dabur).

Volatile Oils Containing Aldehydes

Aldehydes present in volatile oils are divided into two categories:

(i) acyclic aldehyde, and
(ii) cyclic aldehyde

The examples of acyclic and cyclic aldehydes are citral, citronellal and safranal, phellandral, photocitral A, myrtenal, respectively. The aromatic aldehydes include cinnamaldehyde and vanillin. Cinnamon, orange oil, lemon peel, lemon oil, and citronella oil are the important drugs in this group.

Citronella Oil

Synonyms

Citronella grass, Nardus, Mana grass, Nard grass.

Biological source

It is the oil obtained by the steam distillation of fresh leaves of *Cymbopogon nardus* belonging to family Poaceae.

Geographical source

Citronella is native to Southeast Asia and grown commercially in Sri Lanka, India, Mayanmar, Indonesia and Java.

Chemical constituents

The main chemical components of citronella oil are citronellic acid, geraniol, nerol, citral, borneol, camphene, citronellol, citronellal, dipentene, and limonene. It has about 3.0% limonene; 35.3% citronellal; 12.0% citronellol, 24.9% geraniol, 4.3% citronellyl acetate, 6.3% geranyl acetate, and 0.8% linalool.

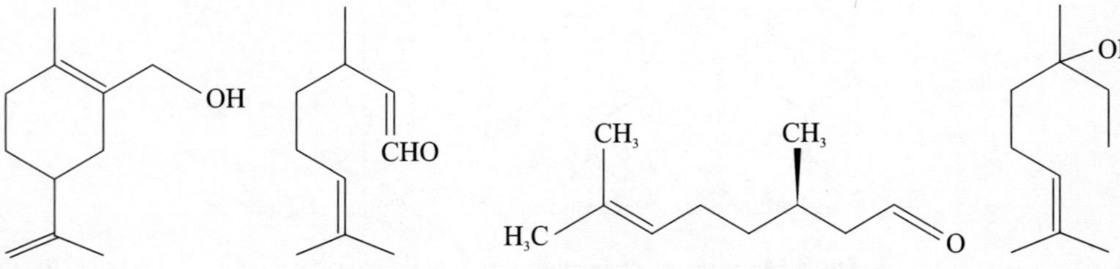

Geraniol Citral Citronellal Linalool

Fig. 4.52 Strucutre of geraniol, citral, linalool

Uses

It is the commercial source of citronella oil, used in perfumery industries. Citronella oil is antiseptic, insect repellent, deodorant, tonic, insecticide, diaphoretic, parasitic, bactericidal, and stimulant.

Volatile Oils Containing Ketones

Ketones present in volatile oils are divided into:

1. **Monocyclic terpene ketones:** Example, menthone, carvone, piperitone, pulegone
2. **Dicyclic ketones:** Example, camphor, fenchone, thujone
3. **Acyclic ketone:** Example, artemisia ketone and tagetone

Camphor, caraway, dill, fennel, and jatamansi, etc. are the important drugs in this class.

Camphor

Synonyms

Gum Camphor, Japan Camphor.

Biological source

Camphor is a solid ketone, obtained from the volatile oil of *Cinnamomum camphora*, belonging to family Lauraceae.

Geographical source

It is found widely in Mediterranean region, Sri Lanka, Egypt, South Africa, China, India, and California. It is successfully cultivated at Dehradun, Saharanpur, Kolkata, Nilgiris, and Mysore.

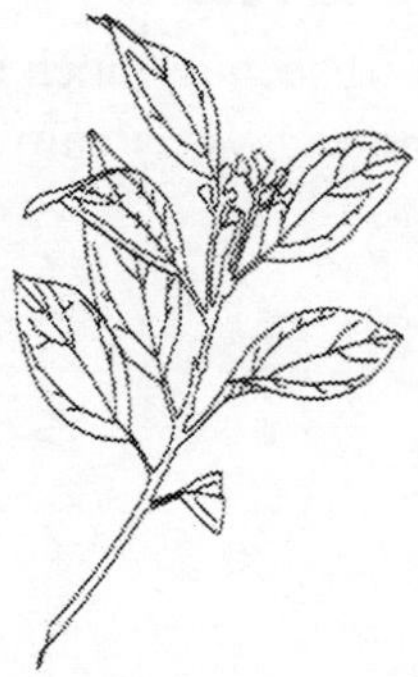

Fig. 4.53 *Cinnamomum camphora*

Chemical Constituents

Camphor oil contains camphor, cineole, pinene, camphene, phellandrene, limonene, and diterpenes. Camphor is entirely a monoterpenic ketone. Its basic carbon framework is related to borneol.

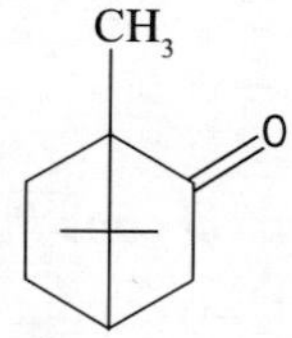

Fig. 4.54 Camphor

Uses

Camphor is used externally as a rubefacient, counterirritant and internally as a stimulant, carminative and antiseptic. It is a topical antipruritic and antiinfective, used as 1–3% in skin medicaments and in cosmetics. It is also used to manufacture some plastics, celluloid, in lacquers, varnishes, explosives, pyrotechnics, as moth repellent, and in embalming fluids.

Marketed products

Ophthacare, Pilex, Rumalaya (Himalaya Drug Company) and Dabur Balm (Dabur)

Volatile Oil Containing Phenol

There are two kinds of phenols found in volatile oils. One present naturally and other produced during destructive distillation of plant products. The examples of naturally found phenols in volatile oils are eugenol, thymol, and carvacrol and on the other hand creosol and guaiacol is the example of volatile oil containing phenol obtained by destrctive distillation from creosote and pine tar. The important drugs containing phenol volatile oils are thyme, clove, myrcia oil, creosote, ajowan, tulsi, pine tar, juniper tar, etc.

Tulsi

Synonyms

Sacred basil, Holy basil.

Biological source

Tulsi consists of fresh and dried leaves of *Ocimum sanctum* belonging to family Labiatae.

Geographical source

It is a herbaceous, much branched annual plant found throughout India. It is propagated by seeds. Tulsi, nowadays, is cultivated commercially for its volatile oils.

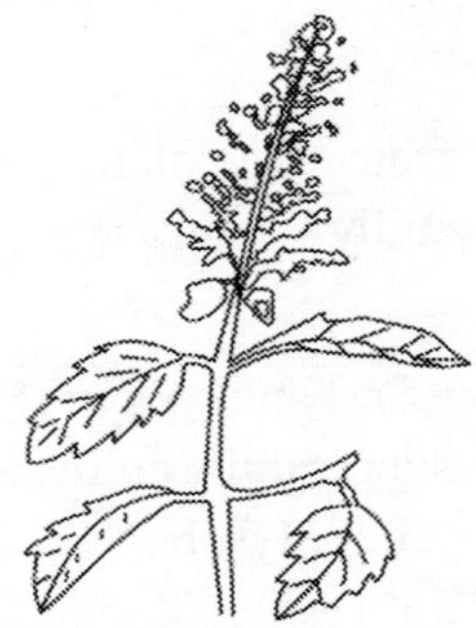

Fig. 4.55 *Ocimum sanctum*

Chemical constituents

Tulsi leaves contain bright, yellow coloured and pleasant volatile oil (0.1 to 0.9%). The oil contains approximately 70% eugenol, carvacrol (3%), and eugenol-methyl-ether (20%). It also contains caryophyllin. Seeds contain fixed oil with good drying properties. The plant is also reported to contain alkaloids, glycosides, saponin, tannins, an appreciable amount of vitamin C and traces of maleic, citric, and tartaric acid.

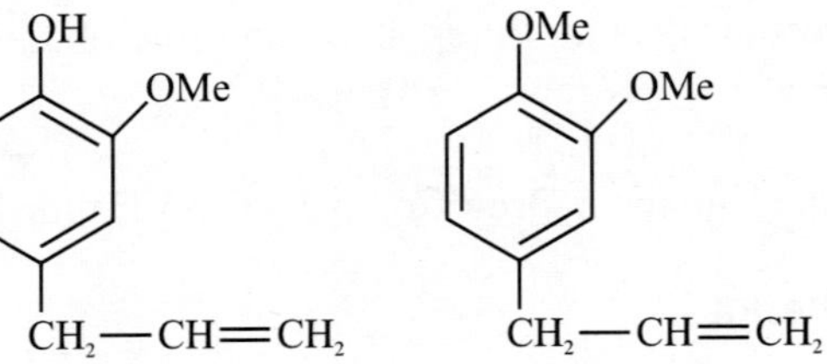

Eugenol Methyleugenol

Fig. 4.56 Strucutre of eugenol, methyleugenol

Uses

The oil is antibacterial and insecticidal. The leaves are used as stimulant, aromatic, spasmolytic, and diaphoretic. The juice is used as an antiperiodic and as a constituent of several preparations for skin diseases and also to cure earache. Infusion of the leaves is used as a stomachic. The drug is a good immunomodulatory agent.

Marketed products

Abana, Diabecon, Diakof, Koflet (Himalaya Drug Company), Respinova (Lupin Herbal Laboratory), Amulcure (Aimil Pharmaceuticals), Nomarks (Nyle Herbals), Sualin (Hamdard), and Kofol syrup (Charak Pharma Pvt. Ltd.).

Volatile Oil Containing Ether

A number of phenolic ethers occur in volatile oils, for example, anethole from anise and fennel, safrole from sassafras and nutmeg. Derivatives of safrole are also often found in volatile oils; for example, myristicin (methoxysafrole) in nutmeg.

Nutmeg

Synonyms

Semen myristicae, Myristica, Nux moschata, *Myristica aromata.*

Biological source

Nutmeg is the kernel of the dried ripe seed of *Myristica fragrans* belonging to family Myristicaceae.

Geographical source:

A native of Molucca islands in Indonesia. It is also cultivated in West Indies, Banda Islands, Archipelago, Malayan, Sumatra, and in Guiana.

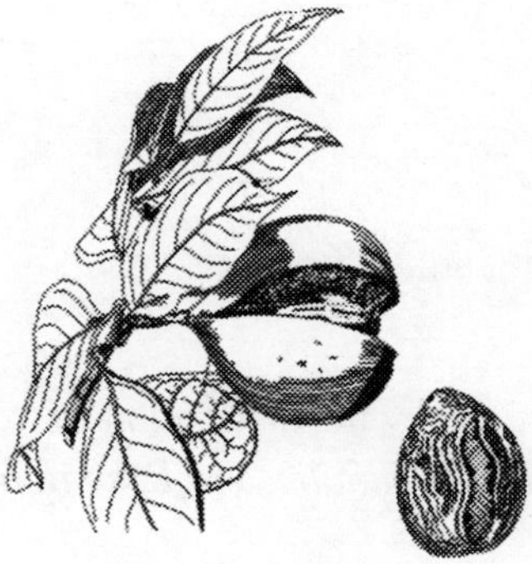

Fig. 4.57 *Myristica fragrans*

Chemical constituents

Nutmeg contains of 5 to 15% volatile oil, lignin, stearin, starch, gum, colouring matter, and 0.08% of an acid substance. The volatile oil contains clemicine, myristicin, geraniol, borneol, pinene, camphene, and dipentene. It also contains eugenol, safrol, p-cymene and isoeugenol in small quantity.

Myristica fragrans

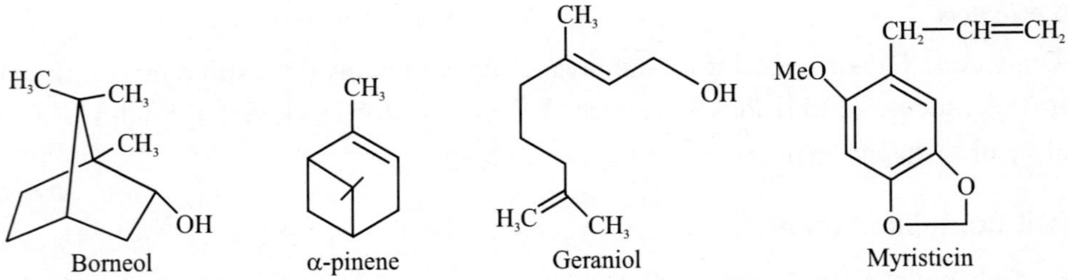

Fig. 4.58 Strucutre of borneol, myristicin

Uses

Nutmeg is aromatic, carminative, flavouring agent. Both nutmeg and mace are used for flatulence, in allay nausea and vomiting. It has narcotic action and peripherally it irritates and produces anesthetics action, since it irritates intestine and uterus it can cause abortion. Oil of nutmeg is used as a local stimulant to GIT.

Marketed products

Diakof, Geriforte, Mentat, Lukol (Himalaya Drug Company), and Kumaryasava (Dabur)

Volatile Oil Containing Oxides

Cineole (eucalyptol) is found in eucalyptus, cajuput, and other volatile oil-yielding drugs. The presence of limonene-l,2-epoxide, pinene oxides, ascaridole (chenopodium oil), and ascaridole epoxide is also reported.

Eucalyptus Oil

Synonyms

Eucalyptus, Stringy Bark Tree, Blue Gum, Blue Gum Tree.

Biological source

Eucalyptus oil is the essential oil obtained by the distillation of fresh leaves of *Eucalyptus globulus* and other species like *E. polybractea, E. viminalis*, and *E. smithii*, belonging to family Myrtaceae.

Geographical source

It is mainly found in Australia, Tasmania, United States, Spain, Portugal, Brazil, North and South Africa, India, France, and Southern Europe.

Chemical constituents

Eucalyptus oil contains volatile oil of which 70 to 85% is 1,8-cineole, also known as eucalyptol. The other constituents present are p-cymene, α-pinene; small quantity of sesquiterpenes like ledol, aromadendrene; aldehydes, ketones, and alcohols. It also has polyphenolic acids like ferulic acid, caffeic acid, gallic acid; flavonoids such as eucalyptin, hyperoside and rutin.

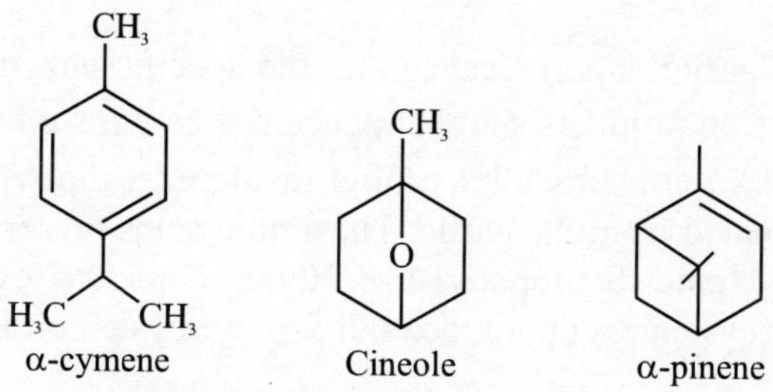

Fig. 4.59 Strucutre of cymene, pinene

Uses

The oil is used as stimulant, antiseptic, flavouring agent, aromatic, deodorant, expectorant, antimicrobial, febrifuge, diuretic, and antispasmodic. It is also used in the treatment of lung diseases, sore throat, cold, as a vapour bath for asthma and various respiratory ailments and in bronchitis.

Marketed products

Cold Balm, Muscle and Joint Rub, Canisep, Erina-EP, Scavon Vet. (Himalaya Drug Company).

Volatile Oil Containing Ester

The most common esters are of terpineol, borneol and geraniol. The perfumes are aged to undergo esterification, thus improving bouquet. Allyl isothiocyanate in mustard oil and methyl salicylate in wintergreen oil are also esters.

The drugs are lavender oil, dwarf pine needle oil, mustard oil and gaultheria oil, garlic, valerian, and rosemary oil.

Garlic

Synonyms

Allium, Lasan (Hindi)

Biological source

Garlic is the ripe bulb of *Allium sativum*, belonging to family Liliaceae.

Geographical source

Garlic occurs in central Asia, Southern Europe, and United States. It is widely cultivated in India.

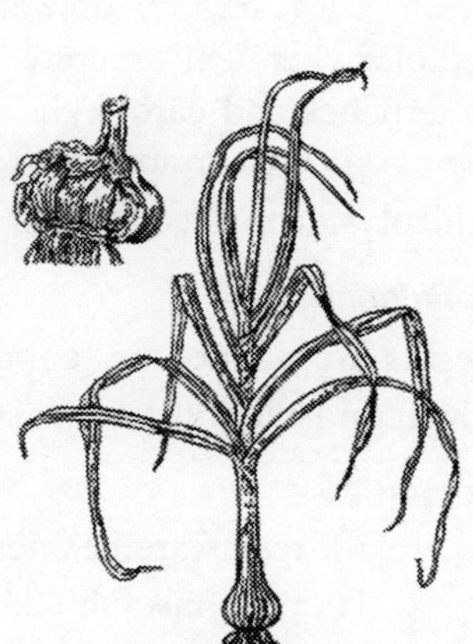

Fig. 4.60 *Allium sativum*

Chemical constituents

Allicin, a yellow liquid responsible for the odour of garlic, is the active principle of the drug. The other constituents reported in garlic are alliin, volatile and fatty oils, mucilage and albumin. Alliin, is the another active principle of garlic. Upon cleavage by the specific enzyme alliinase, an odour of garlic develops, and the fission products show antibacterial action similar to allicin.

Essential oil (0.06–0.1%) contains allyl propyl disulphide, diallyl disulphide, and allicin. γ-Glutamyl peptides are isolated from the garlic. The amino acids present in the bulb are leucine, methionine, S-propyl-L-cysteine, S-propenyl-L-cysteine, S-methyl cysteine, S-allyl cysteine sulphoxide (alliin), S-ethyl cysteine sulphoxide, and S-butyl-cysteine sulphoxide.

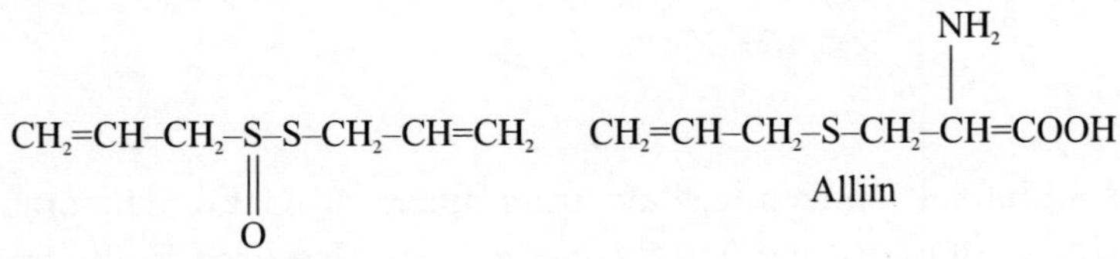

Allicin Alliin

Fig. 4.61 Strucutre of allicin

Uses

Garlic is carminative, aphrodisiac, expectorant, stimulant, and used in fevers, coughs, febrifuge in intermittent fevers, respiratory diseases such as chronic bronchitis, bronchial asthma, whooping cough, and tuberculosis. It is also used in atherosclerosis and hypertension.
Garlic or its constituents exhibit various biological activities, such as antibacterial, antifungal, antiviral, antitumor, and antidiabetic effects.

Marketed products

Lasuna (Himalaya Drug Company) and Lashunadi Bati (Baidyanath).

4.2.6 Resins

Resin is a catergory of water insoluble, crosslinked polymer group by which it may form a complex chemical structure. These are amorphous mixtures of essential oils, oxygenated products of terpenes and carboxylic acids. Resins and resinous products are produced in plants during normal growth or any physical injury to the plants. Usually, resins are found in schizogenous or schizolysigenous cavities or ducts of higher plants.

Definition

Resins are defined as 'complex water insoluble amorphous product with solid characteristics which on heating first sets softened and then melt and burn with sooty flme'.

Properties

1. All resins are heavier than water; they are usually amorphous, hard, and brittle solids.
2. They are insoluble in water and usually insoluble in petroleum ether but dissolve more or less completely in alcohol, chloroform and ether.
3. Chemically, resins are complex mixtures of resin acids, resin alcohols (resinols), resin phenols (resinotannols), esters and chemically inert compounds known as resenes.
4. Many resins, when boiled with alkalis yield soap.
5. By the action of heat they soften yielding clear, adhesive fluids. Resins burn with a characteristic, smoky flame.

6. Resins are often associated with volatile oils (oleoresins), with gums (gumresins) or with oil and gum (oleo-gumresins).
7. Resins may also be combined in a glycosidal manner with sugars.
8. Chemically, resins are not pure substances but complex mixtures of several resinous substances as resin acids, resin alcohols, resin esters, and neutral resins.
9. Resins are non-nitrogenous compounds.

Classification

Resins are classified mostly on the basis of two important features, that is,

(i) Chemical nature or chemical classification.

(ii) Association with the other group of compounds like essential oils and gums or resin combinations.

(i) Chemical classification of resins categorizes according to active functional groups.

- **(a) Resin acids:** Resin acids are the carboxylic acid group containing resinous substances which may or may not have association with phenolic compounds. These compounds are found as the esters derivatives in free state.

  Resin acids are soluble in aqueous solution of alkalies producing frothy solution. It can be derivatized as resonates (metallic salts) and used in soap, paints and varnishes. Colophony and myrrh are the examples of resin acids containing abietic acid and commiphoric acid.

- **(b) Resin esters:** Esterification of resin acids or the other aromatic acids like benzoic, cinnamic, salicylic acids, etc., contributeresin esters. With the influence of caustic alkali, they canbe converted into free acids. The common examples of resin esters are dragon's blood and benzoin.

- **(c) Resin alcohols:** Resin alcohols or resinols are the complex alcoholic compounds of high molecular weight. Like resin acids they are found as free alcohols or as esters of benzoic, salicylic, and cinnamic acids. They are insoluble in aqueous alkali solution but are soluble in alcohol and ether. Resinols are present in benzoin as benzoresinol and in storax as storesinol.

- **(d) Resin phenols:** As like resin alcohol, resin phenols or resinotannols are also havehigh molecular weight, occur in the form of free esters and form phenoxoids (due to presence of phenolic group). It soluble in aqueous alkali solution but basically insoluble in water. Moreover, it can dissolve in alcohol and ether also.

  The sources of resinotannol are balsam of Peru, Tolu balsam and benzoin, etc. It gives a positive reaction with ferric chloride solution.

- **(e) Glycoresins:** Glycoresins are produced by glycosylation of resins combined with sugars. Glycoresins can be hydrolysed by acidic hydrolysis to form glycone and aglycone part. Examples are jalap, resin of Ipomoea.

- **(f) Resenes:** Resenes are a kind of resins which are chemically inert and generally found in free state. They never combine with ester or any other derivatives. Solubility wise resenes are soluble in benzene, chloroform and to some extent in petroleum ether and are completely insoluble in water.

Asafoetida is an example of resene containing drug, which contains drug about 50% of asaresene B.

(ii) Association with the other group of compounds like essential oils and gums or resin combinations.

(a) **Oleoresins:** The homogeneous mixture of resin with volatile oils is called oleoresins. The aromatic essence of oleoresins is due to the presence of volatile oils. An example of oleoresins includes turpentine, ginger, Canada resin, etc.

(b) **Gum resins:** Naturally occurring homogenized mixture of resins with gums are known as gum resins. The separation of gums from oleoresin mixture is somewhat easy because of its high solubility in water. Example of natural gum resin is ammoniacum.

(c) **Oleogum resins:** Oleogum resins are the natural combination of resin, volatile oil, and gum which occurs naturally. Such oleogum resins generally ooz out from the plants due to physical injury, i.e., incisions in the bark and hardens. The examples of such combinations include gum myrrh, asafoetida, gamboage, etc.

(d) **Balsams:** It is a natural resinous mixture containing high proportion of free aromatic balsamic acids, i.e., benzoic acid, cinnamic acid, and their esters. The solubility pattern of such resins also differs from the rest. It is partially soluble in hot water. Few examples of balsams are balsam of Peru, balsam of Tolu, benzoin, and storax. Sometimes few drugs like copaiba and canada are wrongly categorised as balsams which are basically oleogum resins.

Chemical Tests

1. Dissolve the powdered drug in 2-3 mL of acetic anhydride in a test tube and add a drop of con.sulphuric acid.A violet colour is produced which confirms resin colophony.
2. Colophony is dissolved in light petroleum and filtered. To the filtrate 2-3 times its volume, dilute copper acetate solution is added. Emerald green colour is seen in the petroleum layer (upper layer) which identifies the resin colophony.
3. Heat small amount of benzoin slowly in a dry test tube–melts and evolves white fumes on condensation and forms crystalline sublimate.
4. Benzoin heated with potassium permanganate solution–odour of benzaldehyde evolves (Sumatra benzoin).
5. Benzoin is extracted with alcohol and to the extract added with water–milky white solution forms.
6. Digest benzoin with few drops of petroleum ether for 5 minutes. Pour 1 mL of the etherial solution in a porcelain dish containing 2-3 drops of con. sulphuric acid and rotate the dish–reddish brown colour produced (benzoin).
7. Combined umbelliferone test.
8. Drug is boiled with hydrochloric acid for 5 minutes. It is filtered and ammonia is added to the filtrate. A blue fluorescence is produced (asafoetida).
9. Drug is treated with a few drops of 50% nitric acid. Green colour is produced.
10. Drug is treated with a few drops of sulphuric acid. Red colour is produced which changes to violet on washing with water (asafoetida).

Drugs Containing Resins

Asafoetida

Synonyms

Devil's dung; Food of the gods, Asafoda, asant, Hing

Biological source

Asafoetida is an oleo-gum resin obtained as an exudation by incision of the decapitated rhizome and roots of *Ferula asafoetida*, *F. rubricaulis*, and some other species of Ferula, belonging to family Apiaceae.

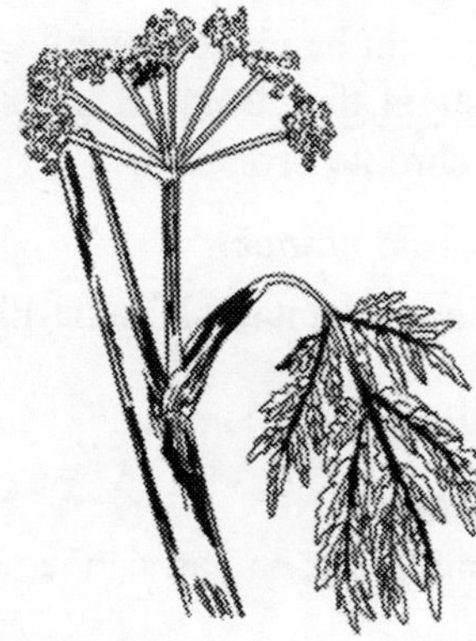

Fig. 4.62 *Ferula asafoetida*

Geographical source

The plant grows in Iran, Turkey and Afghanistan.

Chemical constituents

Asafoetida contains volatile oil (4–20%), resin (40–65%), and gum (25%). The garlic-like odour of the oil is due to the presence of sulphur compounds. The main constituent of the oil is isobutyl propanyl disulphide ($C_6H_{16}S_2$). The flavour is largely due to R-2-butyl-l-propenyl disulphide and 2-butyl-3-methylthioallyl disulphide (both as mixtures of diastereoisomers).The drug also contains a complex mixture of sesquiterpene umbelliferyl ethers mostly with a monocyclic or bicyclic terpenoid moiety. Resin consists of ester of asaresinotannol and ferulic acid, pinene, vanillin and free ferulic acid.

Ferula asafoetida

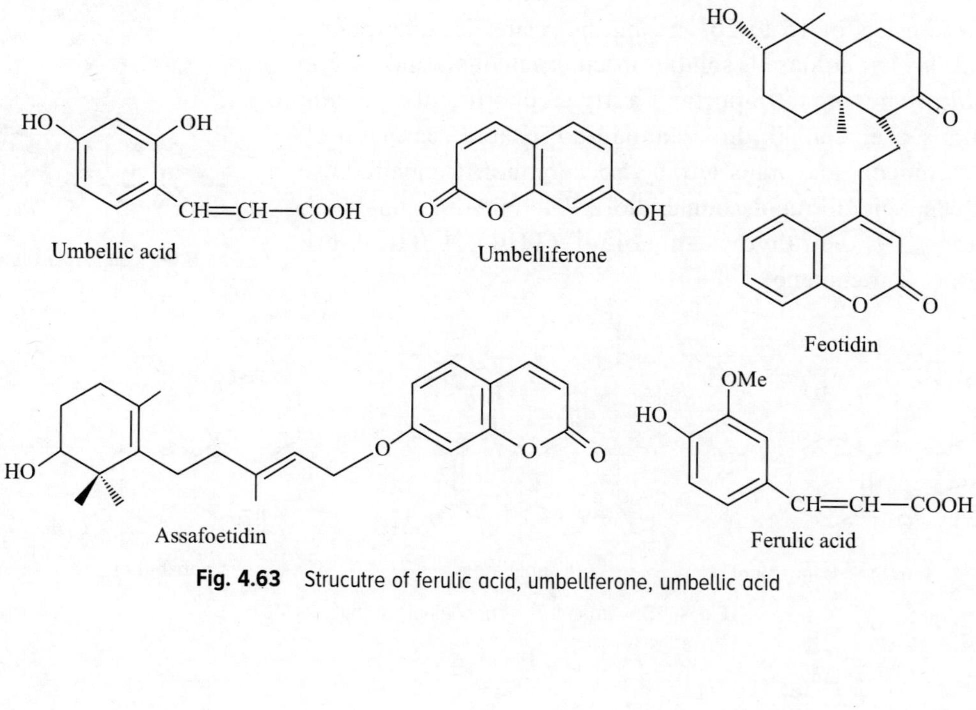

Fig. 4.63 Strucutre of ferulic acid, umbellferone, umbellic acid

Asafoetida also contains phellandrene, geranyl acetate, bornyl acetate, α-terpineol, myristic acid, camphene, myrcene, limonene, fenchone, eugenol, linalool, geraniol, isoborneol, borneol, guaiacol, cadinol, farnesol, assafoetidin, foetidin, etc.

Uses

Asafoetida is used as carminative, expectorant, antispasmodic, and laxative as well as externally to prevent bandage chewing by dogs; for flavouring curries, sauces, and pickles; as an enema for intestinal flatulence, in hysterical and epileptic affections, in cholera, asthma, whooping cough, and chronic bronchitis.

Marketed products

Madhudoshantak (Jamuna Pharma).

Cannabis

Synonyms

Indian hemp, Indian cannabis, hashish, bhang, ganja, charas, *Cannabis indica*, marijuana.

Biological source

Cannabis consists of dried flowering tops of the pistillate plants of *Cannabis sativa*, belonging to family Cannabinaceae.

Geographical source

Cannabis occurs in India, Bangladesh, Pakistan, Iran, Central America, United States, East Africa, South Africa, and Asia Minor.

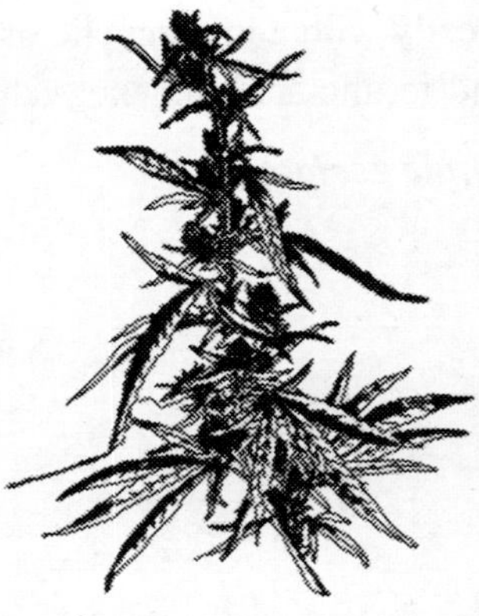

Fig. 4.64 *Cannabis sativa*

Chemical constituents

Cannabis consists of 15 to 20% resin, the resins are amorphous, semisolid, brown coloured, soluble in ether, alcohol, and carbon disulphide. The most important active constituents present in cannabis are: cannabidiol, cannabidolic acid, cannabinol, cannabichromene, and trans-tetrahydrocannbinol. Cannabis also contains cannabidiolic acid, cannabidiol A 9, tetrahydrocannabinol, cannabinol A9, Tetrahydrocannabinol (THC), volatile oil, trigonelline, and cholene.

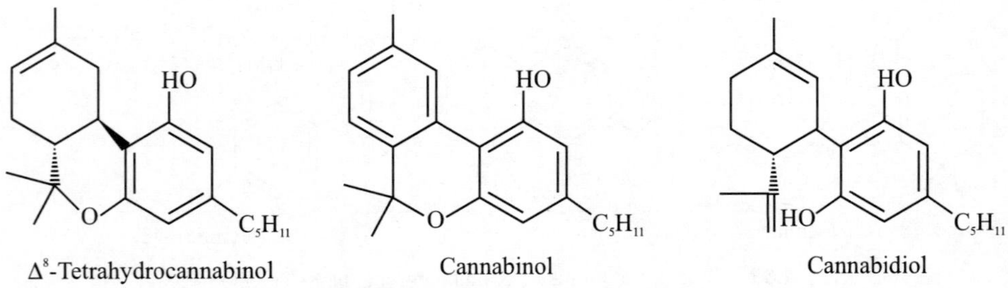

Fig. 4.65 Strucutre of cannabinol, cannabidol

Uses

Cannabis resin is tonic, sedative, analgesic, intoxicant, stomachic, antispasmodic, antianxiety, anticonvulsant, antitussive, and narcotic. Cannabis causes only psycic dependence and acts upon the nervous system.

Marketed Products

Bilwadi Churna (Baidyanath)

EXERCISE

1. Describe the role of pharmacognosy in modern system of medicine.
2. Describe the basic principles of Ayurveda.
3. Explain the key features of diagnosis and treatment of Ayurveda.
4. Briefly explain the fundamental principles of Siddha system of medicine.
5. Classify the drugs used in Siddha system of medicine with their characteristics.
6. Explain briefly the principle and treatment approaches in Unani system of medicine.
7. What is the principle of Yin and Yang theory? Describe in detail the treatment methods in traditional Chinese system of medicine.
8. Describe various laws of Homeopathic treatment based on 'Similia Similibus Curantur'.
9. Define alkaloids. Describe the properties and classification of alkaloids with suitable examples.
10. What is isoquinoline alkaloid? Write the pharmacognosy of any isoquinoline alkaloids containing plant.
11. Define glycosides. Classify them with suitable examples.
12. Write the various chemical tests for identification of glycosides.
13. Describe the pharmacognosy of two drugs containing anthracene and cardiac glycosides.
14. Define flavonoids and classify them with examples.
15. Define tannins, their properties. and classification. Explain Goldbeater's skin test for identification of tannins.
16. Define volatile oils. Classify them with examples.
17. Define resins, their properties, and classification. Write a note on resin combinations.

UNIT V

Plant Fibres, Natural Hallucinogens, Teratogens, Natural Allergens, Primary Metabolites, Oils and Fats & Marine Drugs

Objectives

- To describe the various plants derived fibres and their pharmaceutical utilization.
- To locate the natural source of hallucinogens, teratogens, natural allergens and their effect on human beings.
- To explain the diverse primary metabolites as therapeutic and pharmaceutical agents.
- To understand the chemistry of marine chemicals and their therapeutic effects.

5.1 INTRODUCTION

A number of products made from plants were offered by mother nature. The majority of them are beneficial to humanity, however, certain items made from plants can have some more serious life-threatening side effects. These plants can make people hallucinate, allergic, or teratogenic.

In the production of composite materials, plant fibres are a common option for a variety of industrial applications. Plant fibres including hemp, jute, sisal, kenaf, banana, and ramie are increasingly replacing synthetic fibres in fibre-reinforced composites due to their sustainability. Natural fibres are those that are created by geological, animal, and plant processes. They may be divided into plant fibres, animal fibres, and mineral fibres based on where they came from and are biodegradable over time.

Hallucinogens, which usually originate from plants, have frequently been utilized in ceremonies of faith. The main recognized hallucinogenic plants, with the exception of cannabis, contain alkaloids linked to the neurophysiological transmitters – noradrenaline and 5-hydroxytryptamine (serotonin). Toadstools from the genera Amanita, Psilocybe, and Conocybe are among the toxic fungi that, when consumed orally, can cause hallucinations.

Many proteins have recently been implicated in type 1 allergic responses. Plants, mites, insects, and fungal spores are the principal sources of allergies. Food allergy responses can be brought on by plant-derived allergens that are either ingested through the upper respiratory system or found in a wide variety of plant foods. A person becomes sensitized to an allergen after repeated exposure, which causes an antigen-antibody response that releases histamine or histamine-like substances, which in turn, trigger allergic symptoms. Only a small portion of the tremendous variety of plant proteins that exist have been identified as allergens as of yet. A small number of plant protein families can be related to when looking at the allergen encoding sequences due to sequence similarities. These protein families mostly include of proteins that store seeds, structural proteins, and pathogenesis-related proteins that are engaged in the defence system.

Teratogens typically, but not always, manifest themselves during a brief window of time very early in the gestation cycle. There are 14 main families of plant elements known to have teratogenic effects, in addition to coumarins, lignans, macrolides, nitriles, terpenoids, poisonous amino acids, and other undiscovered chemicals. Most teratogens include nitrogen, much like most hallucinogens do.

Chemicals obtained from aquatic organisms are used in a variety of medical procedures and scientific investigations. Since there are twice as many animal phyla in the sea as on land and a wide variety of microorganisms, the likelihood of discovering novel natural substances suitable for biomedical purposes is significant. Up until now, the majority of medications have been produced from terrestrial creatures. Terpenes, acetogenics, different alkaloids, and polyphenols are among the compounds produced by other species. From usage as antibiotics, painkillers, and anti-inflammatory drugs to sunscreen and anti-cancer compounds, they have either proven or prospective benefit. Several neurotoxins, such as tetradotoxin, block sodium channels in nerve endings and are of great value in biomedical research. Some sponges also produce a substance called Halichondrin B that shows promise in the treatment of ovarian cancer, melanomas, and leukaemia. The futuristic concept of finding new drugs may involve marine pharmaceuticals.

5.2. PLANT PRODUCTS

5.2.1 Natural Fibres

Elongated, very tiny (hair-like) raw materials obtained from natural sources (i.e., animal, vegetable, or mineral) which can be converted into fabrics (felt or paper) or woven cloth after spinning into yarns are generally known as natural fibres.

They are agglomeration of negligible diameter cells against length. Fibres are characteristically cellulosic in nature and abundantly found. Few examples of such fibres includes cotton, wood, grains, straw, etc. where fewer numbers of fibres are being used in fabrics and textile industries.

The length, strength, pliability, elasticity, abrasion resistance, absorbency, and various surface properties of fibres play a detrimental role for its commercial utilization. The fibres used in textile products generally have the better characteristic property such as slender, flexible, and relatively strong. It also possesses greater elasticity either total or partial which retains the original length of fibres.

History of fibres

India has a long history of fibre utilization in terms of spinning of cottons. It dates back to 3000 BCE. The production of silk fibres and silk products was learnt by Chinese and developed the process of sericulture and the methods to spin (dated back 2640 BCE). The flax and wool fabrics might be the oldest reported fibres in the world in 7th and 6th centuries BCE. Presumably, the oldest cultivated fibres plant was hemp, from Southeast Asia and later on spread to China (4500 BCE).

Classification

Natural fibres can be classified according to their origin.

1. **Plant fibres:** These are the cellulose based fibres obtained from plants and vegetables. These fibres are extracted from the plants to make fabrics.

   Cotton: It is one of the plant fibres that is used to make clothes. It is a soft staple fibre that is found as a boll around the seeds in a cotton plant.
2. **Jute:** It is a vegetable fibre that is soft, shiny and is spun into coarse strong threads.
3. **Animal fibres:** These are the protein based fibres obtained from animals. For example: wool, mohair and silk.
4. **Wool:** Wool is a natural textile fibre obtained from sheep, goats and camels. It traps a lot of air. Air is a bad conductor of heat. This makes clothes made from wool useful in winter.
5. **Silk:** It is also a natural textile fibre which is obtained from silkworms. The rearing of silkworm to obtain silk is known as sericulture.
6. **Synthetic fibres:** Synthetic fibres are the manmade polymers designed to make a fabric. Polymers are obtained when many small units are joined together chemically. Some of the examples of synthetic fibres are: nylon, terylene, orlon, viscose, alginate fibres, etc.
7. **Rayon:** It is made from wood pulp. It is also known as artificial silk as it has characteristics resembling silk.
8. **Nylon:** It was the first synthetic fibre. It is used in the making of ropes, sleeping bags, parachutes, different types of clothes, etc. It is one of the strongest fibres known to us.

Another class of fibres obtained from mineral sourcesis known as mineral fibre. Example is asbestos.

The vegetable fibres can be divided into smaller groups, based on their origin within the plant. Cotton, kapok, and coir are examples of fibres originating as hairs borne on the seeds or inner walls of the fruit (trichomes), where each fibre consists of a single, long, narrow cell.

Flax, hemp, jute, and ramie are best fibres, occurring in the inner bast tissue of certain plant stems and made up of overlapping cells.

Abaca, henequen, and sisal are fibres occurring as part of the fibrovascular system of the leaves.

Properties

- Natural fibres chemically consist of cellulose. To some extent it also contains varying amounts of such substances as hemicellulose, lignin, pectins, and waxes.
- The animal fibres consist exclusively of proteins.
- The exception is silk, which constitutes the fur or hair that serves the protective epidermal covering of animals.
- Natural fibres (except mineral fibres) have an affinity towards water both liquid and vapour form, resulting in swelling of the fibres connected with the uptake of water, facilitates dyeing in watery solutions.

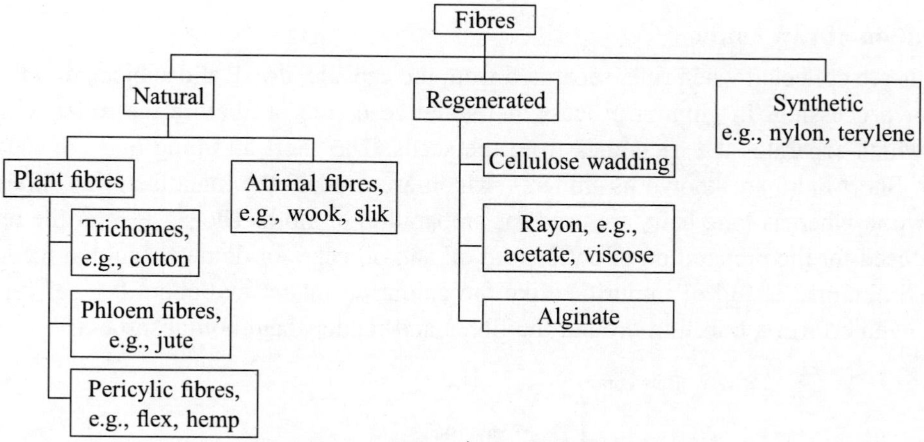

Fig. 5.1 Various classes of fibres

- Natural fibres are non-thermoplastic (unlike synthetic fibres). It does not get soften with applied heat. It does show sensitivity to dry heat but not get shrinkage or high extensibility upon heating. It never becomes brittle when cooled to below freezing temperature.
- At temperatures below a certain point it may decompose.
- Natural fibres tend to yellow upon exposure to sunlight and moisture, and extended exposure results in loss of strength.
- Natural fibres are particularly susceptible to microbial decomposition, including mildew and rot. Cellulosic fibres are decomposed by aerobic bacteria and fungi.
- Wool and silk are subject to microbial decomposition by bacteria and moulds.

5.2.2 Natural Fibres Containing Drugs

Cotton

Synonyms

Raw cotton, Purified cotton, Absorbent cotton, Raw cotton wool.

Biological Source

The natural cotton consists of epidermal trichomes of the seeds of cultivated species of the *Gossypium herbaceum* and other species of *Gossypium* (*G. hirsutum, G. barbadense*) free from impurities, fats and sterilized. It belongs to family Malvaceae.

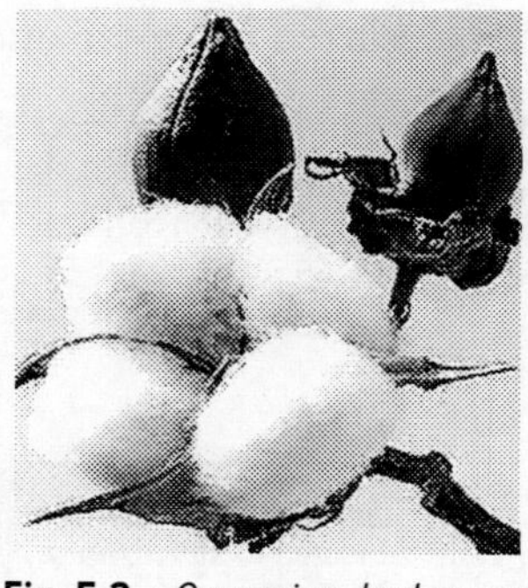

Fig. 5.2 *Gossypium herbaceum*

Geographical distribution

Commercial production of *Gossypium* species are in the United States of America, West Indies, Peru, Brazil, India, China and Egypt. Cotton plants are also now cultivated in Nigeria and Bangladesh.

Preparation of raw cotton

The bolls are collected when ripe, separated from the capsule, dried, and subjected to the ginning press for processing. In ginning process, hairs and seeds are put before the roller with a small space, which separates the trichomes from the seeds. The short and long hair are separated by delinter. Short hairs are known as 'linters', which are used in the manufacturing inferior grade cotton wool, whereas long hairs are used for preparation of cloth. The seeds after the removal of hair are used for the preparation of cottonseed oil and oil cake for domestic animal feed. The raw cotton so obtained is full of impurities like the colouring matter and about 0.6 per cent of wax and oil, which form a thin film around the fibres and render them non-absorbent.

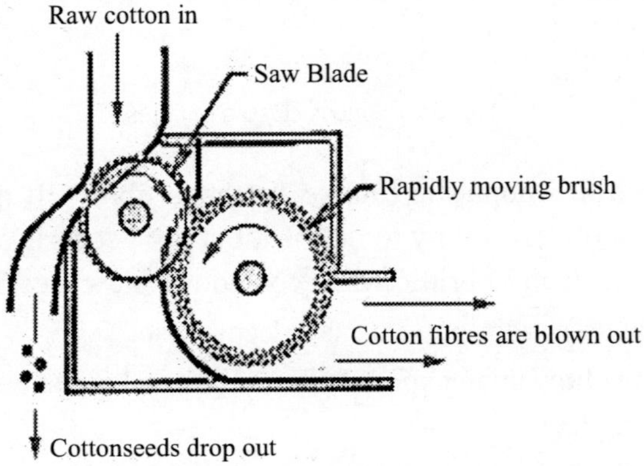

Fig. 5.3 Ginning press

It is then subjected to further purification by treating it with dilute soda ash solution under pressure for about 15 hours. It is then bleached and washed properly, dried, and packed. Spinned to convert it to yarn or thread, which are woven to make fabrics and cloth. The packed cotton is then sterilized using radiations.

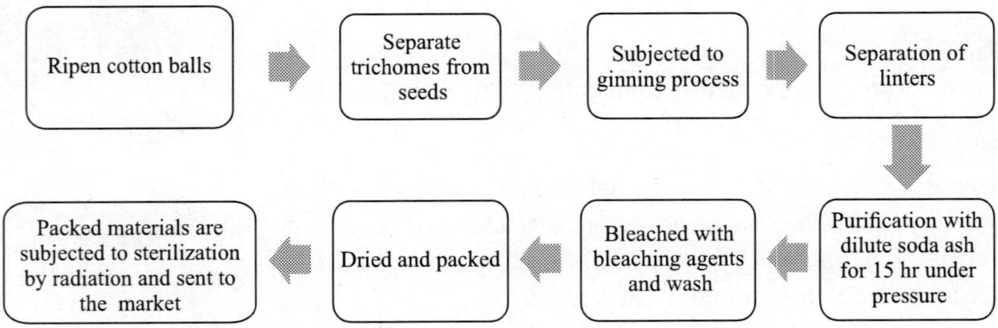

Fig. 5.4 Flow process of surgical cotton preparation

Preparation of Absorbent Cotton Wool

Absorbent cotton wool is prepared from the various cotton wastes obtained during the processing of raw cotton for making yarns. The wastes are loosened and then boiled for 10 to 15 hours under a pressure of about 30 lb in a dilute solution of caustic soda and soda ash. This treatment removes the fatty cuticle and renders the trichomes absorbent. The boiled material is then washed thoroughly with water, bleached with dilute sodium hypochlorite solution and treated with very dilute hydrochloric acid. The bleached mass of fibres is then dried, loosened, scutched, and carded by using appropriate machines. The resultant product is a thin continuous film of absorbent cotton wool. Several such films are superimposed on one another and rolled.

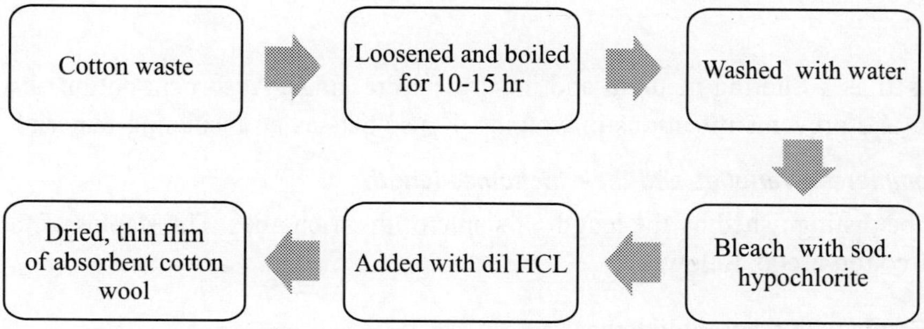

Fig. 5.5 Flow process for absorbent cotton wool

Chemical constituents

It consists of cellulose (90%), moisture (7-8%), wax, fat and oil (0.5%) and cell content about (0.5%). Purified cotton (absorbent cotton) has almost pure cellulose and 6-7% of moisture.

Chemical tests

1. On ignition, cotton burns with a flame, gives very little odour or fumes, does not produce a bead, and leaves a small white ash; distinction from acetate rayon, alginate yarn, wool, silk, and nylon.
2. Dried cotton is moistened with N/50 iodine and sulphuric acid (80% w/w) is added. A blue colour is produced; distinction from acetate rayon, alginate yarn, jute, hemp, wool, silk, and nylon.
3. With ammoniacal copper oxide solution, raw cotton dissolves with ballooning, leaving a few fragments of cuticle. Absorbent cotton dissolves completely with uniform swelling, distinction from acetate rayon, jute, wool, and nylon.
4. In cold sulphuric acid (80% w/w) cotton dissolves; distinction from oxidized cellulose, jute, hemp, and wool.
5. In cold sulphuric acid (60% w/w) cotton, is insoluble; distinction from cellulose wadding and rayons.
6. In warm (40°C) hydrochloric acid it is insoluble; distinction from acetate rayon (also silk, nylon).
7. It is insoluble in 5% potassium hydroxide solution; distinction from oxidized cellulose, wool, and silk.
8. Treat it with cold Shirla stain A for 1 min and wash out. It shows shades of blue, lilac or purple; distinction from viscose, acetate rayons, alginate yarn, wool, silk, and nylon.

9. Treat it with cold Shirla stain C for 5 min and wash out; raw cotton gives a mauve to reddish-brown colour and absorbent cotton a pink one; distinction from flax, jute, hemp. The Shirla stains may be usefully applied to a small piece of the whole fabric under investigation to indicate the distribution of more than one type of yarn.
10. It does not give red stain with phloroglucinol and hydrochloric acid; distinction from jute, hemp, and kapok.

Uses

Cotton is used as a filtering medium and in surgical dressings. Absorbent cotton absorbs blood, pus, mucus, and prevents infections in wounds. It also acts as an insulating material.

Different commercial varieties and their trichomes length

Cotton can be distinguished by the length of staple of the trichomes. The staples of the important varieties of cotton are as follows:

Table 5.1 Cotton with different lengths (size)

Cotton verities	Length of staple of the trichomes
Sea Island	Up to 54.5 mm
Egyptian	31 to 38 mm
Peruvian and Brazilian	29 to 30 mm
Indian	21.4 to 29.2 mm

Silk

Biological Source

Fibres obtained from the cocoons spun by the larvae *Bombyx mori*, belonging to family Bombycidae/Moraceae.

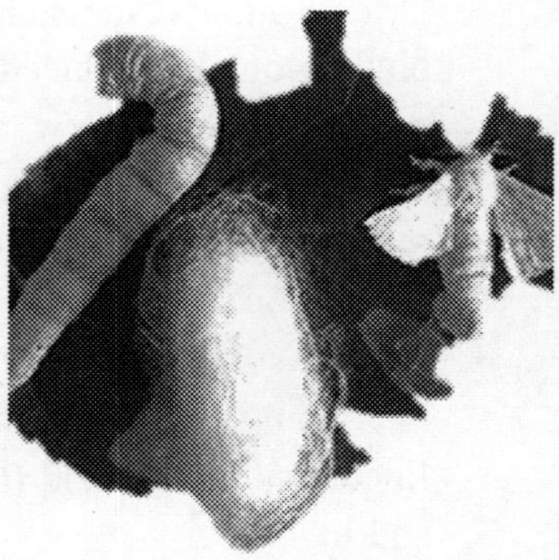

Fig. 5.6 *Bombyx mori*

Geographical Source

The commercial cultivation of silk mostly is done in various countries like China, France, Iran, Italy, Japan, and India.

Preparation

One gramme of silk-worm egg consists of around 15,000 eggs which are kept at 0°C to overcome the immature development. The silkworms eat mulberry leaves day and night and they grow very fast. When the colour of their heads changes darker, it indicates that the time for them to moult has come. It requires almost a month for its development into full size. During this period it takes four moulds and their body turns slightly yellow reaching a size of 4 cm long. The silkworm finally eats a meal which is about twenty to twenty-five times its weight of leaves and attains a size of 9 cm length and 10 mm thick. The skin becomes tight and all these symptoms indicate that it is going to cover itself with a silky cocoon. The process of spinning cocoon continues for almost three days. After 7–8 days, the larvae changes into chrysalides, and the cocoons are collected by throwing them into boiling water, this kills the silkworms and also makes the cocoons easier to unravel. If the caterpillar is left to eat its way out of the cocoon naturally, the threads will be cut short and the silk will be useless. The cocoons are kept in warm water to remove the gum. Since all the eggs hatch almost the same time, the cocoons are collected together and treated at the same period. Some amount of cocoons are retained and allowed to come out for fertilization. The females lay nearly 500 eggs and these eggs are stored till further requirement.

Description

The silk is a fine solid, smooth to touch and yellow in colour. The size of silk fibres is 5-25 micron in diameter and 1200 metres in length. It is soluble in cuoxam and cold dilute sulphuric acid. Silks have good elasticity and tensile strength and are hygroscopic in nature.

Chemical constituents

Silk mainly consists of protein known as fibrion. Fibrion is soluble in warm water and on hydrolysis yields two main amino acids, glycine and alanine.

Uses

Silk is used pharmaceutically in the preparation of sutures, sieves, and ligatures.

The 'stiff silkworm' (dried body in the four to fifth stage of larva, which dies due to infection of the fungus *Beauveria bassiana*) is used in the traditional Chinese medicine.

Chemical Test

1. Silk does not show any reaction with lead acetate solution.
2. Silk is insoluble in water and alcohol but soluble on cuoxam solution (66% H_2SO_4, conc. HCl)

Jute

Synonym

Gunny

Biological source

It consists of phloem fibres from the stem of *Corchorus capsularis*, *C. olitorius*, and other species of *Corchorus*, belonging to family Tiliaceae.

Geographical source

West Bengal and Assam

Preparation

Retting is the process for the preparation of bast fibres. This process is done by three methods, that is, microbial (or water), steam, and mechanical process. The microbial or water retting process is the oldest and the most popular method employed for the breaking of lignin bond present between parenchyma and sclerenchyma. The breaking of this bond facilitates the easy procurement of skin from its core. Then the material is washed, dried to release pectin bond which makes the hard skin to fine thread-like fibres. The jute fibres are graded according to its colour, strength and fibre length. The fibres are of white to brown and 1-4 m. long.

Chemical constituents

Jute is composed of cellulose (50-53%), hemicellulose (20%) and lignin (10-11%) along with other constituents like moisture not more than 12-13%, fats, wax, and ash contributing to 1% each.

Uses

Jute is used chiefly to make cloth for wrapping bales of raw cotton, in the preparation of sacks and coarse cloth. They are also woven into curtains, chair coverings, carpets, Hessian cloth very fine threads of jute can be made into imitation silk and also in the making of paper. It is even used in the manufacture of tows, padding splints, filtering, and straining medium. Jute is used for the preparation of coarse bags.

Chemical Test

1. Fibre with phloroglucinol and concentrated hydrochloric acid produce deep red colour.
2. Fibes with chlorzimc iodide produces yellow stain.

Hemp

Biological source

Hemp is the pericyclic fibre obtained from *Cannabis sativa*, belonging to family Cannabinaceae.

Geographical source

Hemp is grown at any altitude from Norway to the Equator. The raw materials are imported from China, Hungary, America, Germany, Switzerland, Australia, Canada, France, and Norway.

Chemical constituents

Hemp mainly consists of cellulose and lignin.

Uses

Hemp is used in printing inks, paints, varnishes, paper, bank notes, food, textiles and building materials. Due to its high tensile strength, bast fibres are ideal for such specialized paper products as: tea bags, industrial filters, currency paper, cigarette paper, etc.

5.2.3 Natural Hallucinogens

A hallucinogen is a psychoactive substance that works on the brain to affect the senses that powerfully alters perception, mood, and other cognitive processes in brain, generally known as hallucinations. While under the influence of hallucinogens, users might see images, hear sounds or feel sensations that seem to be real but aren't.

Despite the name, they do not necessarily produce true hallucinations. Instead, many hallucinogenic drugs cause users to have experiences that are different from their ordinary reality, but may not involve fullscale hallucinations. Sometimes these drugs are called psychedelics because the conscious mind becomes aware of things that it normally is not aware of. Sometimes they are called entheogens because hallucinogens may provoke intense emotional responses that may be akin to spiritual or religious experiences.

Some natural hallucinogens are plants or fungi that grow naturally in different parts of the world.

Table 5.2 The most common hallucinogenes (with their active ingredients)

Natural source	Chemicals
Peyote cactus	Mescaline, phenethylamine
Magic mushrooms	Psilocybin or psilocin
DMT	N,N-dimethyltryptamine
Salvia divinorum	Salvinorum A
Ayahuasca	Harmaline, N, N-dimethyltryptamine
Cannabis	Tetrahydrocannabinol or THC

Most hallucinogens are alkaloids, a family of perhaps 5000 complex organic molecules that also account for the biological activity of most toxic and medicinal plants. These active compounds may be found in various concentrations in different parts of the plant—root, leaves, seeds, bark and/or flowers—and they may be absorbed by the human body in a number of ways, as is evident in the wide variety of folk preparations. Hallucinogens may be smoked or snuffed, swallowed fresh or dried, drunk in decoctions and infusions, absorbed directly through the skin, placed in wounds or administered as aenemas. To date about 120 hallucinogenic plants have been identified worldwide.

Classification

Hallucinogenic compounds may be divided conveniently into two broad groups: those that contain nitrogen in their structure and those that do not. Those with nitrogen are far more common. The most important of those lacking nitrogen are the active principles of marijuana, terpenophenolic compounds classed as dibenzopyrans and called cannabinols, in particular, tetrahydrocannabinols. The hallucinogenic compounds with nitrogen in their structure are alkaloids or related bases.

Almost all hallucinogens contain nitrogen and are classified as alkaloids. Many hallucinogens have chemical structures similar to those of natural neurotransmitters (acetylcholine-, serotonin-, or catecholamine). They are categorized in distinct categories.

Mechanism of hallucinogens

The hallucinogens are chemically similar to substances (neurotransmitters) that naturally occur in the brain (psilocybin and LSD are similar to serotonin, mescaline is similar to dopamine). The most common brain chemicals are serotonin and acetylcholine, which are responsible for behaviour,

Table 5.3 Categories of hallucinogens

Category 1: Serotonin- like	Category 2: Catecholamine-like	Category 3: Anticholinergic	Category 4: Dissociative Anaesthetics
Structurally resemble 5-HT • Examples include- – LSD (lysergic acid diethylamide) – Psilocybin – DMT (dimethyltryptamine-ayahuasca) etc	Structurally resemble 5-HT, But act on NE, DA, with amphetamine- type effects • Examples include: – Mescaline – DOM (dimethoxy–methamphetamine) – Myristin, elemicin (in nutmeg and mace)	Block muscarinic receptors. • Atropine and Scopolamine works peripherally, causes paralysis and In CNS, respectively, responsible for hallucinatons, delirium, amnesia • Examples: – Belladonna – Jimsonweed	Non-competitiveN- methyl –D -aspartate (NMDA) receptor antagonists. • Binding to PCP site on NMDA receptors blocks calcium channels- Stimulate the release of DA • Example- Ketamine interacts with the opioid receptor.

perception and the body's regulatory systems (mood, hunger, body temperature, sexual behaviour, muscle control). When hallucinogens enter the blood stream, their active ingredients bind to receptors in the brain. As a result, functions of the brain are suppressed, stimulated or otherwise changed, which results in unusual sensory perceptions. The effects of hallucinogens usually begin within an hour of taking a drug, and they can last for 12 hours or more. Hallucinogens are rapidly absorbed in the gastrointestinal tract, through the mucous membranes.

It can be injected directly into the veins. Some can even be inhaled. In low doses, hallucinogens alter a person's mood and change the way they experience the world. In high doses, hallucinogens can significantly affect a person's perception of reality including alternating perceptions of time and space.

5.2.3.1 Sources of Natural Hallucinogen

Amanita Muscaria

Synonyms

Fly agaric mushroom

Biological source

It is a poisonous mushroom with a characteristic red or orange cup, often covered with white flecks of *Amanita muscaria*, belongs to the family Amanitaceae.

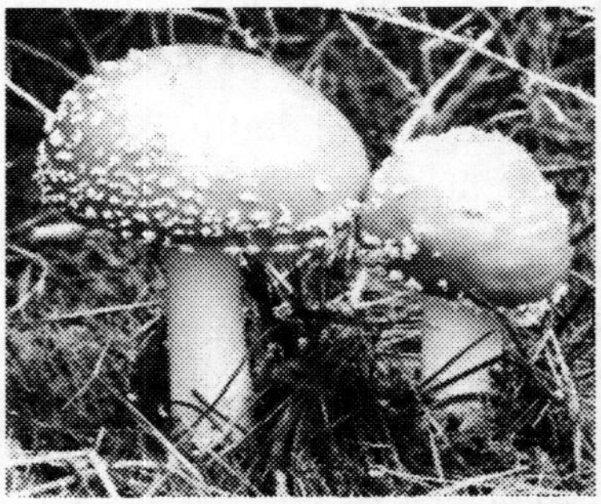

Fig. 5.7 *Amanita muscaria*

Geographical source

It is abundantly found in various parts of northeastern and western Siberia.

Chemical constituents

The main pharmacologically active principle is muscimole (decarboxylation product of ibotenic acid). Other compounds, such as muscazone, are found in lesser concentrations and may contribute to the intoxication. Ibotenic acid (α-amino-3-hydroxy-5-isoazoloacetic acid) as well as muscazone can be regarded as amino acids, while ibotenic acid and muscimole are oxazol derivatives.

Another biomolecule isozasol derivatives (Ibotenic acid and muscimol) present are similar to those of glutamic acid and GABA (γ-aminobutyric acid), products of their enzymatic decarboxylation.

Bioactivity

A larger dose gives more pronounced symptoms of poisoning with spasm and more vivid hallucination. Aggressive attitudes have not been reported. As a result of the poisoning, dryness in the mouth and mydriasis (dilation of the pupils) can occur followed by a period of drowsiness, then a deep sleep with vivid dreams, usually 2 hr after. After the deep sleep, this generally lasts 8 hr, the poisoning ends.

Behavioural changes, like ataxia and sedation, induced by muscimol (agonist of GABAA receptor and partially GABAc receptor) depend on highaffinity binding of this compound to a distinct subtype of GABAA receptor in the cerebral cortex.Moreover, mucimol inhibits GABA uptake by neurons and astrocytes and is a substrate to GABA transaminase.

Myristica Fragrans

Synonym

Myristicae semen

Biological source

Nutmeg is the kernel of the dried, ripe seed of *Myristica fragrans*, belonging to family Myristicaceae.

Geographical source

It is cultivated in Indonesia, Malaysia, Sri Lanka, and the West Indies.

Chemical constituents

Nutmeg contains fats (30 to 40%) and essential oils (10%), which is mostly composed of terpenes (α-pinene, camphene, *p*-cymene, sabinene, β-phellandrene, γ-terpinene, myrcene), terpene derivatives (linalool, geraniol, terpineol), and phenylopropanes (myristicin, elmicin, safrole). Mace oil has a similar composition, but it contains higher levels of terpenes. Both nutmeg and mace are the two major primary products of *M. fragrans* that are commercially used as spices.

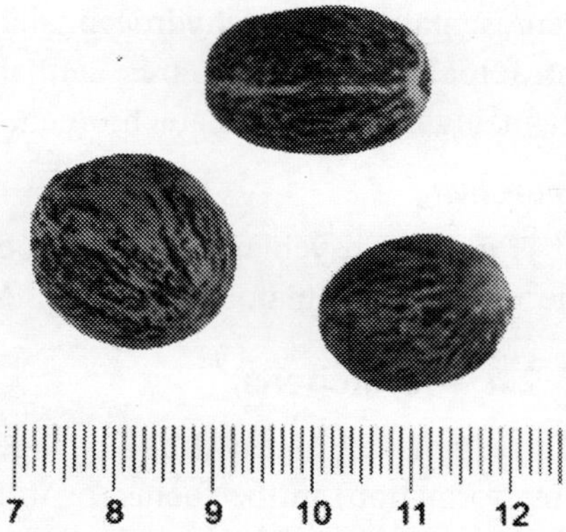

Fig. 5.8 *Myristica fragrans*

Bioactivity

Various extracts and essential oils of nutmeg seeds have been reported with antimicrobial activities against Gram-positive and Gram-negative bacteria, as well as a variety of fungi. Trimyristin and myristic acid are the chief antibacterial principles isolated from *M. fragrans*. It has been reported that myristicin, present in the volatile oil of *M. fragrans*, is a potential chemopreventive agent andsuppressesthe growth of human lymphoid leukemic cells (Molt 4B). Moreover, the dihydroguaiaretic acid from *M. fragrans* mace suppressed the viability of several cancer cell lines, leukemic, colon, and lungs.

Cannabis

Synonyms

Indian hemp, C. sativa herba.

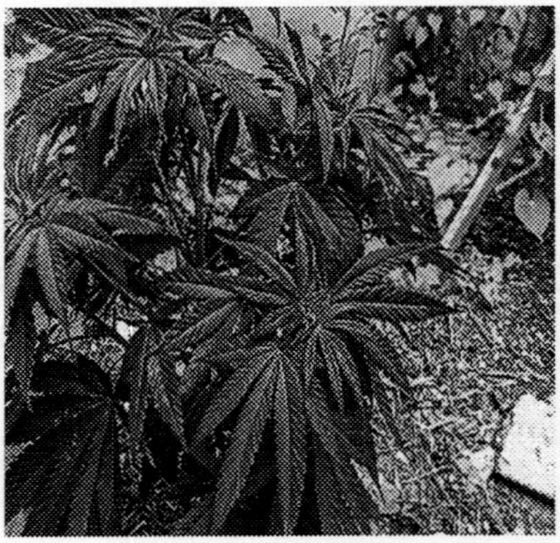

Fig. 5.9 *Cannabis sativa*

Biological source

Cannabis consists of the dried, aerial parts of *Cannabis sativa*, belonging to family Cannabidaceae.

Geographical source

The plant occurs naturally in India, Bangladesh, and Pakistan and is grown in numerous countries with tropical climates suitable for fibre and seed production.

Chemical constituents

Cannabinoids are a group of C21 compounds occurring in resin produced by glandular hairs of C. *sativa*. Among the over 420 known constituents of cannabis, more than 60 belong to cannabinoids, which chemically belong to the terpenophenols. Cannabinoids or phytocannabinoids are accumulated in the glandular hairs, which account for more than 80% of the subcuticular secretion. Generally, they are present in all plant parts, except the seeds.The most important representative is tetrahydrocannabinol (THC), which has hallucinogenic properties. The other principal components are: cannabinol (CBN), cannabidiol (CBD), tetrahydrocannabinol, cannabigerol, and cannabichromene (CBC), etc.

Bioactivity

It is used in psychiatric and neurodegenerative diseases. Also used in multiple sclerosis (MS), nerve pain, rheumatoid arthritis (RA), inflammatory bowel disease (ulcerative colitis), etc.

5.2.4 Teratogens

Teratogens are defined as any agents that result in structural and functional abnormalities (malformation) in the foetus, or in the child after birth, as a consequence of maternal exposure during pregnancy. They can do direct damage to foetus, causing abnormal development. Teratogens may produce physical or functional defects in human embryo or foetus in a variety of ways, such as duration of exposure, amount of teratogenic substance and the stage of development of embryo or foetus during exposure.

Classifications

Teratogens are classified into 4 types:

1. physical agents
2. metabolic conditions
3. infection
4. drugs and chemicals

1. **Physical agents:** The causative agents of hyperthermia also act as physical teratogens. Such agents might be saunas, hot tubs, or infections that raise a pregnant woman's body temperature to 102°F or more. This condition of hyperthermia causes central nervous system malformations, microcephaly, abdominal wall defects, defects of the eye and palate, and limb reduction defects. It is associated with neural tube defects, spontaneous abortions, and various cardiovascular abnormalities basically found in humans. In pregnant women, congenital abnormalities, such as cardiac defects, abdominal wall defects, or a disruption of the enervation of the large intestine called Hirschsprung disease reported due to hyperthermia, in their offspring.
2. **Metabolic conditions:** Its effects in pregnant females such as malnutrition, diabetes, and thyroid disorders are a second category of teratogens. Metabolic conditions are abnormalities in the chemical process of producing energy from food, and thereby affect the development and function of the body. If a pregnant woman is malnourished, then her foetus lacks the nutrients essential for its development. In the case of diabetes, low blood sugar, or hypoglycaemia, may cause foetal malformations. For example:

   Hypoglycaemia interferes with some proteins in the developing foetal heart by increasing the expression of proteins which are regulated by glucose.

   Excessive blood sugar, also seen with diabetes, may cause neural tube defects, or birth defects of the brain and spinal cord, and may also induce the release of free radicals, or damaged cells that are missing an essential molecule, which disrupts foetal development.
3. **Infection:** In fections such as those caused by rubella virus, herpes simplex virus, and syphilis, are a third kind of teratogen. In addition to rubella, herpes simplex virus, and cytomegalovirus—one of the herpes viruses that passes through direct contact with body fluids, congenital abnormalities can be caused by infections of *Toxoplasma gondii*, a parasite often obtained by eating contaminated meat, drinking contaminated water, or coming into contact with infected cat faeces, and *Treponema pallidum*, the bacterium that causes syphilis.
4. **Drugs and chemical:** Such kind of teratogen includes drugs and chemicals that pregnant female ingests.Such as alcohol, cocaine, thalidomide, etc.

Causes of teratogenesis

- Abnormal development may be caused by errors in genetic programming, from environmental agents/ factors or from unknown causes that interfere with the development.
- About 7% of all live birth defects are due to prenatal exposure to radiation, environmental factors and drugs and chemicals.
- Abnormalities caused by genetic events, e.g., mutation in genes, structural changes in chromosomes and aneuploidies, etc., are called malformations.

- Abnormalities caused by environmental agents are called disruptions. The environmental factor may be biological (e.g., viruses and parasites) or non-biological such as physical factors (temperatures, radiations) and chemical factors (drugs and chemical and nutritional imbalance).

Table 5.4 Plants and phytochemicals with teratogenic side effects

Name of the plant	Family	Teratogenicity
Asparagus racemosus	Liliaceae	Gross malformations in foetus, can increase the rate of re-absorption in foetus and may also cause intrauterine growth.
Erythroxylon coca	Erythroxylaceae	Cocaine is metabolized very slowly in the foetus because the foetus has low plasma cholinesterase activity. It may alter the availability and utilization of calcium, and reduce blood flow from the uterus to the placenta leads to prematurity, microcephaly, and sudden infant death.
Coffea arabica	Rubiaceae	Caffeine in combination with alcohol and smoking may cause miscarriages.
Artemisia absinthium	Asteraceae	Ingested in large amounts can cause epileptiform seizures and even abortion. This toxic action is mainly due to the presence of constituents such as the terpenoid thujone
Malus domestica	Rosaceae	Seeds have cyanogenic glycosides that is fatal to even adults.

5.2.5 Natural Allergens

Natural allergens are the antigenic substances made up of protein, lipid or carbohydrate that causes an allergic reaction in body by sensitizing the body's immune system. The word antigen derives from two words "anti" means against and "gen" means genes.

Types of Allergens

Almost any substance may prove to be allergenic. The allergens are categorized as:

(i) Biologic origin (e.g., dust mites)
(ii) Chemical origin (e.g., perfumes)
(iii) Synthetic origin (e.g., fibres cotton linters)

Properties of allergens

- The allergen concerned with the patient's symptoms must be antigenic, that is, it must be capable of eliciting an antibody response.
- Specificity allergenic substances produce specific antibodies and so each type of allergy is constitutionally different from other types.
- Tissues which are affected by antigen are called "shock tissues".
- The antibodies are special protein molecules which help to neutralize the parasitic invaders and protect the person from further exposure.
- The reaction between antigen and antibody is called antigen-antibody reactions.

Mechanism of action of allergens

Generally, allergic reactions take place in the following steps:

1. Primary exposure
2. Secondary exposure and release of mediators

1. **Primary Exposure:** When the body is first subjected to the allergen-antigen the condition is referred to as primary exposure. In this time no symptoms of the allergy are produced because no antibodies has been formed previously.
2. **Secondary Exposure and release of mediators:** During secondary exposures the antigens become attached to the antibody attached on the mast cells white blood cells basophils that form part of our immune system like a key fits into a lock and form a complex. As a result basophils burst due to antigen-antibody reaction causes a liberation of histamine and other mediators of allergic symptoms including leukotriene C or SRS slow reacting substance and bradykin in which are responsible for such symptoms like inflammation swelling redness itching dilatation of blood vessels constriction of the airways and increased mucus secretion.

Types of Allergens

There are different types of allergens:

1. Inhalant allergens
2. Ingestant allergens
3. Injectant allergens
4. Contactant allergens
5. Infectant allergens
6. Infestant allergens

In addition to these material allergens, allergies may be caused by heat or cold physical allergy, changes in climate environmental allergy, anger or frustration psychosomatic allergy, and others.

1. Inhalant Allergens

Allergenic substances that are distributed in the atmosphere and contact the nasal or buccal mucosa during respiration are called inhalant allergens. Inhalant allergens, e.g., cold air, hot air, grains, cotton feathers, volatile oils, etc., become attached to antibodies on mucous membranes and cause allergy. Symptoms of such allergy include: sneezing, itching, lacrimation and swelling of nose and eyes. This condition is known as "sinusitis" or "hayfever". Pollen grains are a potential source of inhalant allergens.

Composition of Pollen Grains

Pollen grains can be distinguished and identified easily due to their heterogeneous nature. They may be oval (e.g., mimosa flower), round (e.g., ragweed), angular (e.g., tilia), square or rectangular in shape. Surrounded by 2 layers, the outer surface of pollen grains is called "exine" while the inner surface is "intine". The surface appearance of exine is characteristic and is a determining factor in identification. It may range from smooth psilate, spiny echinate, with various intervening gradations reticulate granulate lophate. The pollen grains may spread through wind or insects. Atmospheric pollens may be liberated chiefly by anemophilous (wind-pollinated plants) or entomophilous (insect pollinated plants).

Anemophilous: Pollens are usually small in diameter (15 to 45 μ), light,non-adhesive, relatively smooth. *Examples:* Oak trees, walnut, grasses (Bermuda grass and timothy), weeds (ragweed plantain).

Entomophilous: Pollens are usually, larger in diameter (up to 200 μ), heavier, adhesive, spiny. *Examples:* Clover hollyhock, honeysuckle, rose.

2. Ingestant Allergens

The allergenenic substances that are found in foodstuffs and after ingestation or swallow produces allergy in mouth, stomach or intestine are calledingestant allergens. After digestion of foods, the nutrients are absorbed along with allergenic substances which stimulate allergic response in body. These allergens are not localized but produce their effect in the whole body by entering the blood circulation which causes a number of allergic symptoms. Examples: milk, coffee, chocolates, cod liver oil, etc.

Food allergens ordinarily cause GIT symptoms but they may also cause skin rash, puffed lips and tongue, migraine, rhinitis, bronchial asthma. Sometimes severe cases of eczema of hands, atopic dermatitis such as tomato rash, strawberry rash or that caused by eating chocolate shellfish.

Source of Ingestant Allergens

Some of the most common allergens ingested by children are foods considered essential to proper diet and growth such as cow's milk, orange juice, cod liver oil, vitamin containing fish liver oil, etc.

3. Injectant allergens

The allergens that are present in parenteral preparations or injection of insects and cause allergies in a hypersensitive person are called injectant allergens, e.g., penicillin injection, glandular preparations, antitoxins and biting insects.

Source of injectant allergy

Injections and various insects as the source of natural injectants cause allergenic reactions in human.

(i) **Injections:** Penicillin injections induced allergies are well known to most of the lay public. Anaphylactic reactions to penicillin occur with a frequency of 1-5 people in 10,000.

(ii) **Hymenopterous insects:** Insects are the source of natural injectant allergens. Bees, hornets and wasps are the best example of such allergens. Stings of such insects can induce severe reactions. Such patients can be immunized by using injections of antigens. Immunologic comparisons of effects of insects venoms, venom sac extracts, whole insect extracts have been made to determine the optimal method of treatment.

(iii) **Other Insects:** "Biting arthropods" are also subjected to clinical investigations. It includes spiders, mites, lice, chiggers, ticks, sand flies, horse flies, scorpions, centipedes and numerous others indigenous to geographic areas.

4. Contactant allergens

The allergens that produce allergy when coming in contact with the skin epithelium and produce hypersensitivity reactions are called contactant allergens. Examples: plants pollen grains or some clothes. The contactant allergens causes localized reactions in a particular part of the body. The allergic symptoms of the contactant allergens are usually watery blisters and dermatitis.

Sources of contactant allergens

There are many substances and products which are identified as source of contactant allergies These include:

(i) Plants or plant products: Toxicodendrons species is responsible for allergy in hypersensitive individuals, e.g., poison ivy. They contain the same nonvolatile phenolic principle urushiol resin and mainly cause watery blisters. Certain plants such as asparagus, buckwheat, catalpa leaves also cause severe allergic condition like asthma where daffodils, English ivy, ginkgo leaves, lobelia, tobacco, mayapple, osage, orange, smartweeds, etc., plants cause dermatitis.

(ii) Aeroallergens: Occasional contact dermatitis has been caused by aeroallergens such as various pollen grains that contain oils, hairs from different kinds of leaves and flowers and even small fragments of plant tissue carried by smoke emanating from brush fires, grass fires, and burning leaves.

Even though, certain chemicals used in cosmetics industry are also a major source of allergy. For example:

(i) In violet talcum powder "orris root" is used that is a source of allergy.

(ii) In indelible lipsticks "dibromofluorescein" is an allergic ingredient.

(iii) Other Contactant Allergens: Wool clothings and blankets, wool fat, lanolin in cosmetics,perfumes, soaps and soap powders, plain detergents, enzyme detergents, nail polishes, nail polishes removers, hair dyes and hair sprays are the numerous major causes of contact dermititis.

5. Infectant allergens

The bacterial metabolic wastes are considered infectant allergens. Numerous living organisms may cause allergy through the products they release during their metabolism in the human body.

Source of infectant allergens

Many microorganisms or pathogens, certain types of bacteria protozoans molds helminths and other parasitic forms by the presence in the body for long time responsible for chronic illness. Bronchiectasis, an example of infectant allergy: The chronic bacterial infection of the bronchioles where in the constant presence of bacterial wastes may sensitize the allergic individual is the one of the example.

6. Infestant allergens

In a manner somewhat similar to the infectants parasitic organisms may sensitize the human body. Invasions of hookworms, tapeworms, pinworms, threadworms, dermatophytes and other forms have caused allergic response in susceptible individuals. Growth products and metabolic wastes of these parasites are constantly present in the body and referred to as infestant allergens.

Table 5.5 List of plants with their type of allergies

Name of the plant	Family	Type of allergy
Cynodon dactylon	Celastraceae	Hypertension, constipation
Lawsonia inermis	Lythreceae	Chronic inflammation reaction
Ricinus communis	Euphorbiaceae	Erythrocyte agglutination
Cycas circinalis	Cycadaceae	Neurodegenerative disorder
Conium maculatum	Apiaceae	Seizures, respiratory depression
Parthenium hysterophoru	Asteraceae	Dermatitis, respiratory malfunction
Calotropis gigantea	Apocynaceae	Touching the ocular surface causes crown flower keratitis
Blighia sapida	Sapindaceae	Vomiting sickness
Artemisia vulgaris	Asteraceae	Hey fever, allergic asthma

5.3 PRIMARY METABOLITES

Primary metabolites are the substances basically produce during their growth phases. They are directly involved in the metabolic pathways of an organisms necessary for its growth, development, and reproduction. The growth phase associated with the production of primary metabolites is termed 'trophophase'.

Primary metabolites are abundantly found throughout the body commonly known as central metabolites. Some of them are found to be very crucial for various metabolic processes as substrate, while others act as catalysts. Primary metabolites play an essential role in the growth and development of an individual, but do not have any pharmacological action against other factors. The common examples of primary metabolites include proteins, enzymes, carbohydrates, lipids, vitamins, ethanol, lactic acid, butanol, etc.

Generally, primary metabolites are divided into two major groups:

(i) Primary essential metabolites
(ii) Primary metabolic end products

Proteins and carbohydrates belong to the primary essential metabolites which play the main role in the structural and physiological organization of the organism.In the other hand, primary metabolic end-products are those substances which are produced as end-products of various metabolic pathways. It includes lactic acid and ethanol.

Primary essential metabolites are discussed in this topic.

5.3.1 Carbohydrates

Carbohydrates are the most important primary metabolites commonly found in all living organisms. They play the most significant role in development of the structural and physiological components in the living beings. It is a biomolecule structurally made up of carbon, hydrogen, and oxygen. It not only provides the structural support to the plants and bacteria as in the form of cellulose and peptidoglycan respectively but also provides energy in form of ATP after oxidation. Carbohydrates are of various types depending on their length and composition. They are also divided based on their functions. Carbohydrates act as substrates for the important biological processes like Kreb's cycle and glycolysis.

Monosaccharides are also involved in the formation of macromolecules and might even function as reservoirs of energy and fats. Some examples of carbohydrates include glucose, cellulose, glycogen, chitin, peptidoglycan, etc. In phrarmaceutical industries, there is a huge demand for such carbohydrate containing drugs for their use in pharmaceutical formulations. Such carbohydrate includes, acacia, agar, tragacanth, honey, etc.

5.3.1.1 Drugs Containing Carbohydrates

Acacia Gum

Synonyms

Acacia gum, Gum Senegal, Somali Gum, Yellow thorn, Indian Gum, Gum Arabic.

Biological Source

Acacia is the dried gummy exudation obtained from the stems and branches of *Acacia senegal* or *A. arabica* or other African species of acacia, belonging to family Leguminosae.

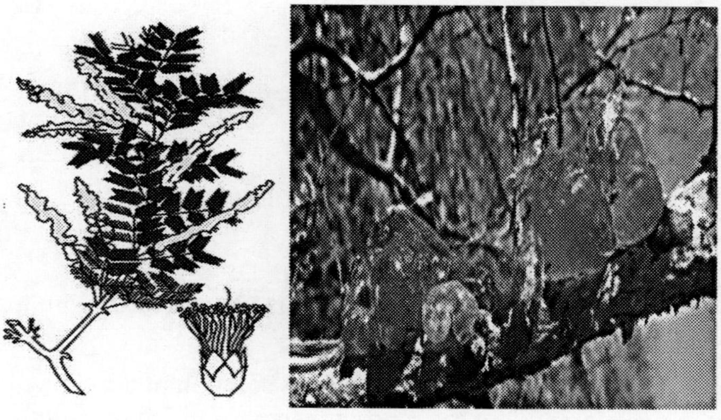

Fig. 5.10 *Acacia senegal*

Geographical source

Acacia trees are abundant in central Sudan, central and West Africa, and tropical and semitropical areas of the world. Sudan is the leading producer of acacia gums worldwide, followed by Nigeria, Chad, Mali, and Senegal. In India it is found chiefly in Punjab, Rajasthan and Western Ghats. Sudan is the major producer of this gum and caters for about 85% of the world supply.

Collection and preparation

Gum is collected by natives from 6 to 8 years old trees, twice a year in dry weather in November or in February/ March. Natives cut the lower thorny branches to facilitate the working and by means of an axe make 2-3 feet long and 2-3 inches broad incision on the stem and branches, loosen the bark by axe and remove it, taking care not to injure the cambium and xylem. Usually they leave a thin layer of bark on xylem. After injury in winter gum exudes after 6-8 weeks while in summer after 3-4 weeks. The exuded gum is scraped off, collected in leather bags and then is cleaned by separating debris of bark and wood and separating sand, etc., by sieving.

Gum is dried in the sun by keeping it in trays in thin layers for about 3 weeks when bleaching takes place and it becomes whiter. This result in uneven contraction and cracks and fissures are formed on its outer surface and as a result original transparent gum becomes opaque. This process is called ripening of the gum.

Chemical constituents

Acacia consists principally of arabin, which is a complex mixture of calcium, magnesium and potassium salts of arabic acid. Arabic acid is a branched polysaccharide that yields L-arabinose, D-galactose, D-glucuronic acid and L-rhamnose on hydrolysis. 1,3-linked D-galactopyranose units form the backbone chain of the molecule and the terminal residues of the 1,6-linked side chains are primarily uronic acids. Acacia contains 12–15% of water and several occluded enzymes such as oxidases, peroxidases and pectinases. The total ash content should be in the range of 2.7-4.0%.

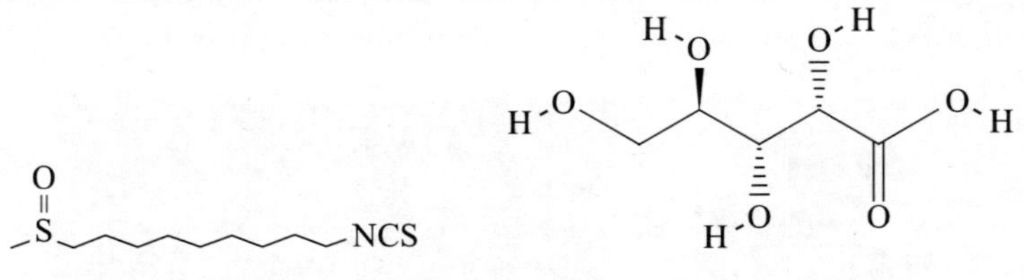

Arabin Arabic acid

Fig. 5.11 Structure of arabin, arabic acid

Chemical Tests

1. **Lead acetate test:** An aqueous solution of acacia when treated with lead acetate solution yields a heavy white precipitate.
2. **Reducing sugars test:** Hydrolysis of an aqueous solution of acacia with dilute HC1 yields reducing sugars whose presence are ascertained by boiling with Fehling's solution to give a brick-red precipitate of cuprous oxide.
3. **Blue colouration due to enzyme:** When the aqueous solution of acacia is treated with benzidine in alcohol together with a few drops of hydrogen peroxide (H_2O_2), it gives rise to a distinct blue colour due to the presence of oxidases enzyme.
4. **Borax test:** An aqueous solution of acacia affords a stiff translucent mass on treatment with borax.
5. **Specific test:** A 10% aqueous solution of acacia fails to produce any precipitate with dilute solution of lead acetate (a clear distinction from agar and tragacanth); it does not give any colour change with iodine solution (a marked distinction from starch and dextrin); and it never produces a bluish-black colour with $FeCl_3$ solution (an apparent distinction from tannins).

Uses

The mucilage of acacia is employed as a demulcent. It is used extensively as a vital pharmaceutical aid for emulsification and to serve as a thickening agent. It finds its enormous application as a binding agent for tablets, for example, cough lozenges. It is used in the process of 'granulation' for the manufacturing of tablets. It is considered to be the gum of choice by virtue of the fact that it is quite compatible with other plant hydrocolloids as well as starches, carbohydrates and proteins. It is used in combination with gelatin to form conservates for micro-encapsulation of drugs. It is employed as colloidal stabilizer. It is used extensively in making of candy and other food products. Gum acacia solution has consistency similar to blood and is administered intravenously in haemodialysis. It is used in the manufacture of adhesives and ink, and as a binding medium for marbling colours.

Marketed product

Dental cream and Eyecare syrup and capsule manufactured by Himalaya Drug Company.

Honey

Synonyms

Madhu, Madh, Mel, Purified Honey.

Biological source

Honey is a viscid and sweet secretion stored in the honeycomb by various species of bees, such as *Apis mellifera, Apis dorsata, Apis florea, Apis indica* and other species of apis, belonging to family apideae.

Geographical source

Honey is available in abundance in Africa, India, Jamaica, Australia, California, Chili, Great Britain and New Zealand.

Collection and preparation

The nectar of the flowers is a watery solution containing 25% sucrose and 75% water. The worker bee sucks this nectar through its hollow tube of mouth (proboscis) and deposits in honeysac located in the abdomen. The enzyme invertase present in saliva of the bee converts nectar into invert sugar, which is partially utilized by the bee and the remaining is deposited into honeycomb. Honeycomb is smoked to remove the bees and honey is obtained by applyng the pressure to it or allowing it to drain naturally. The honey of commerce is heated to 80°C and allowed to stand. The impurities which float over the surface are skimmed off and the liquid is diluted with water to produce honey of 1.35 density. Natural honey has the density of 1.47. Many-a-time, honey is extracted from the comb by centrifugation. It must be free from foreign substances. Honey is liable to fermentation, unless it is suitably processed. Honey is heated to 80°C before it is sent to the market, so as to avoid fermentation. It should be cooled rapidly or else it darkens in colour on keeping. If necessary (and if not prepared by centrifugation method), honey is required to be filtered through wet cloth or funnel.

Chemical constituents

The average composition of honey is as follows: Moisture 14-24%, dextrose 23-36%, levulose (fructose) 30-47%, sucrose 0.4-6%, dextrin and gums 0-7% and ash 0.1-0.8%. Besides, it is found to contain small amounts of essential oil, beeswax, pollen grains, formic acid, acetic acid, succinic acid, maltose, dextrin, colouring pigments, vitamins and an admixture of enzymes, for example, diastase, invertase and inulase. Interestingly, the sugar contents in honey varies widely from one country to another as it is exclusively governed by the source of the nectar (availability of fragment flowers in the region) and also the enzymatic activity solely controlling the conversion into honey.

Chemical tests

Adulteration in honey is determined by the following tests:

1. **Fiehe's test for artificial invert sugar:** Honey (10 mL) is shaken with petroleum or solvent ether (5 mL) for 5-10 min. The upper ethereal layer is separated and evaporated in a china dish. On addition of 1% solution of resorcinol in hydrochloric acid (1 mL) a transient red colour is formed in natural honey while in artificial honey the colour persists for sometime.
2. **Reduction of Fehling's solution:** To an aqueous solution of honey (2 mL) Fehling's solutions A and B are added and the reaction mixture is heated on a steam bath for 5-10 min. A brick red colour is produced due to the presence of reducing sugars.
3. **Limit tests:** The limit tests of chloride, sulphate and ash (0.5%) are compared with the pharmacopoeial specifications.

Uses

Honey shows mild laxative, bactericidal, sedative, antiseptic and alkaline characteristcs. It is used for cold, cough, fever, sore eye and throat, tongue and duodenal ulcers, liver disorders, constipation, diarrhoea, kidney and other urinary disorders, pulmonary tuberculosis, marasmus, rickets, scurvy and insomnia. It is applied as a remedy on open wounds after surgery. It prevents infection and promotes healing.

Honey is an important ingredient of certain lotions, cosmetics, soaps, creams, balms, toilet waters and inhalations. It is used as a medium in preservation of cornea.

Interestingly, potent antibacterial peptides (apidaecins and abaecin) have been isolated and characterized in the honeybee (*Apis mellifera*) itself and a new potent antibacterial protein named royalisin has been found in the royal jelly of the honeybee.

Adulterant and substitutes

Due to the relatively high price of pure honey, it is invariably adulterated ether with artificial invert sugar or simply with cane-sugar syrup. These adulterants or cheaper substituents not only alter the optical property of honey but also its natural aroma and fragrance.

Marketed product

OLBAS Cough Syrup manufactured by Olbas Herbal Remedies, Philadelphia is mainly used for the treatment of cough and sore throat.

Tragacanth

Synonyms

Goat's thorn, Gum dragon, Gum tragacanth, Hog gum.

Biological source

It is the air dried gummy exudates, flowing naturally or obtained by incision, from the stems and branches of *Astragalus gummifer* and certain other species of *Astragalus*, belonging to family Leguminosae.

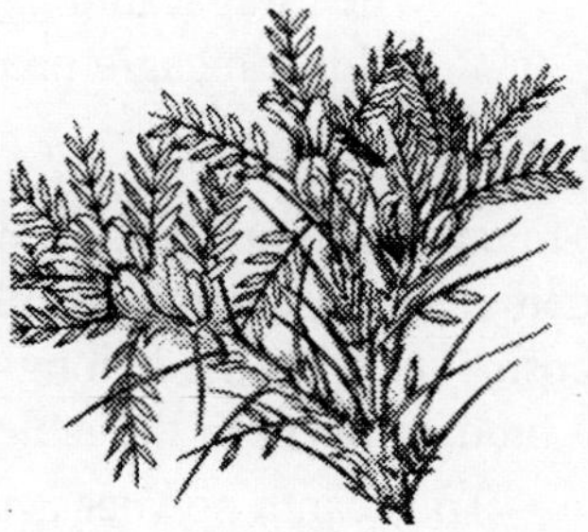

Fig. 5.12 *Astragalus gummifer*

Geographical source

Astragalus species are abundantly found in the mountainous region of Turkey, Syria, Iran, Iraq and the former USSR at an altitude of about 1000-3000 m. In India it is found in Kumaon and Garhwal regions.

Collection and preparation

Collection of gums can be obtained from the plants in their second year. The earth is taken away from the base to a depth of 5 cm, and the exposed part is incised with a sharp knife having a thin cutting edge. The collector has to force opens the incision of a wedge-shaped piece of wood that the gum exudes more freely. The wedge is generally left in the cut for some 12-24 hr before being withdrawn. The gum exudes and is collected 2 days after the incision.

Some of the plants are burned at the top after having had the incision made. The plant then sickens and gives off a greater quantity of gum. The gum obtained after burning is of lower quality than that obtained by incision, and is reddish and dirty looking. The crop becomes available in August-September.

After collection, the gum is graded as ribbons and flakes which are further categorized into various sub-grades on the basis of shape, size and colour. The best grades form the official drug, while the lower grades are used in the food, textile and other industries.

Chemical constituents

Tragacanth gum is composed mainly of sugars and uronic acid units and can be divided into three types of constituents. The acidic constituents tragacanthic acid on hydrolysis yields galactose, xylose and galacturonic acid. A neutral polysaccharide affords galactose and arabinose after its hydrolysis while a third type is believed to be steroidal glycoside. Interestingly, tragacanth comprises two vital fractions: first, being water soluble and is termed 'tragacanthin' (30-40%) and the second, being water insoluble and is known as 'bassorin' (60%-70%). Both are not soluble in alcohol. Bassorin actually gets swelled up in water to form a gel, whereas tragacanthin forms an instant colloidal solution.

Chemical tests

1. An aqueous solution of tragacanth on boiling with conc. HCl does not develop a red colour.
2. It does not produce red colour with ruthenium red solution.
3. When a solution of tragacanth is boiled with a few drops of $FeCl_3$ (10%), it produces a deep-yellow precipitate.

4. It gives a heavy precipitate with lead acetate.
5. When tragacanth and precipitated copper oxide are made to dissolve in conc. NH_4OH, it yields a meagre precipitate.

Uses

Tragacanth is used as a thickening, suspending and as an emulsifying agent. It is used as a demulcent in cough and cold preparations and to manage diarrhoea. It is used as an emollient in cosmetics. It is used along with acacia as a suspending agent. Mucilage of tragacanth is used as a binding agent in the tablets and also as an excipient in the pills.

Tragacanth powder is used as an adhesive. It is also used in lotions for external use and also in spermicidal jellies. It is also used as a stabilizer for ice cream in 0.2-0.3% concentration and also in sauces.

Adulterant and substitutes

Tragacanth gum of lower grades, known as hog tragacanth, is used in textile industry and in the manufacture of pickles. The gum varies from yellowish brown to almost black. Citral gum obtained from *A. strobiliferus* is also used as an adulterant.

Karaya gum which is sometimes known as sterculia gum or Indian tragacanth is invariably used as a substitute for gum tragacanth.

Agar

Synonym

Agaragar, Japanese isinglass, Vegetable gelatin.

Botanical source

It is the dried gelatinous substance obtained by extraction of water from *Gelidium amansii* or various species of red algae like *Gracilaria* and *Pterocladia*, belonging to family Gelidaceae.

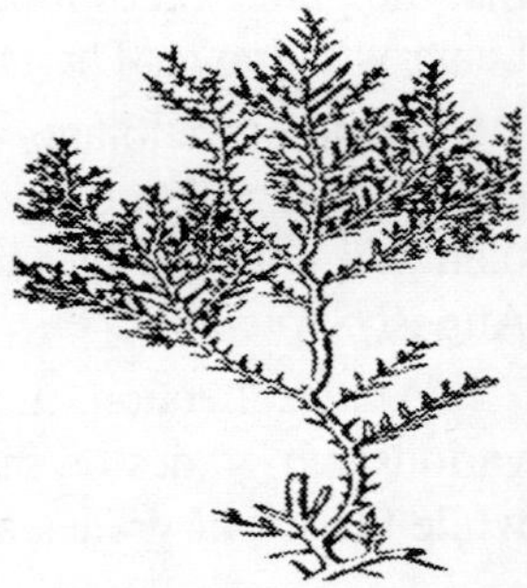

Fig 5.13 *Gelidium amansii*

Geographical source

Commercial production of agar happen in several countries like, Japan (*Gelidium amnasii*), Australia (*Gracilaria confervoldes*), New Zealand (*Pterocladia lucida*), Korea, South Africa, United States, Chile, Spain, Portugal, etc.

Collection and preparation

The red algae are grown in rocks in shallow water or on the bamboos by placing them in the ocean. Collection of the algae is usually made in summer (May and October). The bamboos are taken out and the seaweeds are stripped off. Algae are dried, beaten with sticks and shaken to remove the sand and shell attached to them. Then the entire material is taken to high altitude, washed with water and bleached by keeping them in trays in the sunlight, sprinkling water and rotating them periodically.

The agar is then boiled; one part of algae with 50 parts of water acidified with acetic acid or dilute sulphuric acid. The hot extract is subjected for coarse and fine filtration using cloth to remove the large and small impurities present in them. The filtered extract is then transferred to wooden trough which on cooling forms a jelly-like mass. The mass thus obtained is then passed through screw press to obtain strips of agar. These strips contain water and to remove the water present in them, the agar strips are placed in open air. As a result, the excess water present in them is removed. Then, these strips are again dried in the sunlight in trays.

Modern methods of deep freezing are utilized in the preparation of agar.

Chemical constituents

Agar is a complex heterosaccharide and contains two different polysaccharides known as agarose and agaropectin. Agarose is a neutral galactose polymer and is responsible for the gel property of agar. It consists of D-galactose and L-galactose unit. The structure of agaropectin is not completely known, but it is believed that it consists of sulphonated polysaccharide in which galactose and uronic acids are partly esterified with sulphuric acid. Agaropectin is responsible for the viscosity of agar solution.

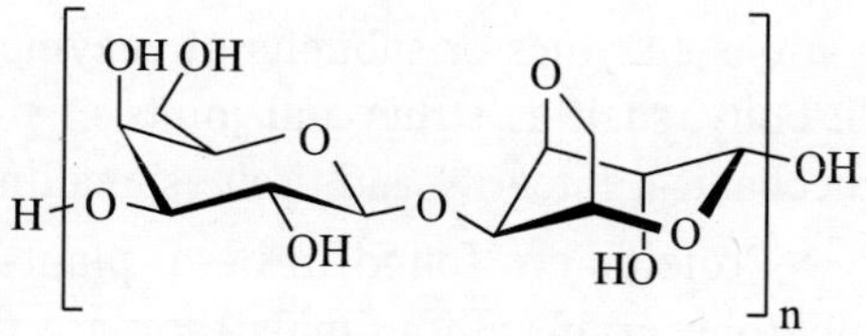

Fig. 5.14 Structure of agarose

Chemical tests

1. Agar responds positively to Fehling's solution test.
2. Agar gives positive test with Molisch reagent.
3. Aqueous solution of agar (1%) is hydrolysed with concentrated HCl by heating for 5–10 min. On addition of barium chloride solution to the reaction mixture, a white precipitate of barium sulphate is formed due to the presence of sulphate ions. This test is absent in case of starch, acacia gum and tragacanth.
4. To agar powder a solution of ruthenium red is added. Red colour is formed indicating mucilage.
5. Agar is warmed in a solution of KOH. A canary yellow colour is formed.
6. An aqueous solution of agar (1%) is prepared in boiling water. On cooling it sets into a jelly.
7. To agar solution an N/20 solution of iodine is added. A deep crimson to brown colour is obtained (distinctive from acacia gum and tragacanth).
8. To a 0.2% solution of agar an aqueous solution of tannic acid is added. No precipitation is formed indicating absence of gelatin.
9. Agar is required to comply with tests for the absence of *E. coli* and Salmonella, and general microbial contamination should not exceed a level of 103 microorganisms per gram as determined by a plate count. It has a swelling index of not less than 10.

Uses

Agar is used to treat chronic constipation, as a laxative, suspending agent, an emulsifier, a gelating agent for suppositories, as surgical lubricant, as a tablet excipient, disintegrant, in the production of medicinal encapsulation and ointment and as dental impression mold base. It is extensively used as a gel in nutrient media for bacterial cultures, as a substitute for gelatin and isinglass, in making emulsions including photographic, gel in cosmetics, as thickening agent in food especially confectioneries and dairy products, in meat canning; sizing for silk and paper; in dying and printing of fabrics and textiles; and in adhesives.

5.3.2 Proteins

Proteins are composed of amino acids joined by peptide bonds characteristically a complex, high molecular weight organic compound. The word protein is derived from greek '*protos*' meaning '*of primary importance*'.

The structural and functional development of all living cells essentially require proteins. Various enzymes or subunits of enzymes are proteins which play structural or mechanical roles in body, such as struts and joints of the cytoskeleton, serving as biological scaffolds for the mechanical integrity and tissue signalling functions, etc.

Proteins are found in both, plant and animals. In plants they are stored in the form of aleurone grains. In animals they are present in structural material in the form of collagen, keratin, elastin, casein and plasma proteins. Some pharmaceutically important proteins are casein, gelatin, heparin, and haemoglobin, etc., from animal source.

Chemistry

Chemically, proteins have a large molecular structure, with molecular masses up to 3,000,000 kDa. For example, the titin (muscle protein) has a single amino acid chain 27,000 subunits. Such long chains of amino acids are referred to as proteins, whereas, shorter strings of amino acids are referred as 'polypeptides', 'peptides', or rarely, 'oligopeptides', etc.

'Polypeptide' usually refers to an amino acid chain lacking of tertiary structure where dividing line is undefined, more likely to act as a hormone (like insulin), rather than as an enzyme.

Twenty amino acids are so far identified where eight of which must be present in the diet. These eight essential amino acids for human beings includes: leucine, isoleucine, valine, threonine, methionine, phenylalanine, tryptophan, and lysine. One more amino acid histidine is also considered to be an essential amino acid for children.

Unlike animal proteins, plant proteins may not contain all the essential amino acids in the necessary proportions. However, a varied vegetarian diet means a mixture of proteins are consumed, the amino acids in one protein compensating for the deficiencies of another.

The structure of protein could be differentiated into four types:

1. Primary structure
The amino acid sequence

2. Secondary structure
Highly patterned substructures–alpha helix and beta sheet– or segments of chain that assume no stable shape.

3. Tertiary structure
The overall shape of a single protein molecule; the spatial relationship of the secondary structural motifs to one another

4. Quaternary structure
Results from the union of more than one protein subunits in this context, which function as part of the larger assembly or protein complex.

Fig. 5.15 Structures of proteins

Properties

- Proteins are sensitive to their environment. They may only be active in their native state, over a small pH range, and under solution conditions with a minimum quantity of electrolytes.
- A protein in its native state is described as folded and that is not in its native state is said to be denatured. Denatured proteins generally have no well-defined secondary structure. They are denatured due to heat, changes in pH, treatment of organic solvents or by ultra violet radiation.

Functions

1. It is plays the most prominent role in growth and repair.
2. They play a crucial role in virtually all biological processes in the body, i.e., body's metabolism as enzymes.
3. Various functions like muscle contraction, immune protection and the transmission of nerve impulses are all dependent on proteins.
4. The proteins of skin and bone provide structural support.
5. Many hormones are nothing but proteins only.
6. Proteins can also provide a source of energy.
7. Excess proteins may also be converted to fat and stored.

5.3.2.1 Protein Containing Natural Products

The important source of proteins includes:

Gelatin

Synonyms

Gelfoam, Puragel, Gelatinum.

Biological source

Gelatin is a protein derivative obtained by evaporating an aqueous extract made from bones, skins, and tendons of various domestic animals. Some important sources are: *Ox, Bos taurus*, and sheep, *Ovis aries* belonging to family Bovidae.

Preparation

The process of manufacture of gelatin may vary. However, the general outline of the process is given below.

1. **Raw material:** Bones, skins, and tendons of Bovideans is collected and subjected to liming operation.
2. **Liming process:** The animal raw materials are first subjected to 'liming' process. In this process, the skins and tendons are steeped for fifteen to twenty and sometimes for 40 days in a dilute milk of lime. During liming process, fleshy matter gets dissolved, chondro proteins of connective tissues gets removed and fatty matter is saponified. The animal skin is further thoroughly washed in running water.

3. **Defattying:** In case of bones, the material is properly ground and defatted in close iron cylinders by treatment with organic solvents such as benzene. The mineral and inorganic part of the bone are removed by treatment with hydrochloric acid.
4. **Extraction:** The treated material from bones, skins and tendons is boiled with water in open pans with perforated false bottom. This process can also be carried out under reduced pressure. The clear liquid runs of again and again and is evaporated until it reaches to above 45 per cent gelatin content.
5. **Setting:** The concentrated gelatin extract is transferred to shallow metal trays or trays with glass bottom. It is allowed to set as a semisolid jelly.
6. **Drying:** The jelly is transferred to trays with a perforated wire netting bottom and passed through series of drying compartments of 30-60°C increasing each time with 10°C. About a month is taken for complete drying.
7. **Bleaching:** In case of darker colour, finished product is subjected to bleaching by sulphur dioxide. Bleaching affords a light coloured gelatin.

Chemical constituents

Gelatin consists of the protein glutin which on hydrolysis gives a mixture of amino acids. The approximate aminoacid contents are: glycine (25.5%), alanine (8.7%), valine (2.5%), leucine (3.2%), isoleucine (1.4%), cystine and cysteine (0.1%), methionine (1.0%), tyrosine (0.5%), aspartic acid (6.6%), glutamic acid (11.4%), arginine (8.1%), lysine (4.1%), and histidine (0.8%). Nutritionally, gelatin is an incomplete protein lacking tryptophan. The gelatinizing compound is known as chondrin and the adhesive nature of gelatin is due to the presence of glutin.

Chemical Tests

1. **Biuret reaction:** To alkaline solution of a protein (2 mL), a dilute solution of copper sulphate is added. A red or violet colour is formed with peptides containing at least two peptide linkages. A dipeptide does not give this test.
2. **Xanthoproteic reaction:** Proteins usually form a yellow colour when warmed with concentrated nitric acid. This colour becomes orange when the solution is made alkaline.
3. **Millon's reaction:** Millon's reagent (mercuric nitrate in nitric acid containing a trace of nitrous acid) usually yields a white precipitate on addition to a protein solution which turns red on heating.
4. **Ninhydrin test:** To an aqueous solution of a protein an alcoholic solution of ninhydrin is added and then heated. Red to violet colour is formed.
5. On heating gelatin (1 g) with soda lime, smell of ammonia is produced.
6. A solution of gelatin (0.5 g) in water (10 mL) is precipitated to white buff coloured precipitate on addition of few drops of tannic acid (10%).
7. Gelatin with picric acid gelatin forms yellow precipitate.

Uses

It is used to prepare pastilles, pastes, suppositories, capsules, pillcoatings, gelatin sponge. It is also usedas suspending agent, tablet binder, coating agent, as stabilizer, thickener and texturizer in food; for manufacturing rubber substitutes, adhesives, cements, lithographic and printing inks, plastic compounds, artificial silk, photographic plates and films, light filters for mercury lamps, clarifying agent, in hectographic matters, sizing paper and textiles, for inhibiting crystallization in bacteriology, for preparing cultures and as a nutrient.

Casein

Biological source

Casein is a proteolytic enzyme obtained from the stomachs of calves. It is extracted from the proteins of the milk. The casein content of milk represents about 80% of milk proteins.

Chemistry

The principal casein fractions are alpha (s1) and alpha (s2)-caseins, β-casein and κ-casein. The distinguishing property of all caseins is their low solubility at pH 4.6. The common compositional factor is that caseins are conjugated proteins, most with phosphate group(s) esterified to serine residues. These phosphate groups are important to the structure of the casein micelle. Calcium binding by the individual caseins is proportional to the phosphate content.

Within the group of caseins, there are several distinguishing features based on their charge distribution and sensitivity to calcium precipitation:

(i) **Alpha (s1)-casein:** (molecular weight 23,000; 199 residues, 17 proline residues).
Two hydrophobia regions, containing all the proline residues, separated by a polar region, which contains all but one of eight phosphate groups. It can be precipitated at very low levels of calcium.

(ii) **Alpha (s2)-casein:** (molecular weight 25,000; 207 residues, 10 prolines).
Concentrated negative charges near N-terminus and positive charges near C-terminus. It can also be precipitated at very low levels of calcium.

(iii) **β-casein:** (molecular weight 24,000; 209 residues, 35 prolines).
Highly charged N-terminal region and a hydrophobia C-terminal region. Very amphiphilic protein acts like a detergent molecule. Self-association is temperaturedependent; will form a large polymer at 20°C but not at 4°C. Less sensitive to calcium precipitation.

(iv) **κ-casein:** (molecular weight 19,000; 169 residues, 20 prolines).
Very resistant to calcium precipitation, stabilizing other caseins. Rennet cleavage at the Phe 105-Met 106 bond eliminates the stabilizing ability, leaving a hydrophobia portion, para- κ-casein and a hydrophilic portion called κ-casein glycomacropeptide (GMP), or more accurately, caseinomacropeptide (CMP).

Uses

It is used in the manufacture of binders, adhesives, protective coatings, plastics (such as for knife handles and knitting needles), fabrics, food additives, and many other products. It is commonly used by bodybuilders as a slow-digesting source of amino acids. There is growing evidence that casein may be addictive for some individuals, particularly those on the autism spectrum or having schizophrenia.

5.3.3 Enzymes

Living organisms produceprotein biocatalystsas primary metabolites which possess catalytic complex chemical reactions of various metabolic pathways that make up life processes, called enzyme. Enzymes are lifeless and when isolated, they still exert their characteristic catalytic effect. Enzymes are formed of polypeptide chains of amino acids that are highly specific for the reaction they catalyze. In the absence of enzymes, the biological reactions would require a long period of time to complete. Enzymes are conservative and do not get spent during chemical reactions. These are involved in almost all forms of metabolic pathways ranging from cellular respiration to internal digestion and absorption. The enzymes produced in various organisms are extracted for their use in industries for processes like fermenting of wine, the leavening of bread, curdling of cheese, and brewing of beer. Some examples of enzymes include lipases, amylases, proteases, etc.

Properties

The chemical property of enzymes vary with type but may show several common properties also.

- They are colloids, soluble in water and dilute alcohol but are precipitated by concentrated alcohol.
- The optimum temperatures of enzymes are between 35-40°C. The deactivation of enzymes may take place at the temperatures above 65°C, especially in the presence of moisture.
- The enzyme activity retardation happens with certain heavy metals, i.e., formaldehyde, free iodine, etc.
- Their activity is markedly affected by the pH. Forexample, pepsin in the stomach has an optimum pH of about 2, whereas salivary amylase has an optimum pH of about 7.
- They are highly selective in their action.
- Enzymes are created in cells but are capable of functioning outside of the cell. This allows the enzymes to be immobilized, without killing them.
- Enzymes only catalyse one reaction, for example, invertase will only produce glucose and fructose, when a glucose solution is passed over beads of enzyme.

Chemistry

The enzymes havehigh molecular weight from about 13,000 to 8,40,000 dalton. They are found in combination with inorganic or organic substances that have an important part in the catalytic action. Non-protein organic compounds are called coenzymes whereas inorganic ions are referred to as activators. Coenzymes are integral components of a large number of enzyme systems. Several vitamins (thiamine, riboflavin, nicotinic acid) have a coenzymatic function.

Classification

At present they are divided according to their action by a complex system established by the Commission on Enzymes of the International Union of Biochemistry (CEIUB). Six major classes are recognized; each has 4 to 13 subclasses, and each enzyme is assigned a systematic code number (BC) composed of 4 digits. The major classes are given in Table 5.6.

Table 5.6 Classification of enzymes

S. No.	Class of enzymes	Reaction catalyzed	Examples
1.	Oxidoreductases	Transfer of electron	Dehydrogenase, oxidase
2.	Transferases	Functional group transfer	Transaminase, Kinases
3.	Lyases	Addition of functional group to double bond	Phospho hexoisomerase, Fumarase
4.	Isomerases	Transfer of groups within molecules to yield isomeric form	Decarboxylases, aldolases
5.	Ligases	Formation of C-C. C-S, C-O and C-N bonds by condensation reaction	Citric acid synthetase

Source and therapeutic role of enzymes

Enzymes are obtained from plant and animal cells and many have been purified.

The enzymes and their therapeutic action is listed below.

Table 5.7 Some enzymes and their therapeutic actions

Name of enzymes	Therapeutic functions
Pepsin, pancreatin, and papain	As digestants.
Hyaluronidase	Facilitates the diffusion of injected fluids.
Streptokinase and streptodornase	Dissolve clotted blood and purulent accumulations
Zymase and rennin	Fermentation and cheese industries
Penicillinase	Inactivates the various penicillins

5.3.3.1 Source of Proteolytic Enzymes

Pepsin

Biological Source

It is the enzyme prepared from the mucous membrane of the stomach of various animals like pig, sheep, or calf. The commonly used species of pig is *Susscrofa* Linn, belonging to family Suidae.

Characteristics

Pepsin binds with protein chains and breaks it up into small pieces preferentially at carboxylic groups of aromatic amino acids such as phenylalanine and tyrosine but does not cleave at bonds containing amino acids like valine or alanine. It mainly cleaves C-terminal to F, L, and E, and it does not cleave at V-, A-, or G-terminals.

Structurally, the active site of pepsin is located in a deep cleft within the molecule. Optimal activity of pepsin is at pH of 1.8-3.5, depending on the isoform. They are reversibly inactivated at about pH 5 and irreversibly inactivated at pH 7-8.

Preparation

By using the process of stripping or scrapping the mucus membrane is separated from the stomach and immediately placed in acidified water for autolysis at 37°C for 2 hours. After autolysis liquid obtained which is composed of both enzyme pepsin and peptone. After filtration liquid mixture is added with sodium or ammonium salts till it get half saturated. At this point only the pepsin separates out, and the peptone remains in the solution. The precipitates are collected and subjected to dialysis for the separation of salts. The pepsin is collected and dried at low temperature.

Table 5.8 Description of pepsin

Physical characteristics	Colour: Pale yellow, Odour: Odourless or with very faint odour, Consistency: Translucent grains Taste: Slightly bitter in taste.
Solubility	Dilute acids, water, and physiological salt (NaCl) solution
pH	Best active at a temperature of 40°C with pH 2–4. Unstable above pH 6
Extra features	Gets denatured at a temperature of 70°C and in the presence of alcohol and sodium chloride.
Storage	1–2 years at 2–8°C.

Uses

Pepsin is also used in the preparation of cheese, and other proteincontaining foods. It is used in laboratory analysis of various proteins. Moreover, it is used in the deficiency of gastric secretion.

Urokinase

Synonym

Uroquinase

Biological source

Urokinase is serine protease enzyme isolated from human urine and from human kidney cells by tissue culture or by recombinant DNA technology.

Preparation

The preparation of urokinase is done by recombinant DNA technology by using genetically manipulated *E. coli* cells. It is a fibrinolytic enzyme produced firstly as prourokinase and then converted to active form by plasmin or kallikrein. Urokinase used medicinally is also purified directly from human urine. It binds to a range of adsorbents such as silica gel or kaolin which can be used to initially concentrate and purify the product. It can be further purified by precipitation with sodium chloride or ethanol or by chromatography. Human urokinase needs sterile filtration, a septic filling and freeze drying.

Chemical constituents

Urokinase enzymes are serine proteases that occur as a single low molecular weight (33 kDa) and double, high molecular weight (54 kDa) polypeptide chain forms. They differ in molecular weight considerably. A single chain is produced by recombinant DNA technique and is known as single chain urokinase plasminogen activator (scuPA).

Uses

Urokinase is used in the treatment of pulmonary embolism, coronary artery thrombosis and for restoring the potency of intravenous catheters. It is generally administered intravenously in a dose of 4400 units/kg body weight per hour for twelve hours.

Streptokinase

Synonym

Estreptokinase, plasminokinase.

Biological source

Streptokinase is an extracellular purified bacterial protein produced from the strains of β-haemolytic *Streptococcus griseus*.

Preparation

Streptokinase is a serine protease group enzyme and its activity lies within the first 230 aminoacid residues at the N-terminal part of the protein that evolves from serine protease due to the replacement of histamine at 57th amino acid by glycine. The amino terminal residue polypeptide chain shows sequence homology to serine protease. Duplication and fusion of gene generate an ancestral streptokinase gene. The streptokinase product of the bacterial culture was preliminary extracted by salt precipitation and then purified by affinity chromatography on plasminogen substituted sepharose-4B in a condition that the plasminogen active site was protected from streptokinase induced activation. The purity of streptokinase was confirmed by SDS-PAGE and its biological activity determined in a specific streptokinase assay. It is produced in the form of a lyophilized powder in sterile vials containing 2,50,000 to 7,50,000 IUs.

Chemical constituents

Streptokinase is the purified bacterial protein with about 484 amino acid residues.

Uses

Streptokinase is the first available agent for dissolving blood clots. Plasmin breaks fibrin clots. Anistreptase or the anisolylated plasminogen streptokinase activator complex (APSAC) can also be used in a similar way for degrading blood clots. Streptokinase and anistreptase are both used in the treatment of pulmonary embolism, venous, and arterial thrombosis and coronary artery thrombosis. It is also sometimes administered along with heparin to counteract a paradoxical increase in local thrombin.

Bromelin

Synonyms

Bromelin, Bromelain.

Biological source

Bromelin is a mixture of proteolytic enzymes isolated from the juice of *Ananas comosus* (pineapple), belonging to family Bromeliaceae.

Geographical source

Pineapple is a native of tropical America. It is grown in almost all parts of the world including India, China, Thai-land, United States, Brazil, Philippines, Mexico, Hawaii, and Taiwan.

Collection and preparation

The ripe fruits are cut off from the plant. The enzyme from fruit and stem are known as fruit bromelin and stem bromelin, respectively. It is isolated from pineapple juice by precipitation with acetone and also with ammonium sulphide.

Chemical constituents

It is a mixture of sulphur containing protein digesting enzymes, called proteolytic enzymes or proteases. It also contains several other substances in smaller quantities, including peroxidase, acid phosphatase, protease inhibitors, and calcium.

Uses

Bromelain is an effective fibrinolytic agent, inhibits platelet aggregation. It is used as a digestive enzyme following pancreatectomy, exocrine pancreas insufficiency and other intestinal disorders.

Bromelain prevents or minimizes the severity of angina pectoris and transcient ischemic attacks (TIA). It is useful in the prevention and treatment of thrombosis and thrombophlebitis. It may even be useful in the treatment of AIDS to stop the spread of HIV. It has no major side effects, except for possible allergic reactions.

Serratiopeptidase

Synonym

Serrapeptase, Serratiopeptidase.

Biological source

Serratiopeptidase is a proteolytic enzyme isolated from nonpathogenic enterobacteria *Serratia E 15*. It is also produced by the larval form of the silk moth.

Preparation

Serratiopeptidase is produced by fermentation technology by using nonpathogenic enterobacteria species such as *Serratia E 15*. The larvae of silk moth produce this enzyme in their intestine to break down cocoon walls. It can thus be obtained from the silk moth larvae.

Chemical constituents

Serratiopeptidase is a proteolytic enzyme of protease type XXVI. The preparation contains 7.1 units/mg solid.

Uses

Serratiopeptidase is the most widely prescribed anti-inflammatory enzyme. It eliminates inflammatory oedema and swelling, accelerates liquefaction of pus and sputum, and enhances the action of antibodies. It is also used as a fast wound healing agent. It is proving to be a superior alternative to the nonsteroidal anti-inflammatory drugs traditionally used to treat rheumatoid arthritis and osteoarthritis. It has wide ranging applications in trauma surgery, plastic surgery, respiratory medicine, obstetrics and gynaecology.

Papain

Synonyms

Papayotin, Vegetable pepsin, Tromasin.

Biological source

Papain is the dried and purified latex of the green fruits and leaves of *Carica papaya*, belonging to family Caricaceae.

Geographical source

The plant is cultivated in Sri Lanka, Tanzania, Hawai, and Florida.

Preparation

It is distributed throughout the plant, but mostly concentrated in the latex of the fruit.

The latex is obtained by making two to four longitudinal incisions, about 1/8 inch deep, on the surface on four sides of nearly mature but green fruits while still on the tree. The incisions are made early in the morning, at intervals of three to seven days. The latex flows freely for a few seconds but soon coagulates. The exudate is collected in nonmetallic containers. The latex is dried as soon as possible after collection. Rapid drying or exposure to sun or higher temperature above 38°C produces dark colour product with weak proteolytic activity. The use of artificial heat yields the better grade of crude papain. The final product should be creamy white and friable.

It is sealed in air-tight containers to prevent loss of activity. If 10% common salt or 1% solution of formaldehyde is added before drying, the product retains its activity for many months.

Chemical constituents

Papain contains several enzymes such as proteolytic enzymes peptidase-I capable of converting proteins into dipeptides and polypeptides, rennin-like enzyme, clotting enzyme similar to pectase and an enzyme having a feeble activity on fats.

The enzymes, papain, papaya proteinase, and chymopapain, have been isolated in crystalline form from the latex. It contains 15.5% nitrogen and 1.2% sulphur. Papain is a protein of 212 amino acids and having a molecular weight of about 23,000 daltons. It is resistant to heat, inactivated by metal ions, oxidants and reagents which react with thiols, and is an endopeptidase activated by thiols and reducing moieties, for example, cysteine, thiosulphate, and glutathione.

Uses

Papain is used to prevent adhesions, infected wounds, protein digestant, anathematic (nematode), episiotomy (incision of vulva).

It is used in dyspepsia, intestinal and gastric disorders, and diphtheria, for dissolving diphtheria membrane; in surgery to reduce incidence of blood clots where thromboplasma is undesirable and for local treatment of buccal, pharyngeal, and laryngeal disorders.

It is used in digestive mixtures, liver tonics, for reducing enlarged tonsils, in prevention of postoperative adhesions, curbuncles, and eschar burns. Also used in meat industry for tenderizing beef, in brewing industry for making chill-proof bear, for degumming natural milk, in preparation of tooth pastes and cosmetics, in tanning industry for bathing skin and hides, and as an ingredient in cleansing solutions for soft contact lenses.

Chemical test

Papain is reacted with a gelatin solution at 80°C in the presence of an activating cysteine chloral hydrate solution for an hour. The solution is cooled to 4°C for long time. The treated solution must not regel in comparison to a blank solution under identical conditions.

Adulteration

Adulterated with arrowroot starch, dried milk of cactus, gutta percha, rice flour and pepsin.

5.3.4 Lipids

The lipids are a large, diverse and naturally occurring organic heterogeneous group of components related to the fatty acids. Characteristically, it is insoluble in water but soluble in non-polar organic solvents, i.e., ether, chloroform and benzene. Chemically, lipids are hydrocarbon compounds present as structural components of cell membranes and act as barrier for polar molecules. Fats and fixed oil, waxes, phospholipids, steroids, etc., belongs to the group of lipids. They occur widely in plant and animal kingdoms.

Types of lipids

These are broadly classified as simple lipids, complex lipids and derived lipids.

1. **Simple lipids:** It is made up of esters of fatty acids with various alcohols. It includes:
    1. **Fats:** They are esters of fatty acids with glycerol. Oils are fats in the liquid state.
    2. **Waxes**: They are esters of fatty acids with higher molecular weight monohydric alcohols.
2. **Complex lipids:** Such lipids consist of esters of fatty acids in addition to alcohol and a fatty acid. These further classified as:
    - (i) **Phospholipids: Phospholipids** are lipids containing a phosphoric acid residue with addition to fatty acids and alcohol, they have nitrogen containing bases and other substituents, e.g., in glycerophospholipids the alcohol is glycerol and in sphingophospholipids the alcohol is sphingosine.

(ii) Glycolipids (glycosphingolipids): They contain lipids with a fatty acid, sphingosine and carbohydrate.

(iii) Other complex lipids: Lipids such as sulfolipids and amino lipids. Lipoproteins may also be placed in this category.

3. **Precursor and derived lipids:** They are uncharged, acylglycerols (glycerides), cholesterol, and cholesteryl esters are known as neutral lipids and are produced by the hydrolysis of simple and complex lipids. These include fatty acids, glycerol, steroids, other alcohols, fatty aldehydes, and ketone bodies, hydrocarbons, lipid-soluble vitamins, and hormones.

Some of the different types of lipids are described below in detail.

Fatty acids

Fatty acids are carboxylic acids (or organic acid), usually with long aliphatic tails (long chains), either unsaturated or saturated.

- **Saturated fatty acids:** Lack of carbon-carbon double bonds indicate that the fatty acid is saturated. The saturated fatty acids have higher melting points compared to unsaturated acids.
- **Unsaturated fatty acids:** Unsaturated fatty acid is indicated when a fatty acid has more than one double bond."Often, naturally occurring fatty acids possess an even number of carbon atoms and are unbranched."

Chemical tests for lipid

1. **Salkowski test:** Sample dissolves in chloroform and adds equal volume of concentrated H_2SO_4. To produce bluish-red to cherry to cherry-red colour.
2. **Liebermann-Burchard test:** Sample is dissolve in chloroform in a dry test tube. Add few drop of acetic anhydride and few drop of concentrated H_2SO_4. The solution turns red, then blue and finally bluish-green.

5.3.4.1 Fixed Oils and Fats

Fixed oils and fats are obtained from plants or animals. They differ only according to their melting points but eventually they belong to the same group in terms of chemical properties. If a substance is liquid at 15.5-16.5°C it is called fixed oil and solid or semisolid at the above temperature, it is called as fat. They are made of two kinds of molecules: glycerol (a type of alcohol with a hydroxyl group on each of its three carbons) and three fatty acids joined by dehydration synthesis. Since there are three fatty acids attached, these are known as triglycerides.

Fats have all single bonds between the carbons in their fatty acid tails, thus all the carbons are also bonded to the maximum number of hydrogens possible. The hydrocarbon chains in these fatty acids are, thus, fairly straight and can pack closely together, making these fats solid at room temperature.

Oils mostly have some double bonds between some of the carbons in the hydrocarbon tail. These oils are called unsaturated fats because of the kinks in the hydrocarbon tails.

Examples of saturated and unsaturated fatty acids are given in the figure below.

Saturated fatty acid	Unsaturated fatty acids
Butyric acid (Butter fat)	Oleic acid (Safflower oil, corn oil)
Palmitic acid (Arachis oil, Sesame oil)	Arachidonic acid (Arachis oil)
Myristic acid (Palm oil)	Linoleic acid (Sunflower oil)
Lauric acid (Coconut oil)	Linolenic acid (Linseed oil)

Fig. 5.16 Saturated and unsaturated fatty acids

Properties

- Fixed oils and fats are insoluble in water and alcohol and are soluble in light petroleum, ether, chloroform, and benzene (exception in solubility is castor oil that is soluble in alcohol because of its hydroxy group of ricinoleic acid).
- They float on water since their specific gravity is less than one.
- They produce a permanent translucent stain on the paper and are called fixed oils.
- Fixed oils and fats cannot be distilled without their decomposition.

Analytical parameters for fats and oils

Following are the parameters to analyse the fats and oils.

1. **Iodine value** is the mass of iodine in gm that is consumed by 100 g of fats or oil. It is a measure of the extent of unsaturation and higher the iodine value, the more chance for rancidity.
2. **Saponification value** is the number of mg of potassium hydroxide required to saponify 1 g of fat under the conditions specified. It is a measure of the average molecular weight of all the fatty acids present.
3. **Hydroxyl value** is the number of mg of potassium hydroxide (KOH) required for neutralizing acetic acid combined with hydroxyl groups, when 1 g of a sample is acetylated.
4. **Ester value** is the number of mg of potassium hydroxide (KOH) required to saponify the ester contained in 1 g of a sample.
5. **Unsaponifiable matter:** The principle is the saponification of the fat or oil by boiling under reflux with an ethanolic potassium hydroxide solution. Unsaponifiable matter is then extracted from the soap solution by diethyl ether. The solvent is evaporated and then the residue is dried and weighed.

6. **Acid value** is the amount of free acid present in fat as measured by the mg of potassium hydroxide needed to neutralize it. As the glycerides in fat slowly decompose the acid value increases.
7. **Peroxide value** is a measure of the concentration of peroxides and hydroperoxides formed in the initial stages of lipid oxidation. Milliequivalents of peroxide per kg of fat are measured by titration with iodide ion. High peroxide values are a definite indication of a rancid fat, but moderate values may be the result of depletion of peroxides after reaching high concentrations. It is widely used to test for oxidative rancidity.

5.3.4.1.1 Fixed oil containing drugs

Castor Oil

Synonyms

Castor bean oil, Castor oil seed, Oleum ricini, Ricinus oil.

Biological source

Castor oil is the fixed oil obtained by cold expression of the seeds of *Ricinus communis*, belonging to family Euphorbiaceae.

Geographical source

It is mainly found in India, Brazil, America, China, Thailand; in India it is cultivated in Gujarat, Andhra Pradesh, and Karnataka.

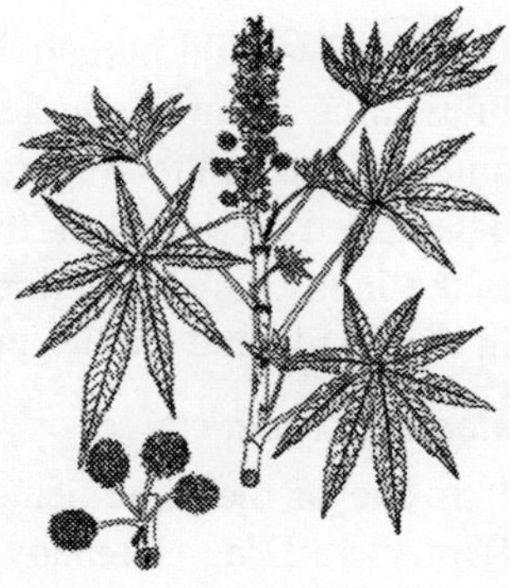

Fig. 5.17 *Ricinus communis*

Preparation

Castor oil is obtained from castor seeds. The oil is obtained in two ways; either after the removal of the seed coat or with the seed coat. Seed coats are removed by crushing the seeds under the grooved rollers and then they are subjected to a current of air to blow the testas. The kernels are fed in oil expellers and at room temperature they are expressed with 1 to 2 tonnes pressure per square inch till about 30% oil is obtained. The oil is filtered, steamed 80-100°C to facilitate the coagulation and precipitation of poisonous principle ricin, proteins and enzyme lipase present in it. Oil is then filtered and this oil with 1% acidity is used for medical purpose.

The oil cake which remains contains of ricin, lipase and about 20% oil. The cake is grounded, steamed to 40° to 80°C, and 3 tonnes pressure per sq. inch is applied. This yields the second quality of oil with 5% acidity and is used for industrial purpose.

The residual cake which remains after the expression of the second quality oil still contains about 8 to 10% oil. This oil is obtained by subjecting it to extraction in soxhlet with lipid solvents. This oil obtained is also used in industry. The residual cake is used as manure and not fed to animal due to the presence of ricin. The cake is also used for the production of lipase.

Chemical constituents

Castor oil consists of glyceride of ricinoleic acid, isoricinoleic, stearic, and dihydroxy stearic acids. Ricinoleic acid is responsible for laxative property. Castor oil also contains vitamin F.

90% of the fatty acid content is ricinoleic acid. The ricinoleic acid is an 18-carbon acid having a double bond in the 9-10 position and a hydroxyl group on the 12th carbon. This combination of hydroxyl group and unsaturation occurs only in castor oil.

Identification tests

About 5 mL of light petroleum (50° to 60°) when mixed with 10 mL of castor oil at 15.5° shows a clear solution, but if the amount of light petroleum is increased to 15 mL, the mixture becomes turbid. This test is not shown by other oils.

Uses

Castor oil is mild purgative, fungistatic, used as an ointment base, plasticizer, wetting agent,and lubricating agent. Ricinoleic acid is used in contraceptive creams and jellies. It is also used as an emollient in the preparation of lipstick, in tooth formulation, as an ingredient in hair oil. The dehydrated oil is used in the manufacture of linoleum and alkyl resin. The main use of castor oil is the industrial production of coatings, also employed to make pharmaceuticals and cosmetics in the textile and leather industries and for manufacturing plastics and fibres.

Marketed Products

It is one of the ingredients of the preparations known as Lip Balm and Muscle and Joint Rub (Himalaya Drug Company).

Chaulmoogra Oil

Synonlyms

Hydnocarpus oil, Gynocardia oil.

Biological source

Chaulmoogra oil is a fixed oil obtained by cold expression from ripe seeds of *Hydnocarpus wightiana*, *H. anthelminticta*, *H. heterophylla*, and other species of Hydnocarpus, belonging to family Flacourtiaceae.

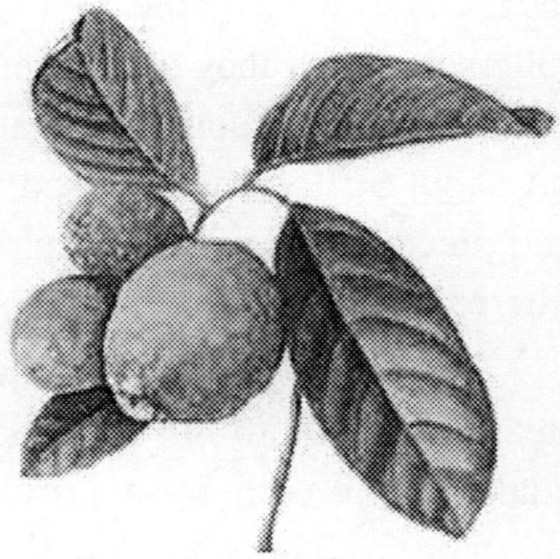

Fig. 5.18 *Hydnocarpus wightiana*

Geographical source

The native of this plant is Burma, Thailand, eastern India, and Indo-China.

Chemical constituents

Chaulmoogra oil contains glycerides of cyclopentenyl fatty acids like hydnocarpic acid (48%), chaulmoogric acid (27%), gorlic acid with small amounts of glycerides of palmitic acid (6%), and oleic acid (12%). The cyclic acids are formed during last 3–4 months of maturation of the fruit and are strongly bactericidal towards the micrococcus of leprosy.

The seed contains a flavonolignan hydnocarpin; isohydnocarpin, methoxy hydnocarpin, apigenin, luteolin, chrysoeriol, hydnowightin, epivolkenin, and cyclopentenoid cyanohydrin glycosides.

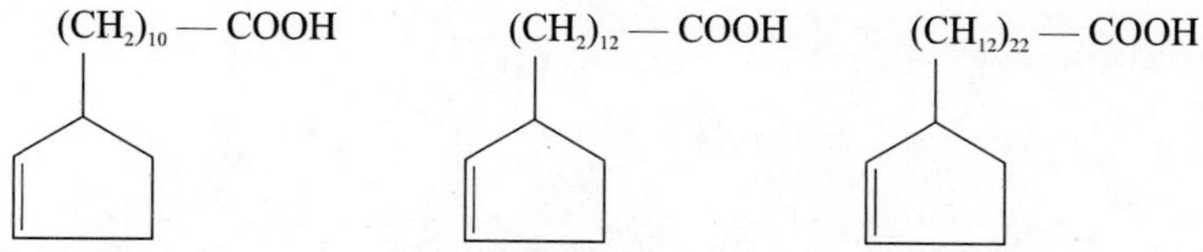

Hydnocarpic acid Chaulmoogric acid Gorlic acid

Fig. 5.19 Chemicals from *Hydnocarpus* species

Uses

The oil is useful as anti-leprotic and skin diseases. The cyclopentenyl fatty acids of the oil responsible for this anti-leprotic potentials. The oil has now been replaced by the ethyl esters and salts of hydnocarpic and chlumoogric acids.

5.3.4.1.2 Fat containing natural products

Lanolin

Synonyms

Wool fat, oesipos, agnin, alapurin, anhydrous lanolin, adeps lanae, laniol

Biological source

Lanolin consists of fat-like purified secretion of the sebaceous glands which is deposited into the wool fibres of sheep, *Ovis aries*, belonging to family Bovidae.

Preparation

Wool obtained from sheep is washed with a soap or alkali solution. An emulsion of wool fat, called wool grease, takes place in water. Raw lanolin is separated by cracking the emulsion with sulphuric acid. Wool grease floats on the upper layer and fatty acids are dissolved in the lower layer. Lanolin is purified by treating with sodium peroxide and bleaching with reagents.

Chemical constituents

The chief constituents of lanolin are cholesterol, isocholesterol, unsaturated monohydric alcohols ($C_{27}H_{45}OH$), lanoceric ($C_{30}H_{60}O_4$), lanopalmitic ($C_{16}H_{22}O_3$), carnaubic and other fatty acids. Lanolin also contains esters of oleic and myristic acids, aliphatic alcohols, such as cetyl, ceryl and carnaubyl alcohols, lanosterol, and agnosterol.

It is a complex mixture of esters and polyesters. There are 33 high molecular weight alcohols, and 36 fatty acids are constituents of Lanolin. The alcohols are of three types; aliphatic alcohols, steroid alcohols, and triterpenoid alcohols. Even though the fatty acids are of three types: saturated non-hydroxylated acids, unsaturated non-hydroxylated acids, and hydroxylated acids.

Liquid lanolin is rich in low molecular weight, branched aliphatic acids, and alcohols, whereas waxy lanolin is rich in high molecular weight, straight-chain acids, and alcohols.

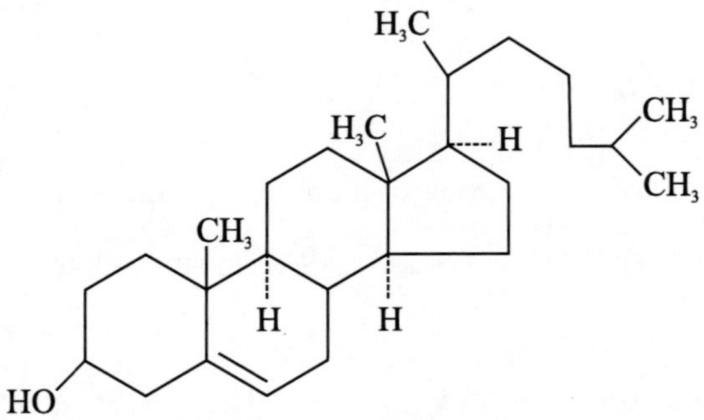

Fig. 5.20 Structure of cholesterol

Identification tests

Dissolve 0.5 g of lanolin in chloroform, and to it add 1 mL of acetic anhydride and two drops of sulphuric acid. A deep green colour is produced, indicating the presence of cholesterol.

Uses

It is used as an emollient, as water absorbable ointment base in many skin creams and cosmetics and for hoof dressing.

5.3.4.2 Waxes

Esters of long-chain fatty acids and alcohols are known as wax. The basic difference between wax and fat is their variation of saponification values. Wax can be saponified with alcoholic alkali where fats may be saponified by alcoholic alkali or by aqueous alkali. Like fatty acids, it also contains monohydroxy alcohols of high molecular weight (e.g., cetyl alcohol, melissyl alcohol, myricyl alcohol, etc.). Cholesterol or phytosterols are also present intermittently. Due to lack of hydrolysing enzymes of wax in body, wax is not edible.

The wide distributions of waxes are found in nature. Many plants contain waxy layer or coating in leaves and fruits, which may defend from dehydration and from small predators too. Spermaceti, beeswax, carnuba wax, etc., are the examples of waxes which have great impact in pharmaceutical industries.

5.3.4.2.1 Wax containing natural products

Beeswax

Synonyms

White beeswax, Yellow beeswax, Cera alba.

Biological source

Beeswax is the purified wax obtained from honeycomb of hive bee, *Apis mellifera* and other species of *A. dorsata, A indica* etc. belonging to family Apidae.

Geographical Source

It is mainly found in Jamaica, Egypt, Africa, India, France, Italy, etc.

Preparation

The wax is secreteed from last four segments of abdomen on the ventral surface of worker bees in honeycomb due to maintaining a high temperature. Just below the sterna it has a smooth porous layer of cells form the chitinous area that secretes the wax. While passing through mouth via front leg, it gets mixed with the saliva, which is then built on the comb. This wax forms a capping on the honey cells.

Honeycomb or the capping is melted in boiling water soon after removal of honey. The melted wax gets solidified on cooling and floats on the water. In the meantime the impurities settle below and honey leftovers get dissolved in water. The pure wax is then poured into earthen vessels wiped with damp cloth and the wax so obtained is yellow beeswax.

White beeswax generally obtained from yellow beeswax. The yellow beeswax is run on a thin stream of spinning wet drum, from which long ribbon like strips are scrapped off. The ribbon strips are placed on cloth in thin layers, rotated from time to time and bleached in sunlight till the outer layer becomes white. White beeswax is obtained by treating yellow beeswax chemically with potassium permanganate, chromic acid or chlorine or charcoal.

Chemical constituents

Beeswax contains myricin, which is melissyl palmitate; melting point 64°C, free cerotic acid ($C_{26}H_{52}O_2$), myricyl alcohol ($C_{30}H_{61}OH$) is liberated when myricyl palmitate is saponified. Melissic acid, some unsaturated acids of the oleic series, ceryl alcohol, and 12 to 13% higher hydrocarbons are present.

Uses

Beeswax is used in the preparation of ointments, plaster, and polishes.

Adulterants

Beeswax is adulterated by solid paraffin, ceresin, carnauba wax, or other fats and waxes of animal or mineral origin.

In yellow wax the iodine value is also of use as a test for detection of adulterants but in white wax the bleaching process has altered the bodies which absorb the iodine.

Marketed products

Saaf Organic Eraser Body Oil and Jatyadi tel (Dabur).

5.4 MARINE DRUGS: NATURAL BIOACTIVE COMPOUNDS

Almost three-fourths of the earth's surface is covered by sea and oceans; where almost 5,00,000 species of marine organisms like invertebrates and algal species are residing over there. Only a miniscule portion of this mysterious water world has been explored.

The marine flora and its residential living world are a great source of biologically potent compounds. The animals, plants and other microorganisms living in this extreme environment in the deep waters may produce different metabolites (secondary metabolites) compared to teristerial living organisms.

Ancient civilizations of Greece, Japan, China and India have explored some sea living as a potent source of drugs, like alginic acid, spermaceti, agar, carrageenan, protamine sulphate, cod liver oil, halibut liver oils, etc. All these products have a huge market value.

Simultaneous distributions of major organic matter produced by the marine organisms are found in different habitats; they are coral reefs, mangrove swamps and sea grass meadows. Different habitats produce, different yield of products which may have symmetric action.

In he last half of the twentieth century numerous novel marine compounds have been isolated and evaluated for their pharmacological activities like antineoplastic or antitumour, anticoagulants, antimicrobial, anti-inflammatory, antiparasitic, antibacterial, antiviral, etc. A large number of chemical classes are explored from the ocean womb mainly terpenes, shikimates, alkaloids, peptides, acctogenin, polyketides, etc. These chemicals are mixed biosynthetic products and also have their own chemical structure, differing from others. It may be believed that those differentiations occur due to vast diversity of marine world and their variety of habitats. All marine compounds possess a unique chemical structure. Strong variation is also observed in the nutrients and their level of concentration for the plant of sea origin at seasonal or of successional characters. The extreme condition like low temperature and low intensity light may be the key factor for different component deposition like high nitrate concentration in winter session and comparatively low at spring. Moreover different micronutrients like trace elements and vitamins variations are frequently observed on those marine organisms.

If you look around the various parts of the world, the traditional uses or utilization of marine products is not that much rare. Ocean derived seaweeds have been undoubtedly used in several kinds of human ailments or treatment of anaemic conditions in pregnancy, in iodine deficiency, even as vitamin supplement. Other marine species like *Cystoseria barbata*, *Sargassum conusam*, *Jania rubens*, etc., have also been utilized for the treatment of intestinal problems, worm infections, reduction of high cholesterol level, reduction of glucose in blood (hypoglysemic), etc.

In New Zeland, scabies has been treated with seaweeds (*Durvillaea antractica*) where as burns and wounds are dressed with seaweed (*Prophyra atropurpurea*) in Hawaii.

Historical Perspective and Current Status

Seaweedbased recipes for a number of disorders such as pain, abscesses, menstrual difficulties and cancer are recommended in Chinese pharmacopoeia. Seaweed remedies are also used by the San Blas Indians in Panama and Romans attributed medicinal effects to some marine animals. Natural products derived from marine organisms have been the focus of many investigations in the last quarter of this century. Representative examples of marine derived therapeutics include Manoalide, a non-steroidal sesterpenoid, a novel marine compound that might be considered a prototype with therapeutic potential as anti-inflammatory and as analgesic. Manoalide is the first inhibitor of phospholipase A2 and is being explored in a number of disorders. Discodermolide is a novel polyhydroxylated lactone with potent immunosuppressive activity being, *in vivo*, 100-1000 times more potent than cyclosporine-A and that also harbours cytotoxic activity. The available data with the antimalarial compound axinositrile 3 indicates activity in resistant strains and anticipates an important potential in the clinical setting. Also, new polyesters with antifungal activity have been discovered from the marine dinoflagellate

Gambierdiscus toxicus. These chemical entities are the most potent antifungal agents discovered, with *in vitro* potency 2000-fold higher than anfotericin-B and with moderate toxicity against mammalian cells. Such data gives evidence of a positive therapeutic index and indicates a favourable tolerability profile in the clinical setting. In addition, a number of approaches incorporating targeted based discovery models are yielding to the identification of novel entities with therapeutic potential in a number of diseases; for instance, conotoxins are selective peptide antagonists/agonists of ionic channels and G-proteinreceptors that have shown relevant activity in chronic pain and potential in other conditions.

Marine natural products have been discussed on the basis of their source, chemical characterization and specific pharmacological uses. By using this concept marine obtained drugs are classified to two classes:

1. Based on phytochemical structures
2. Based on pharmacological uses.

5.4.1. Based on Phytochemical Structures

5.4.1.1 Marine Derived Alkaloids

Heterogeneous group of basic nitrogen containing compounds are called alkaloids or alkali-like substances. They contribute a vast number of classes of natural products and are synthesized in almost all the evolutionary levels in terrestrial plants, microorganisms and marine organisms. Alkaloids usually exist as a mixture of several major and a few minor compounds of the same biosynthetic origin and differ only in functional groups in an organism. They usually contain one or two nitrogen atoms on their structure but sometimes it may increase to five, for example, ergotamine from ergot. Alkaloids possess a highly potent pharmacological data and some often high toxic molecule against various pathogens by apparently evolving in the defence mechanism.

Marine derived alkaloids closely resemble the endogenous amines like serotonin, dopamine or histamine. Their potential pharmacological action on neurological targets and consequential impact on animal behaviour is virtually unexplored. Indole alkaloids are one of the most promising classes of alkaloids identified so far.

Recent and potential pharmaceuticals belong to the marine derived indole alkaloid group has been discussed in this part of this topic including small molecule natural indole alkaloids with their biological actions, and their potential to treat different human ailments.

The alkaloids found in marine algae may be divided into three groups.

(a) Phenylethylamine alkaloids,
(b) indole and halogenated indole alkaloids, and
(c) other alkaloids.

According to the structural similarity, the marine algae derived alkaloids mostly belong to the two different chemical groups, i.e., phenylethylamine and indole. The proper investigations of their biological activities have not been fully investigated. The characteristics of marine derived alkaloids are very uncommon and rare comparatively existent terrestrial plant alkaloids. Most of the marine alkaloidal drug research has been primarily focused on finding drugs for treatment of cancer.

The first alkaloid isolated from marine algae was hordenine in 1969. Till date, approximately it reached up to two thousand alkaloids which were extensively found from marine floras and especially in marine algae. For example, two derivatives: lophocladine A and lophocladine B isolated from a red alga *Lophocladia* sp., and their anticancer activity has been proved successfully in various cancer cell lines.

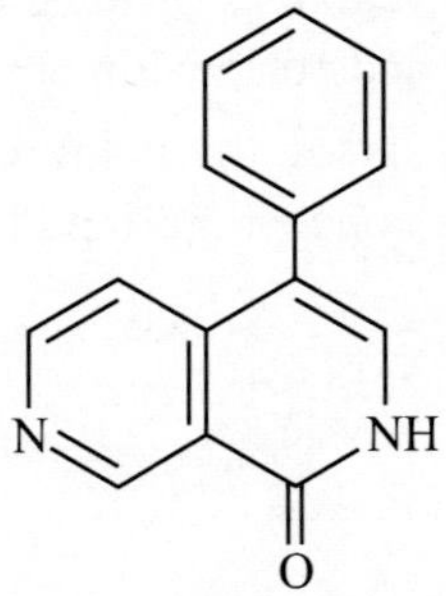

Fig. 5.21(a) Lophocladine A

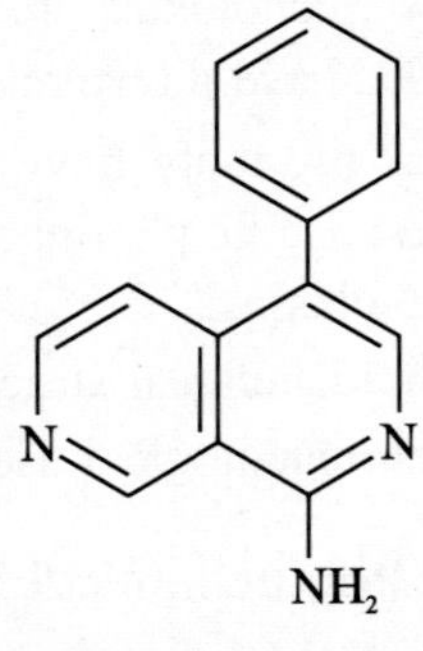

Fig. 5.21(b) Lophocladine B

Coastal mangroves do contain alkaloids of anticancer activity. Brugine a sulphur containing alkaloid; in *Bruguiera sexangula*, and benzoquinones in *Aegiceras corniculatum* and *Kandelia kandel* have been recorded.

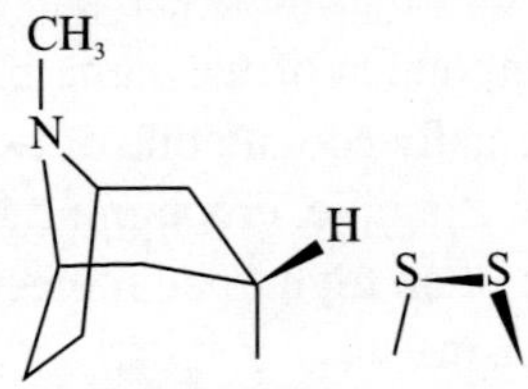

Fig. 5.22 Brugine

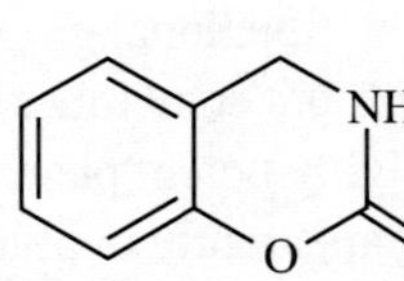

Fig. 5.23 Benzoxazolinone

Cribrostatin 3

A bis-tetrahydroquinoline alkaloid was isolated from the sponge *Cribrochalina* sp. and found to be a potent antimicrobial activity against *Neisseria gonorrheae*, in microgramme quantity and also very strongly active against penicillin-resistant, *N. gonorrheae*. Another nitrogen heterocyclic sponge constituent cribrostatin 6 was isolated later and found to be more promising lead antibiotic for Gram-positive bacteria, particularly *Streptococcus pneumoniae*, including multidrug-resistant strains.

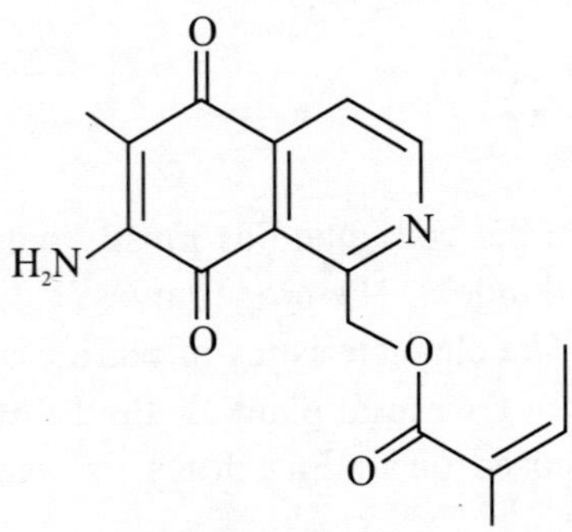

Fig. 5.24 Cribrostatin 3

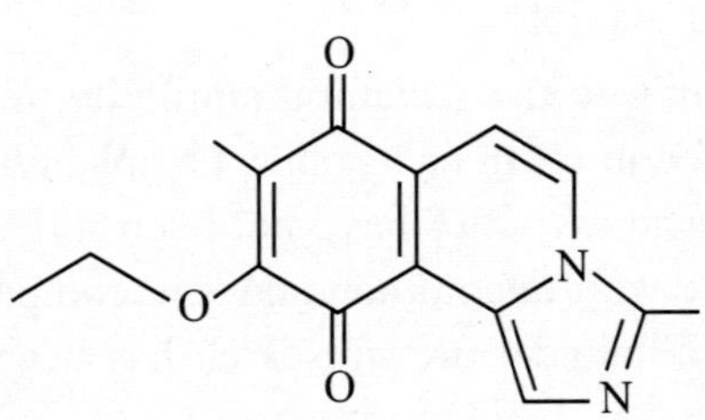

Fig. 5.25 Cribrostatin 6

Alkylpiperidine and alkylpyridine alkaloidal class of alkaloids are contributed by marine sponge species. In this context four alkylpiperidine alkaloids, i.e., Haliclonacyclamine E and Arenosclerins A, B, and C were isolated from a sponge, *Arenosclera brasiliensis*, which displayed a strong antimicrobial activity against different strains of pathogenic bacteria. The length of the alkyl chain, the presence of charged pyridinium moiety, and bromine atom in the structure of the tested substance are important factors that determine its bioactivity. Both, natural poly-APS and synthetic derivatives, were chemically stable in water, showed a broad-spectrum activity against both Gram-positive and Gram-negative bacteria. These sponge derived substances are in structural modifications found as alkylpyridines and related pyridinium salts.

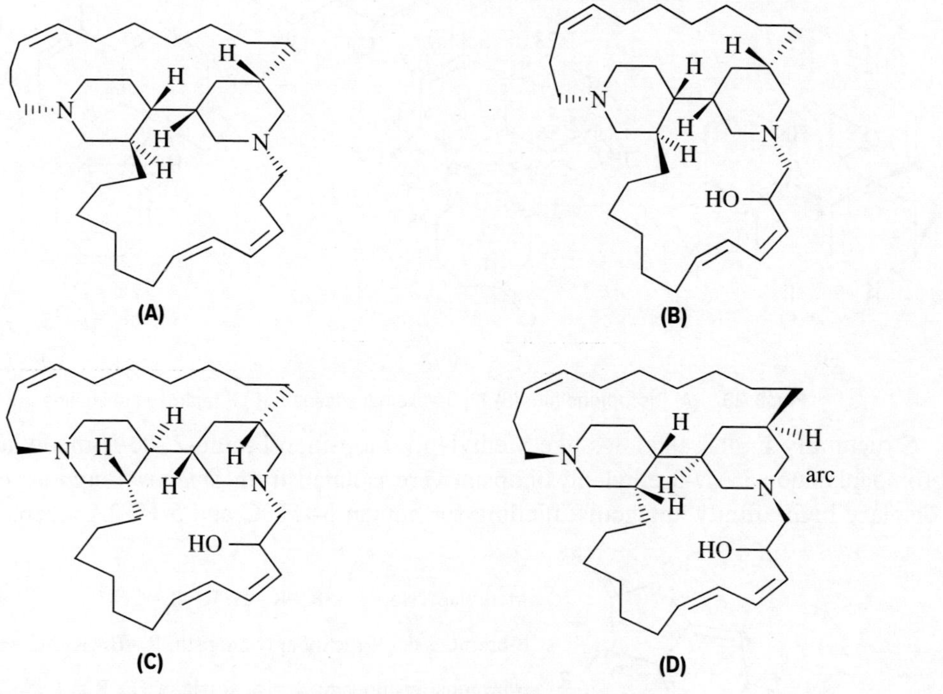

Fig. 5.26 (A) *Haliclonacyclamine E*, (B) *Arenosclerin A*, (C) *Arenosclerin C*, (D) *Arenosclerin B*

Another compound from this group of alkaloids, Haliclonacyclamine A was isolated from the Haliclona sponge which acts as a powerful in vitro and in vivo anti-plasmodial agent against the chloroquine-resistant *Plasmodium falciparum* strain FCB1and *Plasmodium vinckei petteri*.

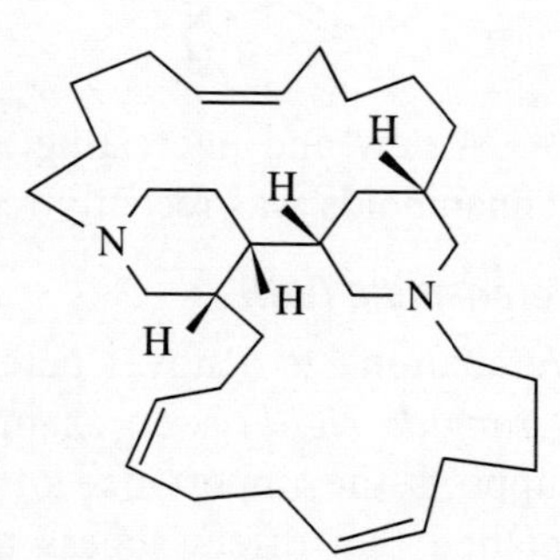

Fig. 5.27 Haliclonacyclamine A

Manzamine alkaloids

Three manzaminetype alkaloids, 12,34-oxamanzamine E, 8-hydroxymanzamine J, and 6-hydroxymanzamine E, were isolated from an *Acanthostrongylophora* species. All three manza-mines were active against mycobacterium tuberculosis with minimum inhibitory concentration and these substances show very promising anti-parasitogenic activity, but they cannot be obtained in a large amount from the sponges.

Discorhabdin R

Discorhabdin R, an antibacterial pyrroloiminoquinone alkaloid, was isolated from the southern Australian sponges *Negombata* sp. and an antarctic *Latrunculia* sp.

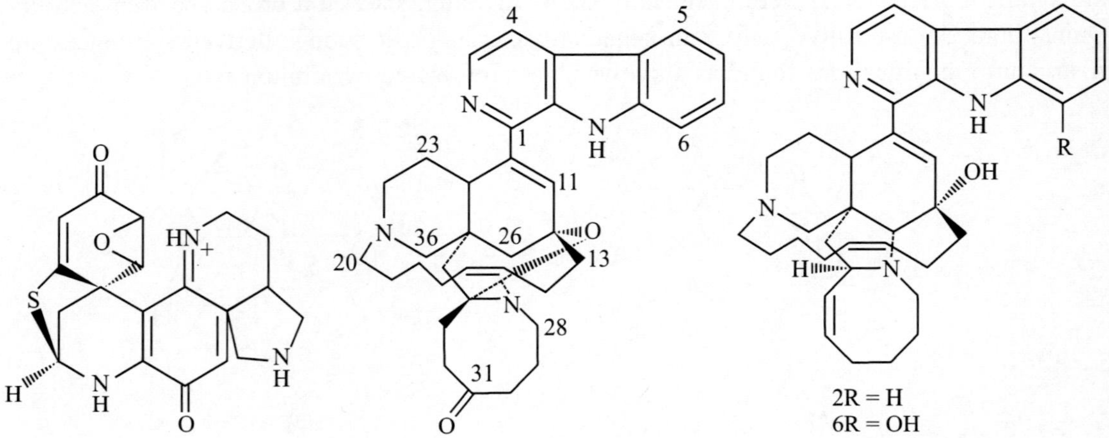

(A) (B) (C)

Fig. 5.28 (A) Discorhabdin R, (B) 12, 34-oxamanzamine E (C) 8-hydroxymanzamine J

Structurally similar alkaloids like Methylaplysinopsin, 6-bromo-2′-de-*N*-methylaplysinopsin, 6-bromoaplysinopsin, *N*-3-ethylaplysinopsin were isolated from *Smenospongia aurea* which act as displace high-affinity antagonist binding for human 5-HT2C and 5-HT2A receptors

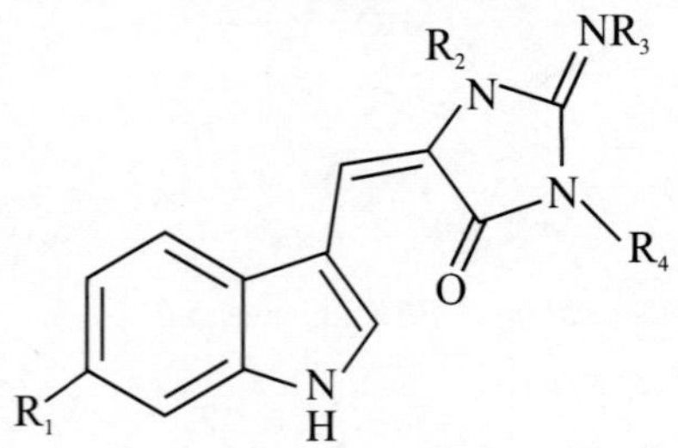

Methylaplysinopsin, R_1=R_3=H, R_2=R_4=CH_3

6-bromo-2′de-N-methylaplysinopsin, R_1=Br, R_2=R_3=H, R_4=CH_3

6-bromoaplysinopsin: R_1=Br, R_2=R_4=CH_3, R_3=H

N-3-ethylaplysinopsin: R_1=H, R_2=R_4=CH_3, R_3=CH_2CH_3

A new and interesting marine metabolite, sharing structural similarities with indoles and cannabinoids was recently reported to possess promising antidepressant activity.

Veranamine (VRI)

Veranamine is a novel patented compound, isolated from *Verongida rigida* is an example of an unusual structure and supports the importance of isolation often being the only method that offers access to structurally new and unique molecules which could not be readily synthesized for a biological evaluation. Chemically, VRI is 8-bromo-4,5,5-trimethyl-5,6-dihydrobenzo[c][2,7]naphthyridine and used

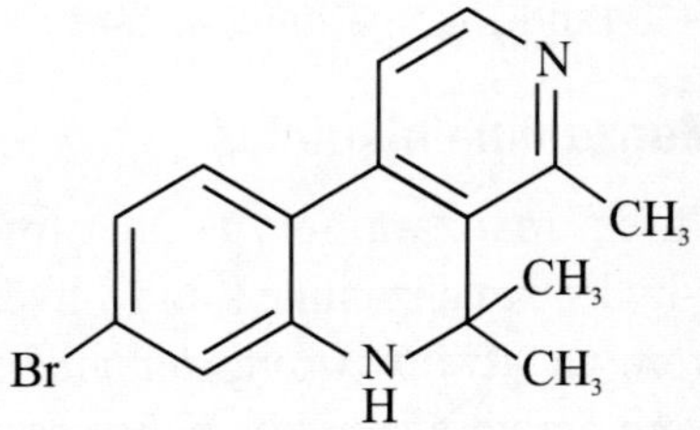

Fig. 5.29 VRI

to treat mental disturbances and neurotic and psychic origin or neurological disorders such as depression.

5.4.2 Marine Derived Polysaccharides

Polysaccharides or glycans are chemically a group of chemical compounds consisting of monosaccharide D-glucose. But simultaneously other monosaccharide like D-fructose, D-galactose, L-galactose, D-mannose, L-arabinose, and D-xylose are also present on them. Some monosaccharide derivatives found in polysaccharides including the amino sugars like D-glucosamine, D-galactosamine, etc., or as their various derivatives like *N*-acetylneuraminic acid and *N*-acetylmuramic acid or as simple sugar acids like glucuronic and iduronic acids, etc.

The interest about marine seaweed derived polysaccharides in various medical and pharmaceutical fields is not much older approach; may be only few years early with its increasing popularity and demand. Various pharmaceutical significant polysaccharides from algal origin include alginates, agar, and carrageenans, etc.

The algal polysaccharides contain active principals, mainly sulphated polysaccharids which are capable to enhance the innate immune response by promoting the tumoricidal activities of macrophages and natural killer cells. Recent studies have implicated that sulphated polysaccharides recognize a range of cell adhesion systems. It can bind to CD_2, CD_3, and CD_4 in T lymphocytes and enhance the proliferative response of T lymphocytes. Sulphated polysaccharides can enhance the adaptive immune response by promoting such process.

Agar

Agar is primarily obtained from red algae which belongs to the genera *Gelidium* and *Gracilaria*. It is an unbranched polysaccharide and chemically, it is constituted by galactose sugar molecules. Agar present in the cell membranes of red algae provides the primary structural support for the algal cell walls.

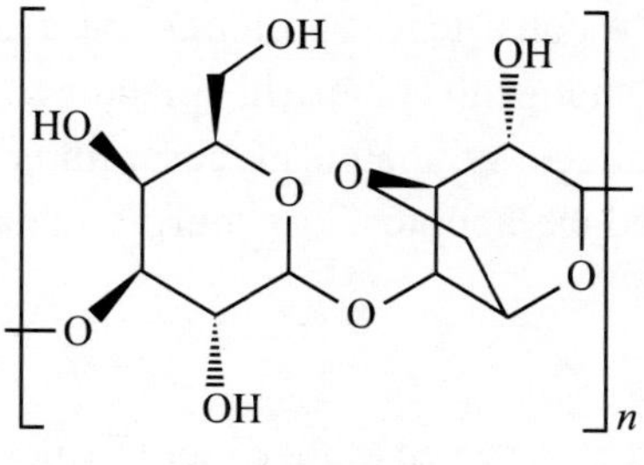

Fig. 5.30 Agar

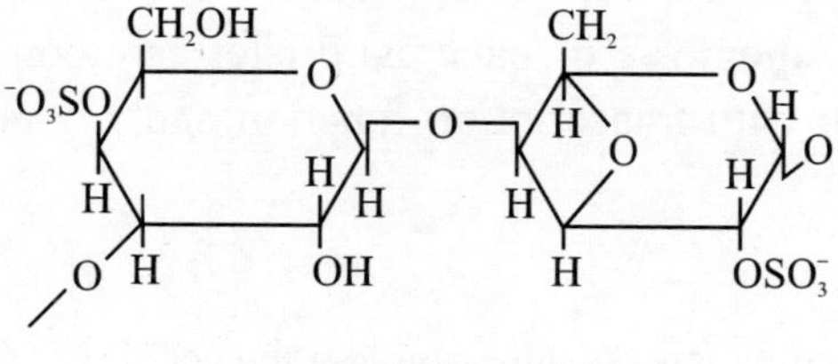

Fig. 5.31 Carrageenan

Carrageenans

Carrageenans are high molecular weight sulphated D-galactans composed of repeating disaccharide units with alternating 3-linked D-galactopyranose (G-units) and 4-linked galactopyranose (D-units) or 3,6-anhydro-galactopyranose (AnGal-units) obtained from red seaweed *Kappaphycus alvarezii*. Carrageenans are normally classified according to their structural characteristics, including their sulphation patterns and the presence or absence of AnGal on D-units. The most industrially relevant carrageenans are κ, ι and λ forms.

B-1

B-1, a sulphated polysaccharide composed of a trisaccharide (galactose, glucose and suphate at a molar ratio 2:1:2) repeating unit, isolated from the marine bacterium culture filtrate of *Pseudomonas* strain WAK-1 which was originally isolated from the brown seaweed *Undaria pinnatifida* produced extracellular sulphated B-1. It can induce apoptosis of human leukaemic cells.

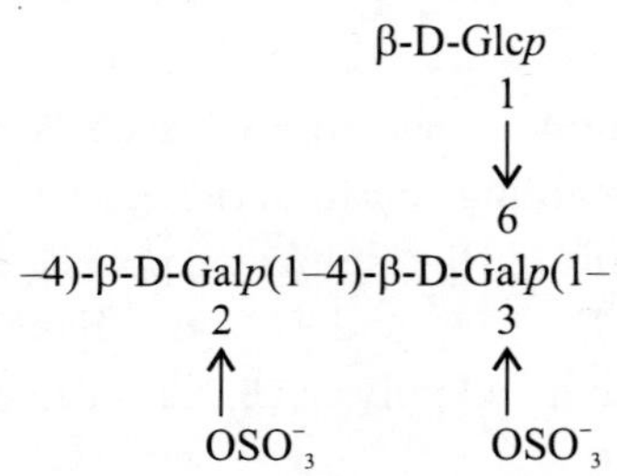

Fig. 5.32 B-1

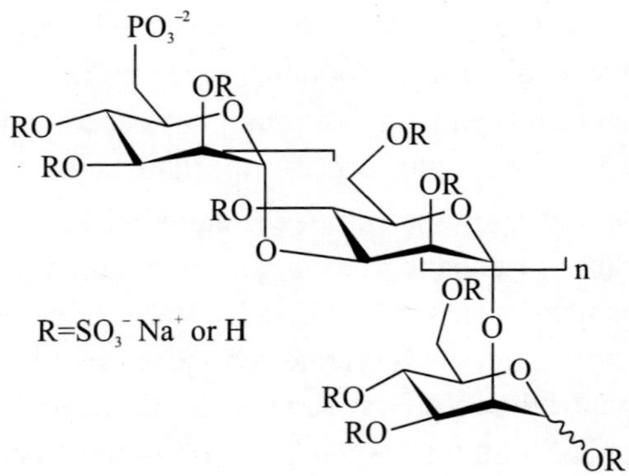

Fig. 5.33 PI-88

PI-88

PI-88 is a highly sulphonated oligosaccharide obtained as a randomly, but reproducibly, sulphated mixture with an average sulphation of three sulphates per mannose residue and a molecular weight of 2100-2585 Da. PI-88 inhibits heparanase activity and competes with heparan sulphate binding of peptide growth factors involved in angiogenesis. PI-88 consistently prolongs the activated partial thromboplastin time (APTT) through activation of endogenous heparin cofactor II. PI-88 induces apoptosis of pancreatic islet carcinoma. Internalized sulphated glycosaminoglycans interfere with transcription function and subsequently induce apoptosis of murine melanoma cells.

Ulvan

Ulvan is the major water-soluble polysaccharide found in green seaweed of the order Ulvales (*Ulva* and *Enteromorpha* sp.) that has sulphate, rhamnose, xylose, iduronic and glucuronic acids as main constituents. Ulvan structure shows great complexity and variability as evidenced by the numerous oligosaccharides repeating structural units identified in nativeand chemically modified. The main repeating disaccharide units reported areulvanobiouronic acid 3-sulphate types containing either glucuronic or iduronic acid. Additionally, minor repeat units have been reported that contain sulphated xylose replacing the uronic acid or glucuronic acid as a branch on *O*-2 of the rhamnose-3-sulphate.

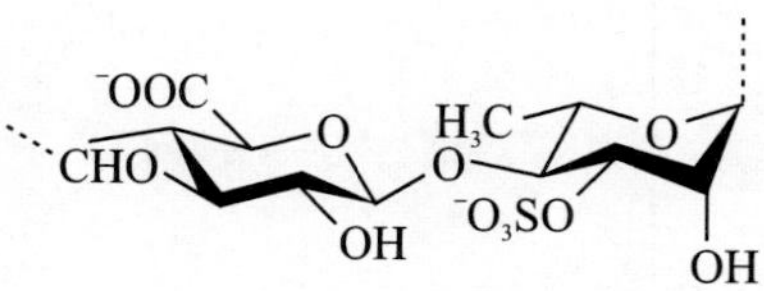

Fig. 5.34 Ulvan A

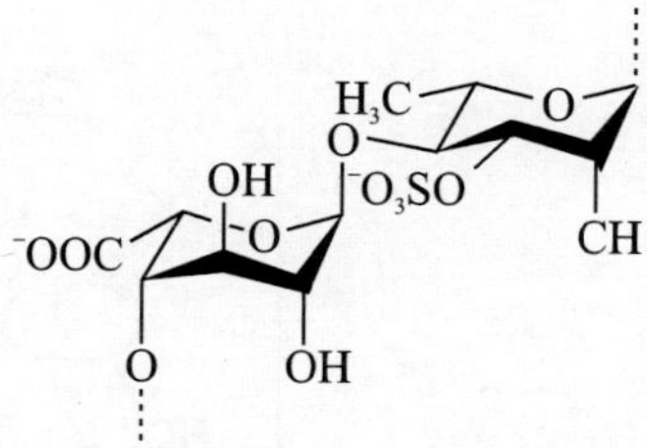

Fig. 5.35 Ulvan B

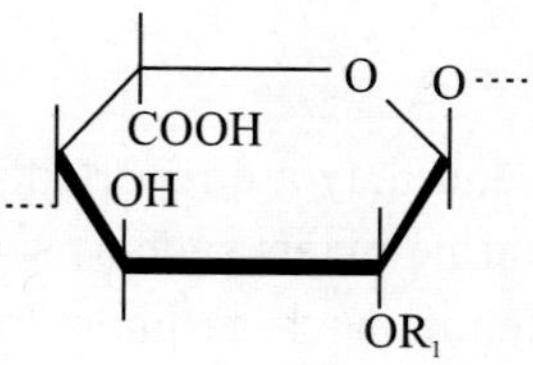

Fig. 5.36 Iduronic acid

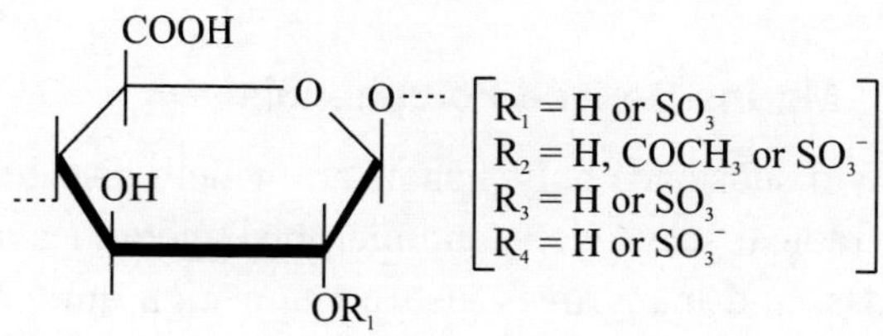

Fig. 5.37 Glucuronic acid

Fucoidan

Fucoidan is one of the sulphated polysaccharides (sulphated L-fucose) derived from cell wall of brown algae. Its sulphation and molecular weight, and the conformation of its sugar residues vary with the seaweed species.

Fucoidans have diverse biological properties, on cellular processes and binding proteins such as adhesion proteins, growth factors, cytokines, and a variety of enzymes, including coagulation proteases. They can also modulate clinically relevant phenomena such as angiogenesis, tumour metastasis, and atherosclerosis. Furthermore, heparan sulphate, pentosan sulphate and chondroitin sulphate, which exhibit anticoagulant activities, inhibit angiogenesis.

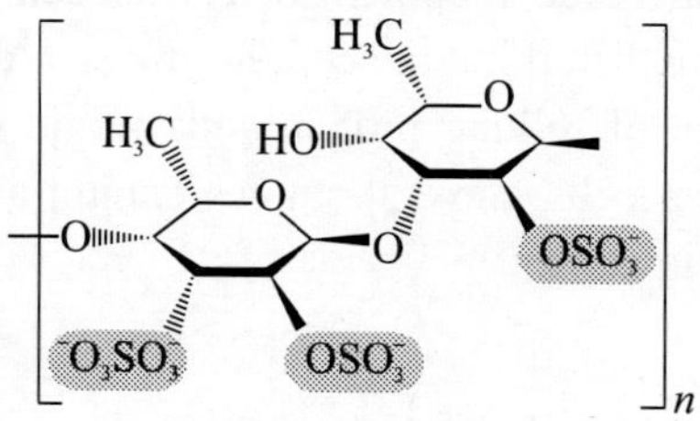

Fig. 5.38 Fucoidan

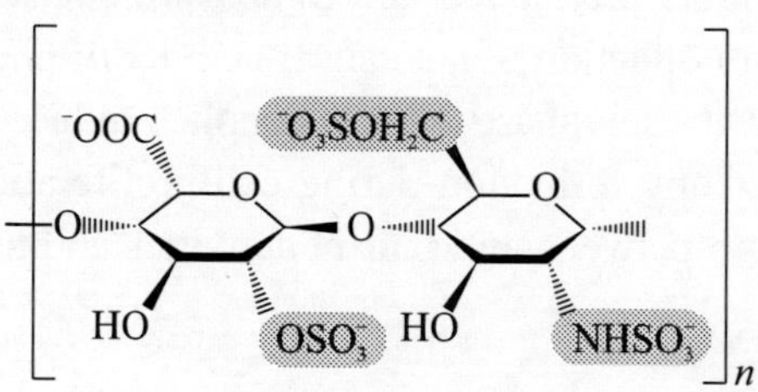

Fig. 5.39 Heparan sulphate

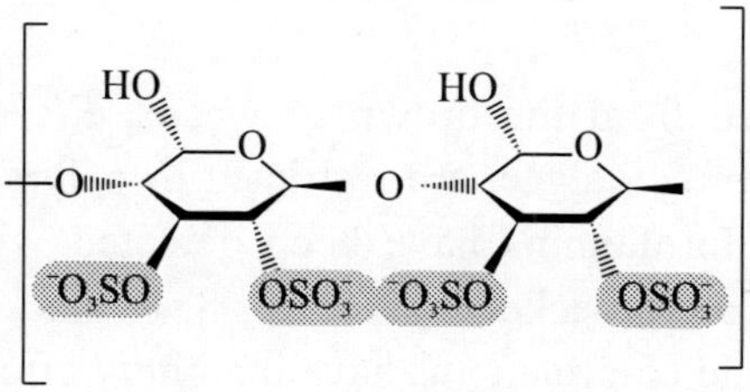

Fig. 5.40 Pentosan sulphate

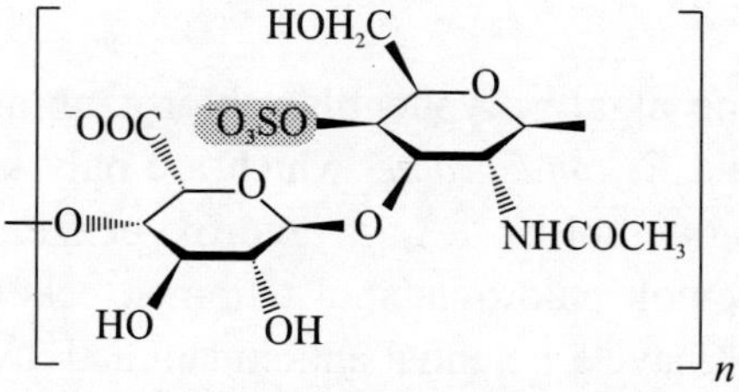

Fig. 5.41 Chondroitin 4 sulphate

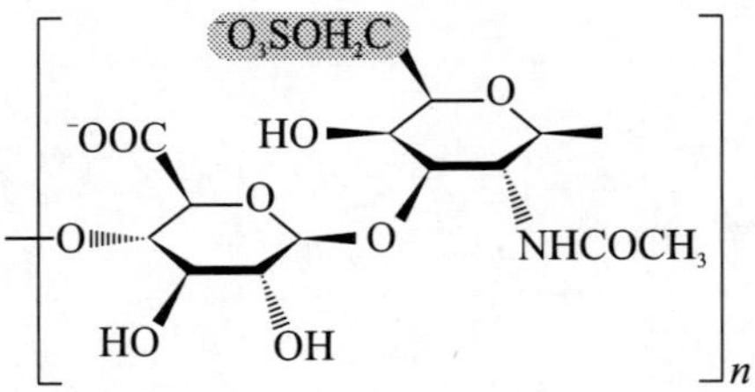

Fig. 5.42 Chondroitin 6 sulphate

5.4.3 Marine Derived Polyphenols

The phyto substance polyphenols are widely distributed in plants and they are reportedly acting as free radical scavengers, antimicrobial and anticancer agents. Marine plants such as seaweeds, sea grass, and mangroves also contain high amounts of polyphenols such as phenolic acids, flavonoids, anthocyanidins, lignin, tannins, catechin, epicatechin, epigallocatechin, and gallic acid.

These polyphenolic compounds have shown many health benefiting bioactivities, such as antioxidant, anticancer, antiviral, anti-inflammatory, and an ability to inhibit human platelet aggregation. Some studies have shown a positive correlation between the increased dietary intake of natural antioxidants and the reduced coronary heart disease, cancer mortality, as well as longer life expectancy. Moreover, they are natural metal chelators with high antioxidant activity that may be successfully used to prevent a variety of toxic metal ion-induced organ dysfunctions. Polyphenols may regenerate α-tocopherol through reduction of the α-tocopheroxyl radical. A close association between anticarcinogenic activity and antioxidant activity has been reported with low-molecular weight polyphenols. Polyphenolic compounds inhibit cancer cells by xenobiotic metabolizing enzymes that alter metabolic activation of potential carcinogens, while some flavonoids can also alter hormone production and inhibit aromatase to prevent the development of cancer cells. The mechanism of action of anticancer activity of phenolics is by disturbing the cellular division during mitosis at the telophase stage. Phenolics reduce the amount of cellular protein and mitotic index, and the colony formation during cell proliferation of cancer cells. Several studies exhibit a close relationship between antioxidant activities and total phenolic content.

Scutellarein

The red alga *Osmundea pinnatifida* (Hudson) Stackhouse, led to the isolation of a flavone, which was assigned as Scutellarein 4'-methyl ether that possess antiallergic, anticancer and anticytotoxic activities.

Marine algal polyphenols, phlorotannins, obtained from the brown seaweeds, *Eisenia bicyclis* and *Ecloniakurome*, which are only known in brown algae, are restricted to polymers of phloroglucinol or 1,3,5-trihydroxybenzene. Six phlorotannins have been detected, viz., phloroglucinol, phloroglucinol tetramer, eckol, phlorofucofuroeckol A, dieckol, 8, 8, bieckol, etc., which have a potential antioxidant activity. The crude phlorotannins have inhibitory effects on HAase. The half maximal inhibition (IC_{50}) values of crude phlorotannins inhibit four times stronger than that by an anti-allergic drug.

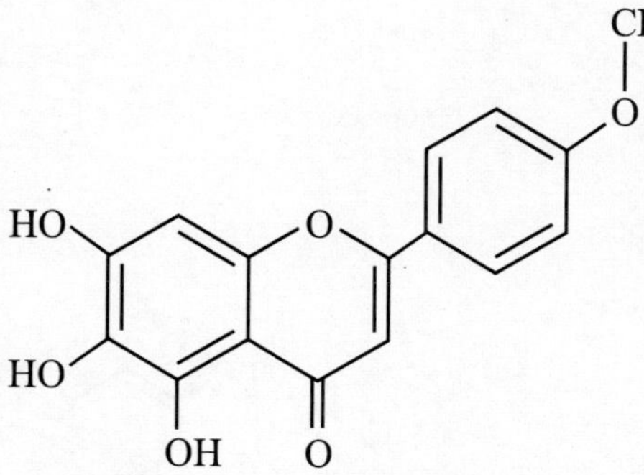

Fig. 5.43 Scutellarein 4′-methyl ether

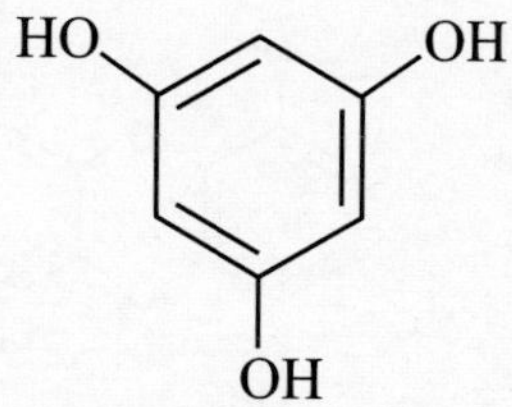

Fig. 5.44 Phloroglucinol

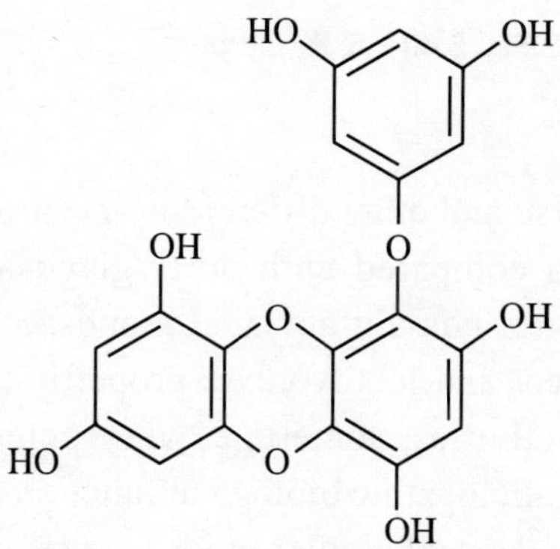

Fig. 5.45 Ecol

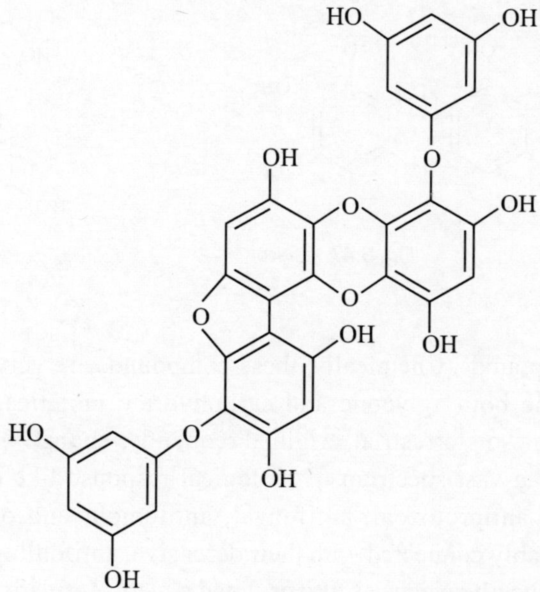

Fig. 5.46 Phlorofucofuroecol A

5.4.4 Marine Derived Glycosides

Widely found secondary metabolites like triterpene and steroid glycosides are also derived from numerous marine animals. Triterpene glycosides were also isolated from sea cucumbers like (Holothurioidea, Echinodermata), in which they have been found in all the orders of this class. Steroid glycosides from starfish (Asteroidea, Echinodermata) compose another well-known group of bioactive marine glycosides, some of them were partly reviewed along with different bioactive sesterterpenes and triterpenes isolated from sponges. There are almost 170 unusual sponge glycosides were isolated from the species of Astrophorida and Poecilosclerida.

Different sponge glycosides have aglycones of a great diversity with alicyclic bi-, tri- or tetracyclic aglycones. There is not only mono- and biosides, but also oligoglycosides among

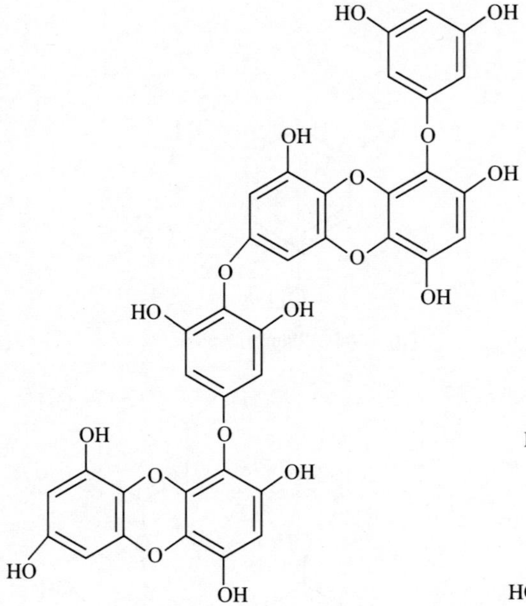

Fig. 5.47 Diecol

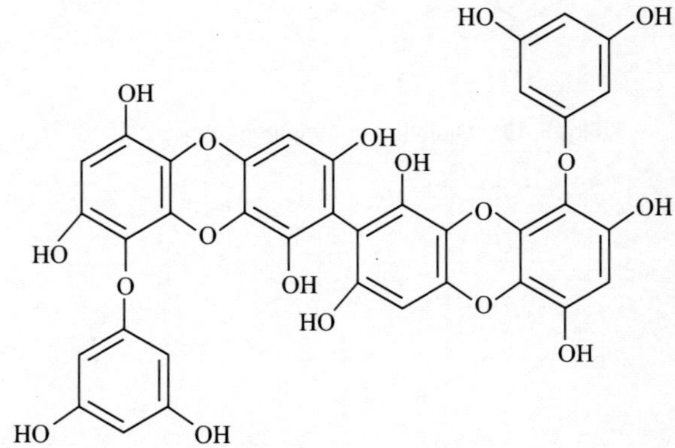

Fig. 5.48 8, 8′- Biecol

compounds. Chemically, these compounds are very diverse and quite different in the structures of the both aglycone and carbohydrate moieties, when compared with other glycosides of marine or terrestrial origin. Frequently, sponge glycosides contain acylated monosaccharide units a vast spectrum of biological response like deterrent and ichthyotoxic properties, along with antiprotozoal, antifungal, antitumour and other activities, sometimes very potent and probably connected with their defensive, antifouling, and allelopathic biological functions. Such sponge glycosides as glycosylated acyclic derivatives and unusual bipolar lipids are presumably membrane constituents of sponge cells, modulating their membrane properties.

Sarasinosides A

Sarasinosides are the tetracyclic triterpene glycosides widely obtained from a sponge species Melophlus *sarasinorum*, belongs to the family Ancorinidae. It is also known in literature as *Asteropus sarasinorum*, *Melophlus isis* and *Stellettinopsis isis* as junior synonymic names of the same species. The glycoside fraction of *Melophlus sarasinorum* contains complicated mixture of 14-nor-methyl-lanostane (or 30-norlanostane) triterpene glycosides.

Thus, totally 23 sarasinosides were isolated from *Melophlus sarasinorum*. Most of these glycosides are pentaosides and their carbohydrate chains may differ in the third monosaccharide unit (glucose or xylose) only. Sarasinoside A possesses strong activity against the yeast *Saccharomycescerevisiae*, but it is inactive against the bacteria *Bacillus subtilis* and *Escherichia coli*. It can be used in the treatment of HIV.

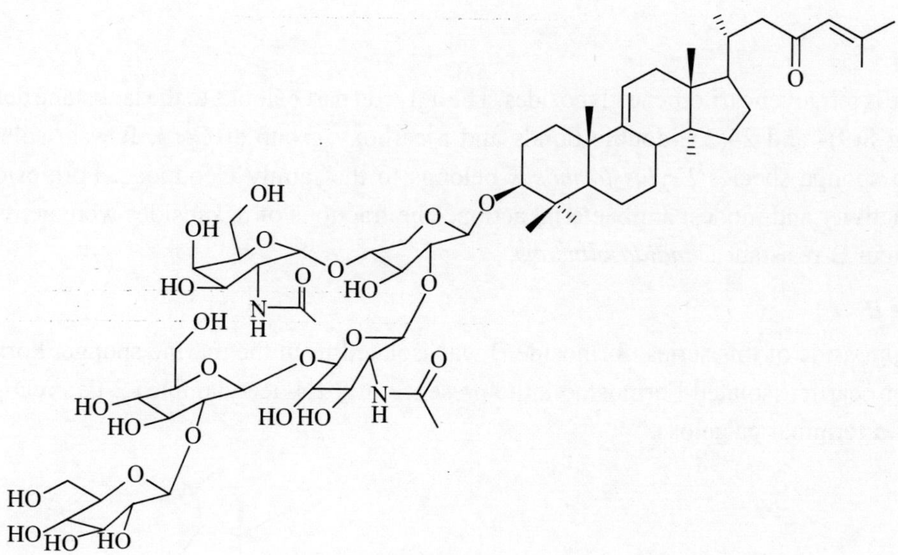

Fig. 5.49 Sarasinosides A

Pseudopterosins and Fuscosides

Pseudopterosins and fuscosides are chemically diterpene glycosides. Fuscosides A, has been isolated from Caribben gorgonians. Pseudopterosins and Fuscosides exhibit extremely promising anti-inflammatory activity.

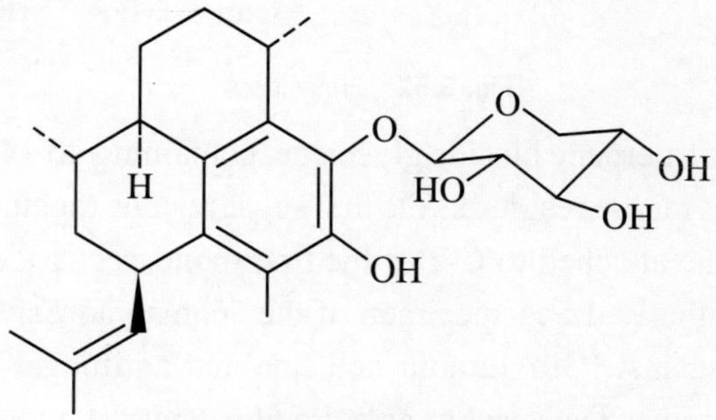

Fig. 5.50 Pseudopterosins

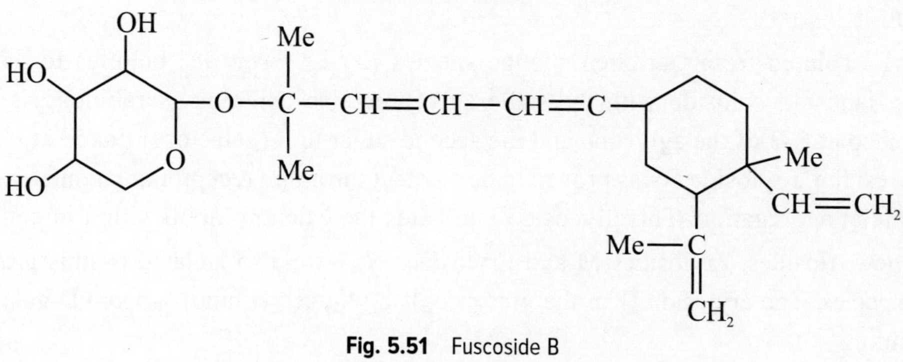

Fig. 5.51 Fuscoside B

Formoside

Formoside is tetracyclic triterpene glycosides. The aglycon part belongs to the lanostane derivatives, containing 8(9)- and 24(25)-double bonds and a carboxy group at C-14. It was isolated from Caribbean sponge species *Erylus formosus* belongs to the family Geodiidae. Formoside shows antiviral activity and modest antibacterial action. The fractions of hexaosides were active against amphotericin B-resistant *Candida albicans*.

Formoside B

Another glycoside of this series, formoside B was isolated from the marine sponge. Formoside B differs from earlier isolated Formoside inthe presence of 2-(N-acetylamino)-2-deoxyD-galactose instead of a terminal galactose.

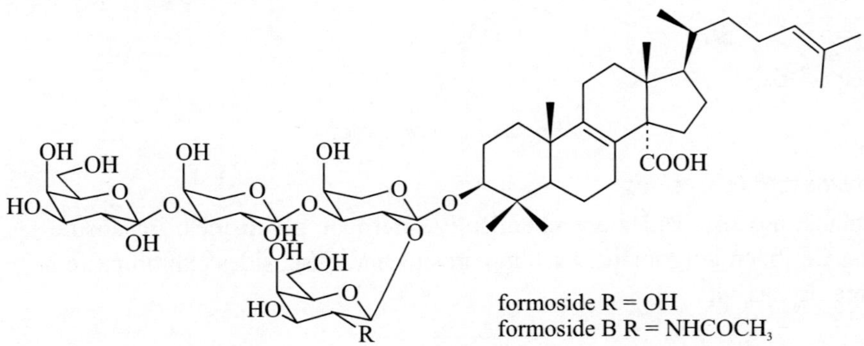

Fig. 5.52 Eryloside A

Eryloside Aisa bis-nor-triterpene bioside glycoside, containing 4ß,14-di-nor-methyl-lanostane aglycone and ß-D-galactopyranose residue as the first sugar residue together with another (terminal) ß D-galactopyranose residue attached to C-2 of the first monosaccharide residue in carbohydrate moiety, was isolated from the Red Sea specimen of the sponge, an *Erylus lendenfeldi* species. It shows cytotoxic activity against P388 tumour cell line and antifungal activity against *Candida albicans* and also active against *Escherichia coli*, *Bacillus subtilis* and *Candida albicans.*

Eryloside F

Eryloside F, isolated from Caribben sponge species *Erylus formosus*, belongs to the family Geodiidae, lanostane bioside with the same aglycone, also containing arabinose as the first sugar attached at C-3 of the aglycone and the second sugar unit (galactose) linked at C-2 of the arabinose residue. Eryloside F was proved to be a potent thrombin receptor antagonist, inhibiting human platelet aggregation. This glycoside facilitates the calcium mobilization in cells.

Two new triosides, Erylosides M and Erylosides N, were also isolated by this group from the same species. The eryloside H in the presence of 2-(N-acetylamino)-2-deoxyD-galactose on their structure.

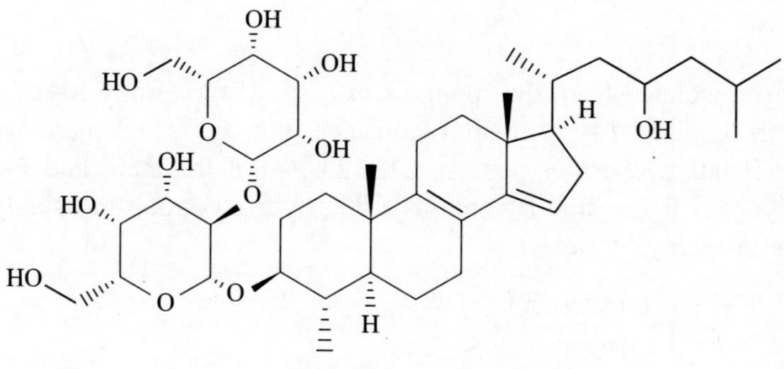

Fig. 5.53 Eryloside A

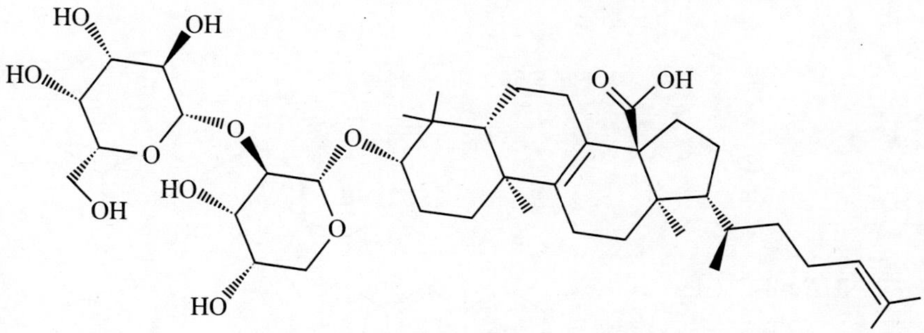

Fig. 5.54 Eryloside F

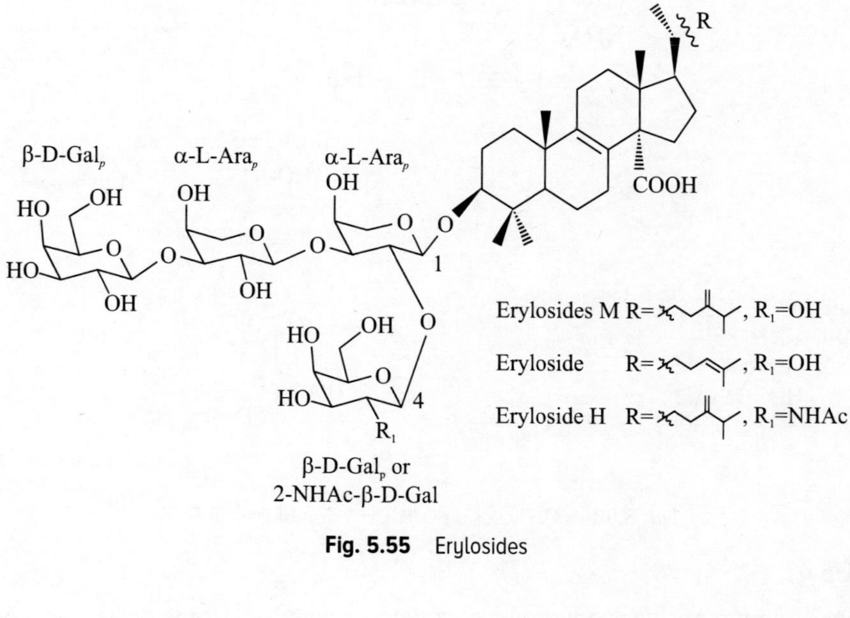

Fig. 5.55 Erylosides

Ulososides

Ulososides have been isolated from the sponge *Ulosa* sp. of the family Mycalidae. It is total of five glycosides with oxidized 14-nor-methyl-lanostane type aglycones, namely, ulososides A-E. except Ulososides B, all Ulososides possess 22S, 23 R-diol fragment and 24S-methyl in side chains of their aglycones. Ulososide B contains a 23ξ-hydroxy group in its aglycone side chain, but not containing 24-methyl group.

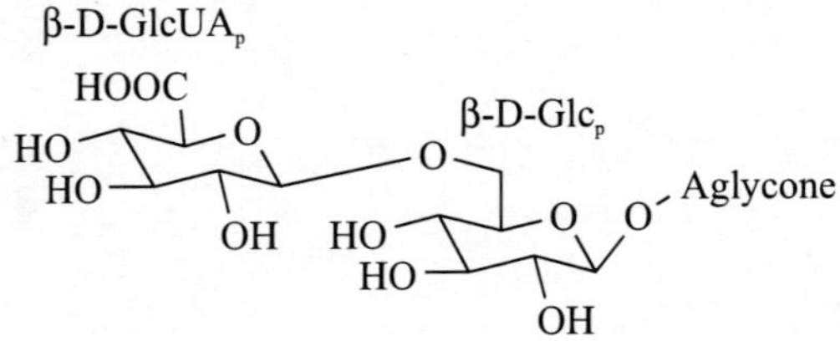

Fig. 5.56 Ulososides A

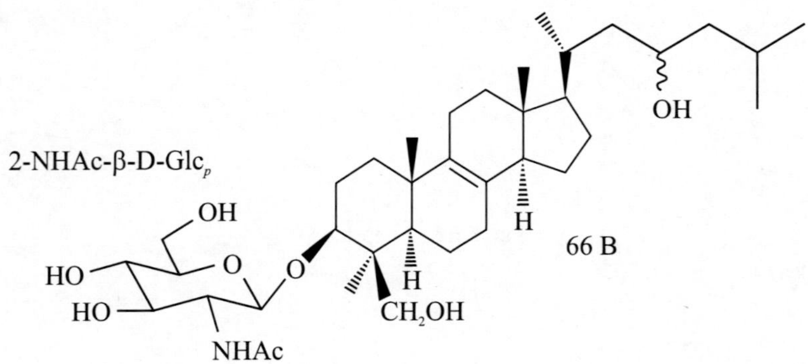

Fig. 5.57 Ulososide B

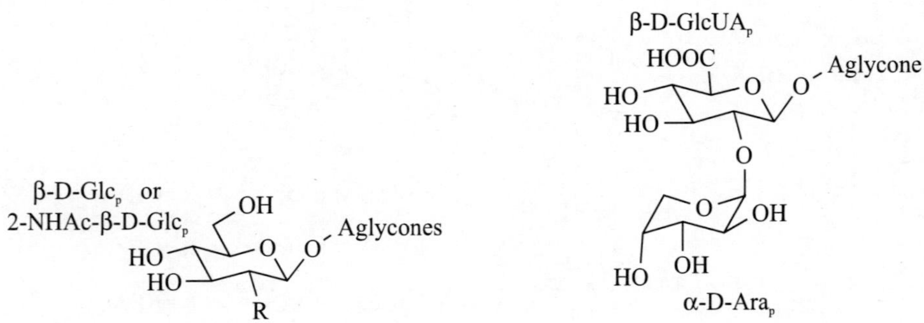

(A) (B)

Fig. 5.58 (A): Ulososide C (R=OH) (B): Ulososide E

Rhabdastoside A

It is triterpene xylopyranoside, containing a skeleton related to isomalabaricanes system, was isolated along with several new isomalabaricane derivatives from the methanol extract of the sponge *Rhabdastrella globostellata* belongs to the family Ancorinidae. It may demonstrate potent antiproliferative properties and promotion of DNA polymerase β binding to DNA.

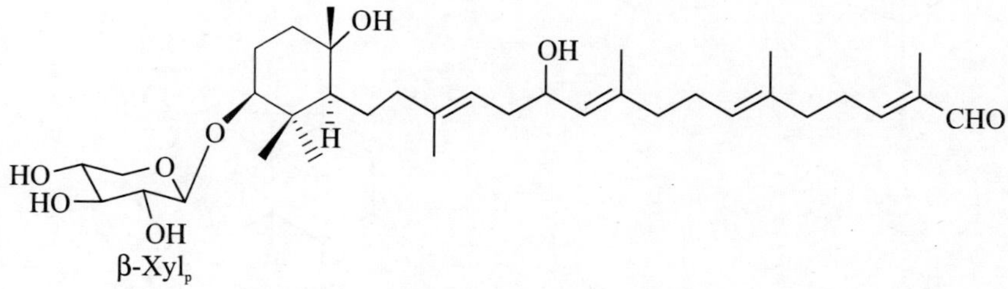

Fig. 5.59 Rhabdastoside A

Xestovanin A and Secoxestovanin A

Two triterpene glycosides, xestovanin A and secoxestovanin A with new skeleton systems were found in Xestospongia. *Vanilla*. Aglycone moiety in xestovanin A is formed by unusual 11, 15- and 9, 17-squalene cyclizations. Both xestovanin A and secoxestovanin A belong to triterpene biosides and contain carbohydrate chains with 1,2-bonded D-fucose and L-rhamnose.

Xestovanin A shows antifungal activity against *Phytium ultimum*.

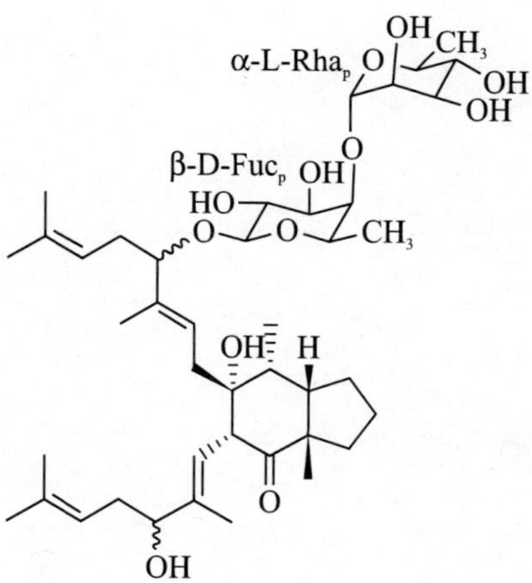

Fig. 5.60 Xestovanin A

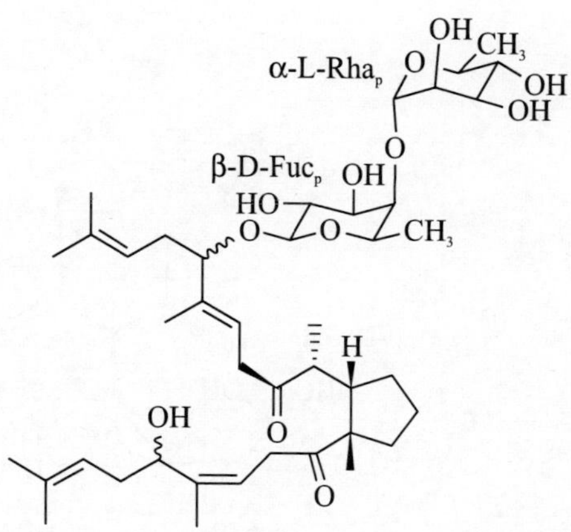

Fig. 5.61 Secoxestovanin A

5.4.5 Marine Derived Terpenoids and Steroids

Astrogorgiadiol and Astrogorgin

Astrogorgiadiol, chemically a 9,10-secosterol and astrogorgin, a new eunicellin based diterpenoid, were isolated from the gorgonian *Astrogorgia* sp., both the compounds were found to display activity to inhibit cell division of the fertilized eggs.

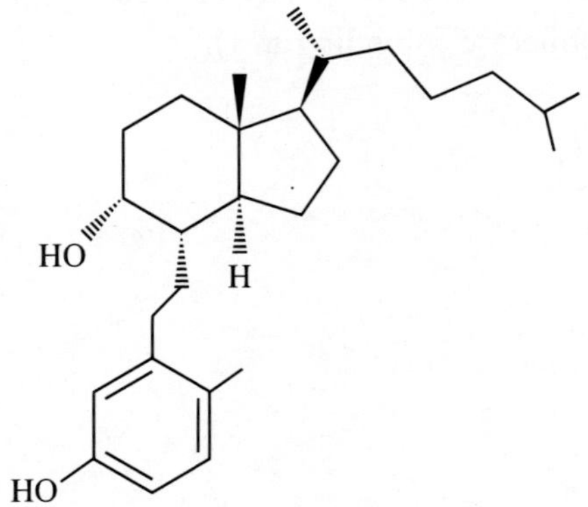

Fig. 5.62 Astrogorgiadiol

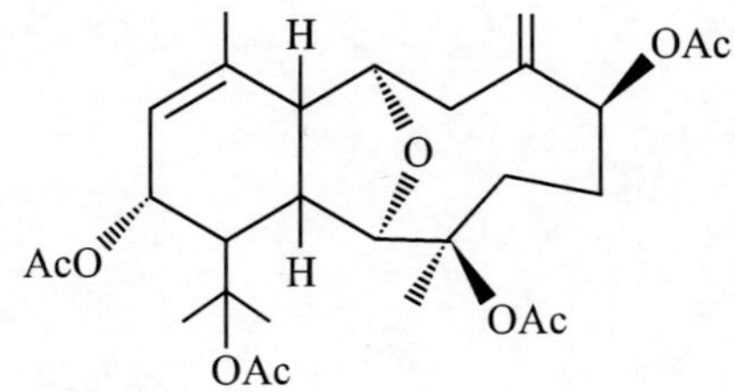

Fig. 5.63 Astrogorgin

Pachastrelloside A

It is a steroidal bioside obtained from the marine sponge *Pachastrella* sp. *Bebryce grandicalyx* belongs to the family of Pachastrellidae. Pachastrelloside A has the sterol aglycone, oxidized in the rings A and B, with two monosaccharide residues like D-galactopyranosyl and 4-*O*-acetyl-β-D-xylopyranosyl which are linked to C-4 and C-8 of its aglycone which induces the formation of multinucleated, unicellular embryos at the action on fertilized eggs of sea urchins.

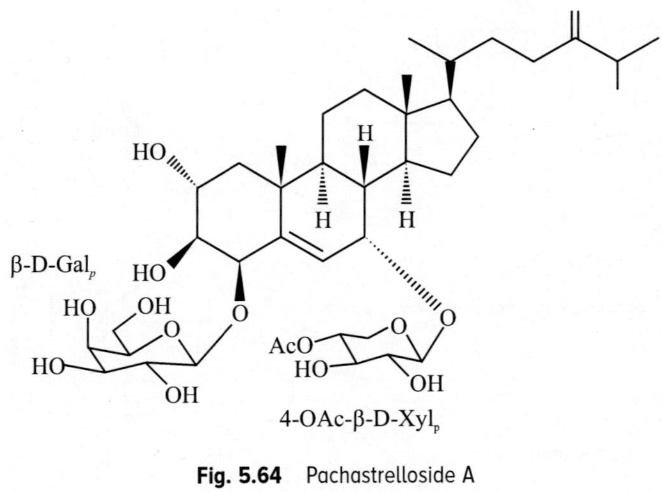

Fig. 5.64 Pachastrelloside A

Acanthifolioside

It is a group of steroid glycosides from the same sponge were, Acanthifoliosides A-F. Acanthifoliosides are structurally related to pandarosides steroid saponins, Acanthifoliosides A-C were proved to be mono-β-D-xylopyranosides, acanthifoliosides D and E are mono-α-L-rhamnopyranosides, while acanthifolioside F contains a branched trioside carbohydrate chain. Acanthiofoliosides exhibit moderate antiprotozoal activities.

Euplexides A

Euplexides are farnesyl hydroquinone glycosides, of moritoside class. Euplexides A has been isolated from the gorgonian *Euplexaura anastomosans*. The compound exhibited moderate cytotoxicity and antioxidizing activity as well as inhibitory activity against PLA2.

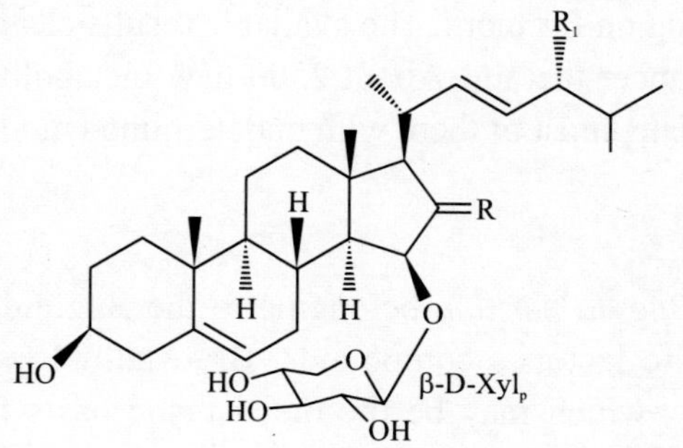

Fig. 5.65 Acanthifolioside A, R=O, R_1 = CH_3
Acanthifolioside B, R=β–OH, R_1 = CH_3

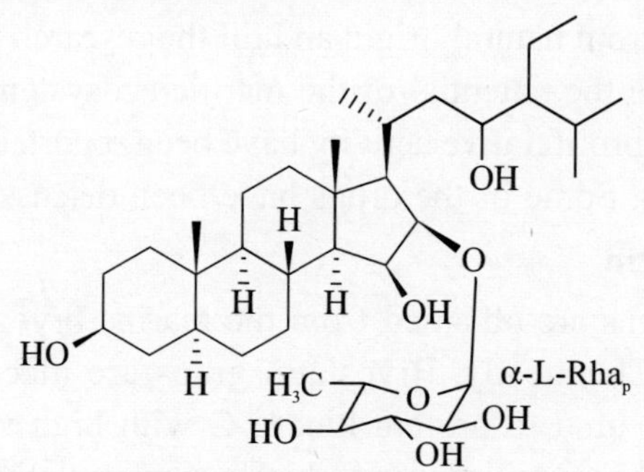

Fig. 5.66 Acanthifolioside D

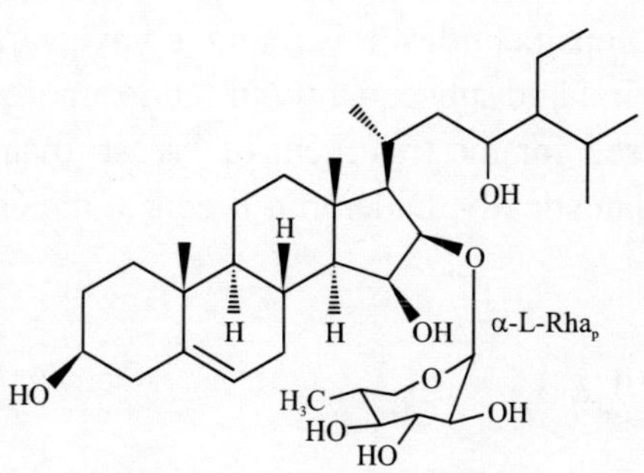

Fig. 5.67 Acanthifolioside E

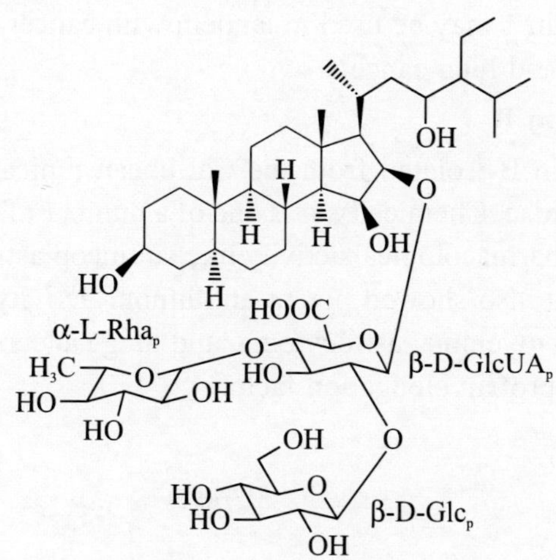

Fig. 5.68 Acanthifolioside F

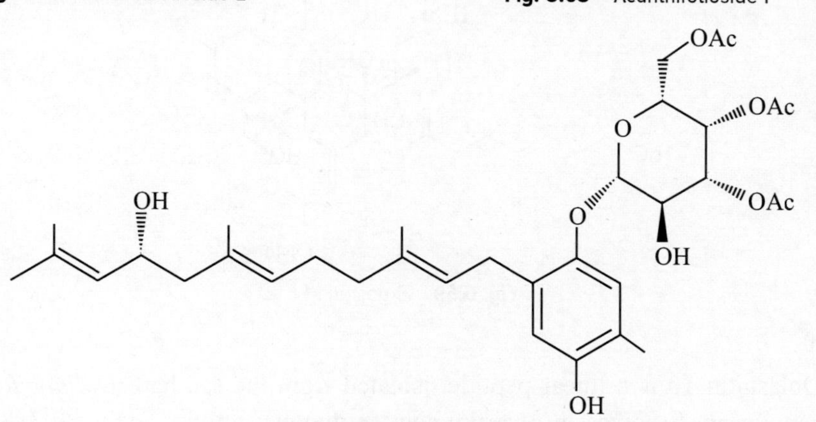

Fig. 5.67(i) Euplexides A

5.4.6 Based on Pharmacological Use

5.4.6.1 Marine Derived Anticancer Drugs

In cancer treatment, the lion share of anticancer drugs, almost 60% commercial drugs have been derived from natural origin and till the research is going on for more. The available results clearly anticipate the potential of the marine ecosystem in cancer therapy. About 2500 new metabolites with antiproliferative activity have been reported till date, most of them with undetermined modes of action. Some of the drugs have been discussed.

Bryostatin

Bryostatins are obtained from the marine bryozoan *Bugula neritina* belonging to the Bugulidae family. Chemically, Bryostatin grups are macrocyclic lactones compounds. Bryostatin 1 was found to bind to protein kinase C with high affinity, which may be the mechanistic basis for both observed anticancer and immunostimulating activities. It is not effective in cancer treatment by itself but it believes to enhance the activity of such chemotherapies as taxol and cisplatin. Bryostatin 1 may be used in tandem with cancer treatments that respond to taxol, such as breast, ovarian and lung cancers.

Didemnin B

Didemnin B isolated from the Caribbean tunicate *Trididemnum solidum* belongs to the family Didemnidae. Chemically, it is one of a number of related depsipeptides. It is found to have various potent pharmacological activity like; antineoplastic, antiviral and subsequently immunosuppresive action. It also showed potent antitumour activity and used for the treatment of breast, ovarian, cervical, myeloma, astrocytoma, and lung cancers. Mechanistically, Didemnin B acts at the GTP-binding protein elongation factor.

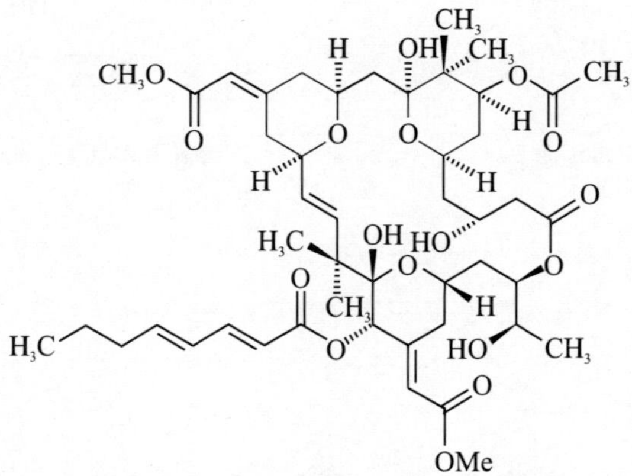

Fig. 5.69 Bryostatin 1

Dolastatin 10

Chemically Dolastatin 10 is a linear peptide, isolated from the sea hare *Dollabella auricularia* from the Indian Ocean. It possesses a very potent antitumour activity against P 388 cells. It can be use in the treatment of breast and liver cancers, solid tumours and leukaemia.

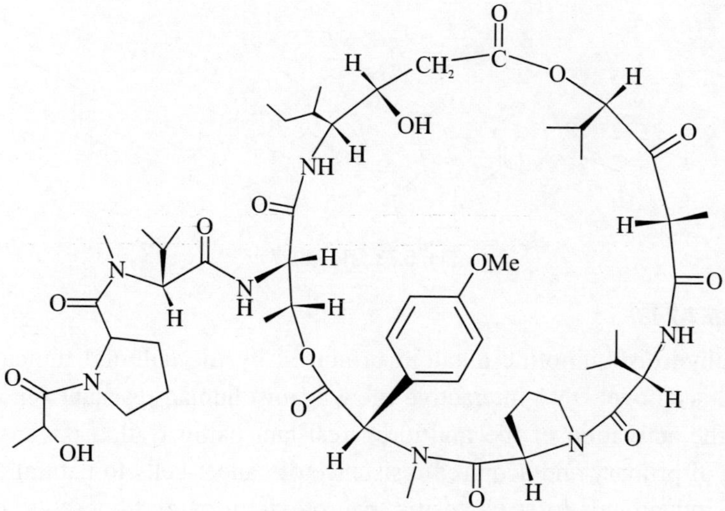

Fig. 5.70 Didemnin B

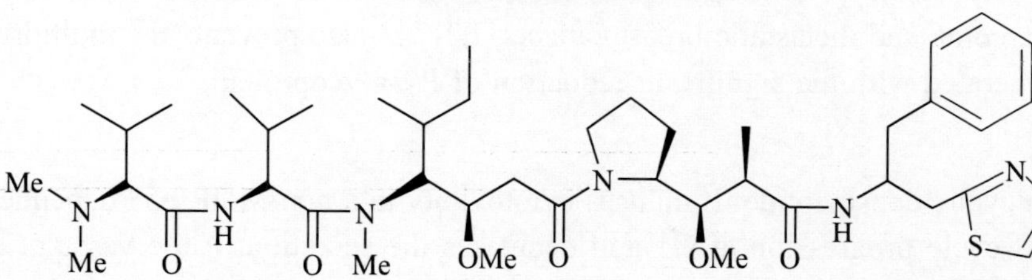

Fig. 5.71 Dolastatin 10

Dolastatin 15

Dolastatin 15, another cyanobacterial peptide isolated from a sea hare *Dolabella auricularia* in trace amounts also possesses a potent anticancer properties.

TZT-1027 (Soblidotin)

TZT-1027 is a newly synthesized dolastatin 10 derivative. Its structure differs from dolastin 10 only in the absence of the thiazole ring from the original dolaphenine residue, resulting in a terminal benzylamine moiety. TZT-1027 has a potent antitumour activity which inhibits microtubule polymerization and perturbs microtubule dynamics and also inhibits the growth of various human cancer cells.

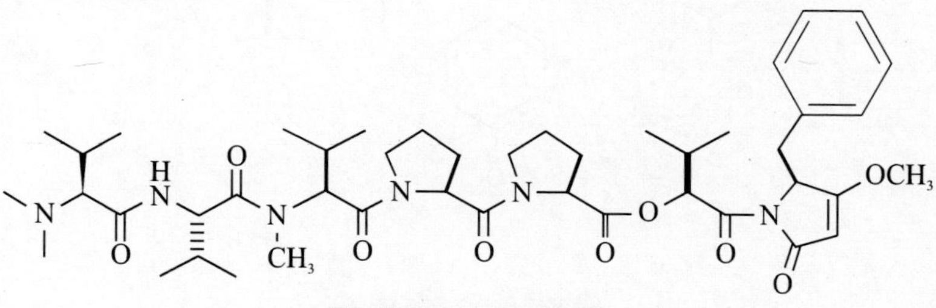

Fig. 5.72 Dolastatin 15

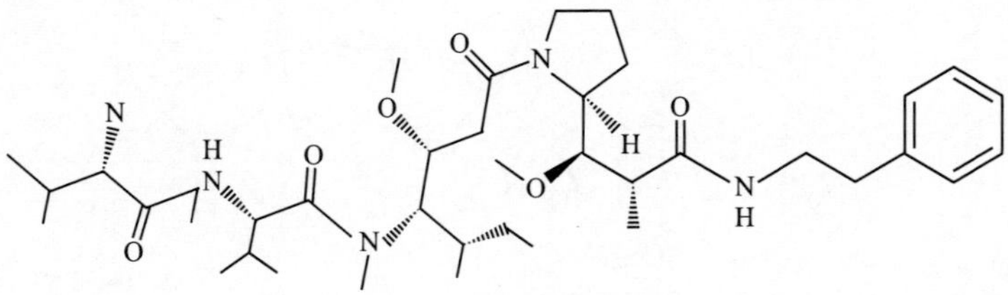

Fig. 5.73 TZT-1027

Ecteinascidin-743(ET-743)

ET-743 is a tetrahydroisoquinoline alkaloid produced by the colonial tunicate *Ecteinascidia turbinate*. ET-743 is a novel DNA interactive agent against human-resistant xenografted tumours. ET-743 inhibits the activation of the multidrug resistant pathway that is considered to be the main mechanism of primary and acquired resistance of cancer cells to natural anticancer drugs. ET-743 does not induce hair loss, mucositis, neurotoxicity or diarrhoea like other anti-cancer drugs. It has been found promising activity in the treatment of advanced soft tissue sarcoma (STS), osteosarcoma and metastatic breast cancers. ET-743 also prevents the multidrug resistant tumours incorperated with the significant reduction of P- \glycoprotein.

AplidinR (APL)

Aplidin R is a cyclic depsipeptide. It induces cytotoxicity in a non-MDR/p53 dependent manner, blocks the cell cycle progression at G1 and decreases the secretion of the vascular endothelial growth factor (VEGF) and the expression of the VEGF-r1 receptor. It has a positive therapeutic index in patients harbouring pretreated solid tumours and lymphoma. Apladin was more selective towards leukaemia and lymphoma cells than towards normal cells, thus it selectively targets and preferentially kills human leukemic cells.

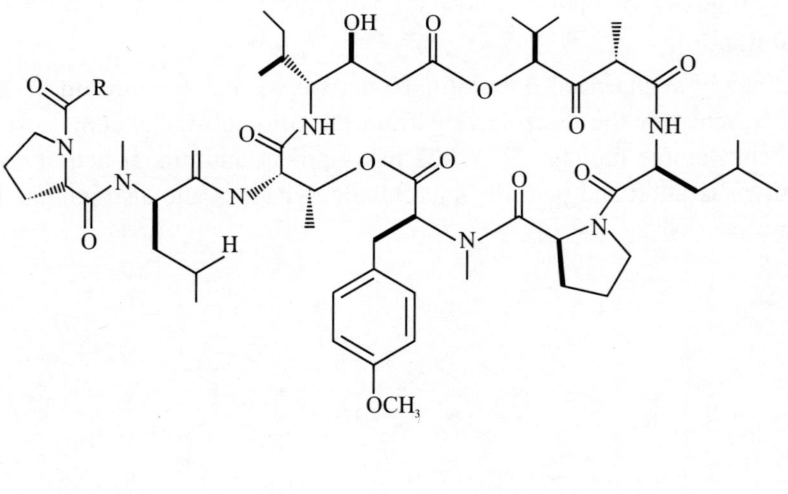

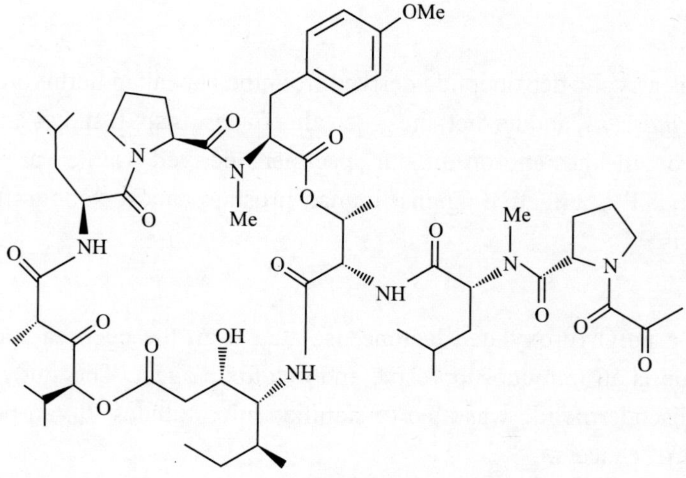

Aplidin

Fig. 5.74 Didemnin B

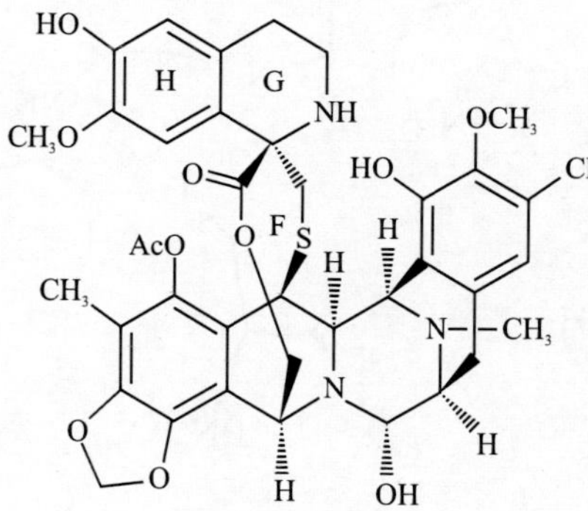

Fig. 5.75 Ecteinascidin-743

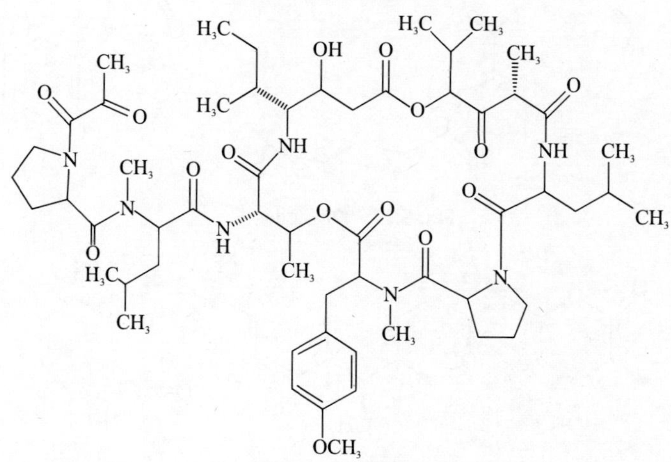

Fig. 5.76 Aplidin R (APL)

Kahalalide F (KF)

Kahalalide F (KF) is a cyclic depsipeptide derived from the Hawaiian herbivorous marine species of *Mollusc, Elysia rufescens*, and its diet, the green alga *Bryopsis* sp. It shows antitumour activities both on transformed cell lines and on tumour specimens derived from a variety of solid human tumours. Moreover, KF is effective against human prostate cancer xenografts, and in patients with severe psoriasis.

Discodermolide

Discodermolide is a polyhydroxylated lactone, isolated from the deepsea sponge *Discodermia* ssp. Descodermolide is an immunosuppresive and cytotoxic agent. The study of its mechanism has revealed that discodermolide was able to stabilize microtubules. It can be used as a potent agent for treatment of cancers.

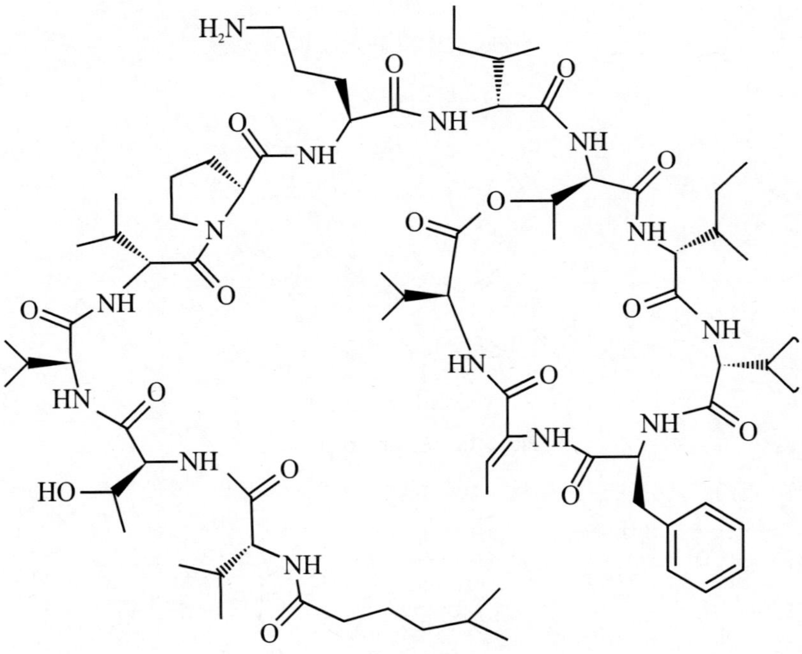

Fig. 5.77 Kahalalide F

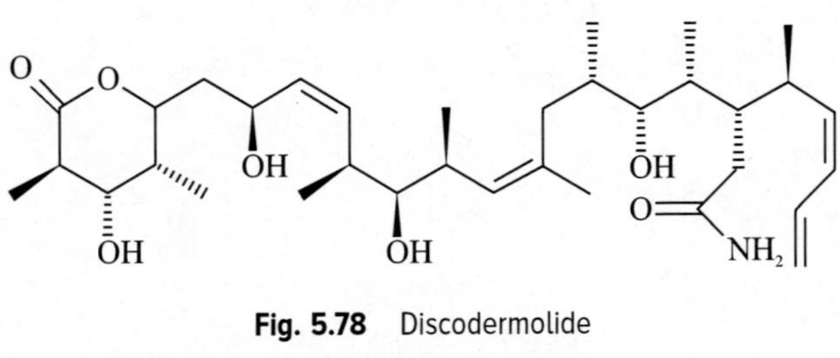

Fig. 5.78 Discodermolide

5.4.6.2 Marine Derived Analgesic and Anti-Inflammatory Drugs

More than 300 species of cone snails residing in marine environment, act as a good source of analgesic compounds. The snail's gland biosynthesizes hundreds of different peptide toxins. They have the action to immobilize a victim by affecting the neuromuscular transmission in its organism.

Manoalide

Manoalide is a sesquiterpenoid isolated from the sponge *Luffariella variabilis*. It is a potent analgesic and anti-inflammatory agent. Manoalide is by far the best characterised PLA_2 inhibitor from natural sources.

Pseudopterosins

The pseudopterosins (A-D) are a group of tricyclic diterpene glycosides isolated from the Caribbean Sea whip (gorgonian) *Pseudopterogorgia elisabethae* belongs to Gorgoniidae. They are potent anti-inflammatory and analgesic agents and appear to inhibit eicosanoid biosynthesis by inhibition of both PLA2 and 5-lipoxygenase.

Ziconitide

Ziconitide is a 25 amino acid peptide. This drug is obtained from the venom of a predatory snail *Conus magnus*. It acts by binding to and inhibiting presynaptic calcium channels, thereby preventing neurotransmitter release. Ziconitide is 50 times more potent than morphine, is so exquisitely precise and does not cause the adverse effects of opiates. So it can be best used in pain management

ω-conotoxin

ω-conotoxin is a linear peptide composed of 25 amino acid residues, which was isolated from the Pacific mollusc *Conus magnus*. Six cysteine residues form three disulphide bridges exist in this compound. The disulphide bridges provide ω-conotoxin with a well-formed and unique space structure, as well as the ability to specifically block the work of N-type voltage-sensitive calcium channels.

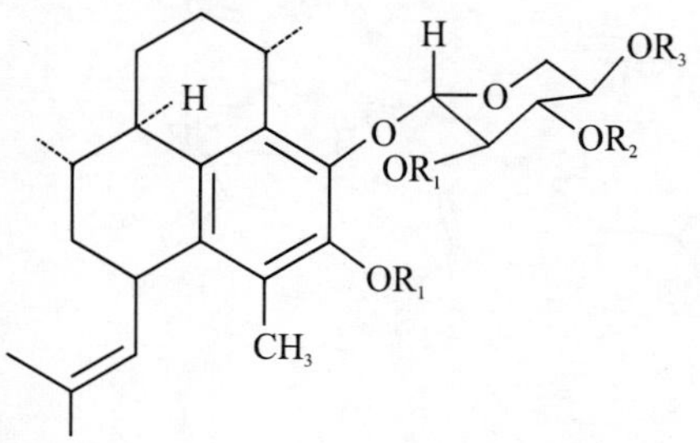

Fig. 5.79 Pseudopterosins A, R_1=R_2=R_3=R_4=H
Pseudopterosins B, R_1=Ac, R_2=R_3=R_4=H
Pseudopterosins C, R_2= Ac, R_1=R_3=R_4=H
Pseudopterosins D, R_3= Ac, R_1=R_2=R_4=H

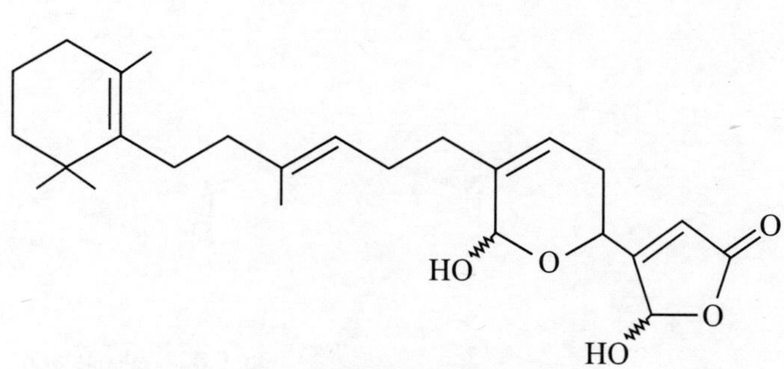

Fig. 5.80 Manoalide

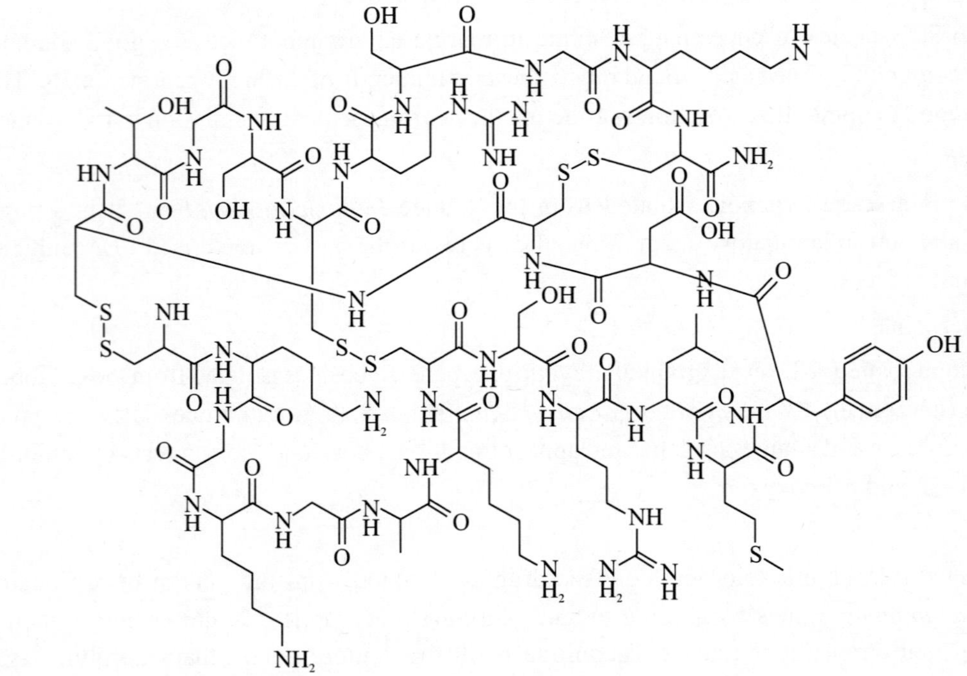

Fig. 5.81 Ziconitide

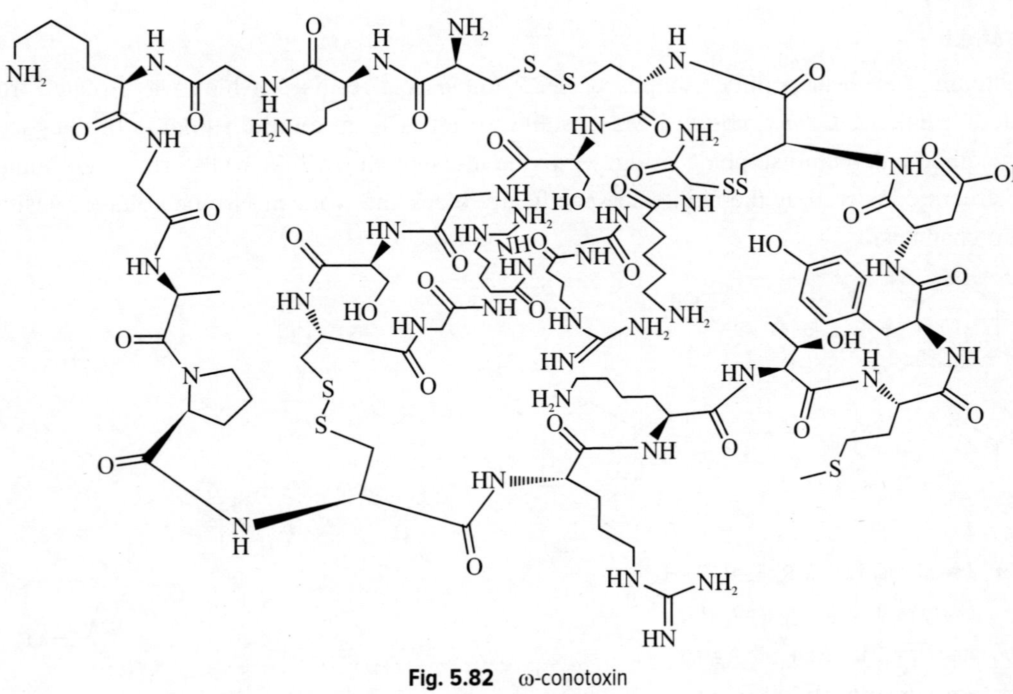

Fig. 5.82 ω-conotoxin

Contignasterol

Contignasterol is a steroid, characterized by a cis-junction of the C and D cycles, obtained from the sponges *Petrosia contignata*. It was found as an anti-inflammatory agent. In contrast to a drug with analogous action, this compound is not an inhibitor of A_2 phospholipase, but it inhibits the excretion of histamine by leukocytes and is referred to as a leukocyte-selective anti-inflammatory agent.

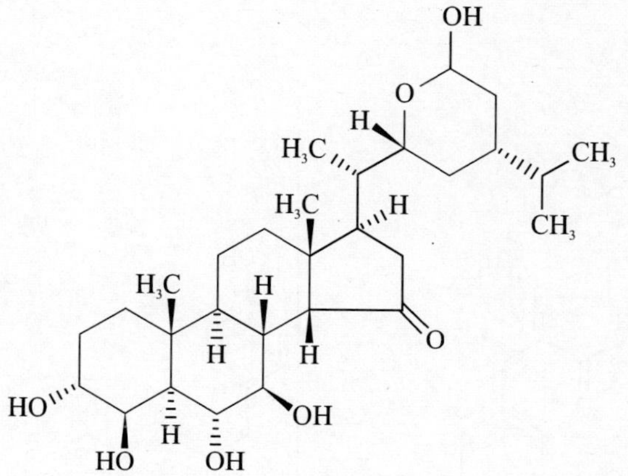

Fig. 5.83 Contignasterol

5.4.6.3 *Marine Derived Antimicrobial and Antiviral Drugs*

Mycalamide B

Mycalamide B is obtained from Mycale species of antiviral metabolite from marine sponges. Mycalamide B is a strong inhibitor of protein synthesis, which shows inhibiting activity along with less toxicity.

Pseudopteroxazol

Chemically, pseudopteroxazol is a benzoxazole diterpene alkaloid. It was isolated from the gorgonian coral *Pseudopterogorgia elisabethae*, which have a potent antimicrobial property against mycobacterium. It inhibits the growth of this mycobacterium without any toxic effects.

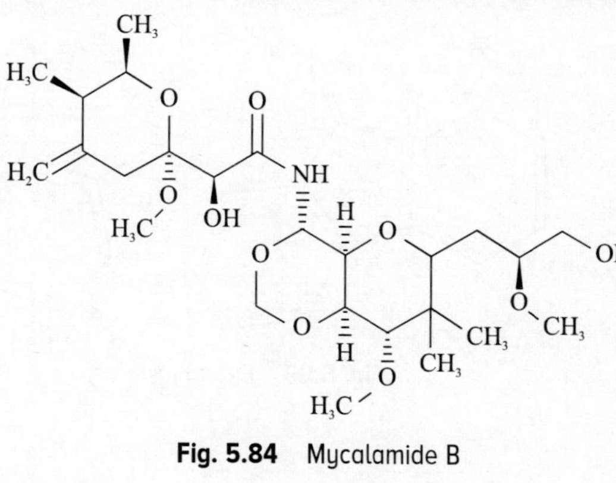

Fig. 5.84 Mycalamide B

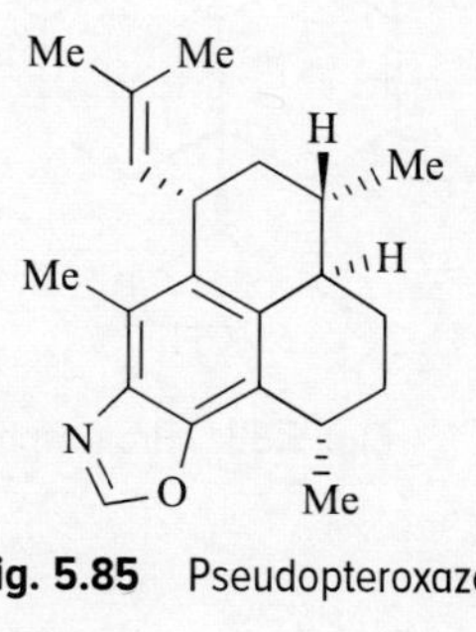

Fig. 5.85 Pseudopteroxazol

Psammaplin A

Psammaplin A is a symmetrical bromotyrosine disulphide. This drug was obtained from Psammaplysilla sp. which possesses oxime moieties, was found to have potent cytotoxicity to P388 cells. Several of these were found to possess potent antibacterial activity. Another compound also found from the same with dimeric metabolite, called biprasin, which has similar activity.

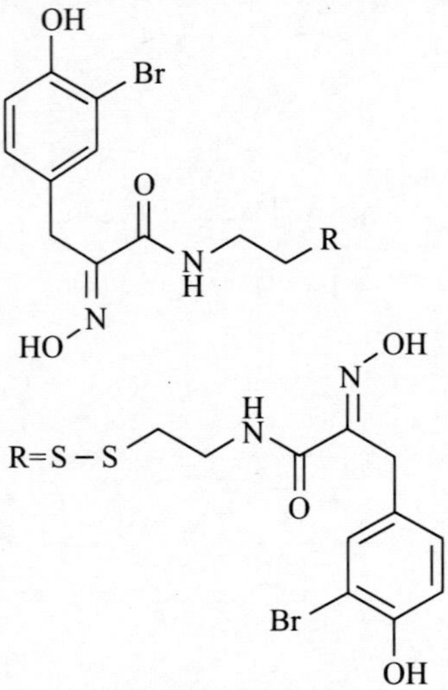

Fig. 5.86 Psammaplin A

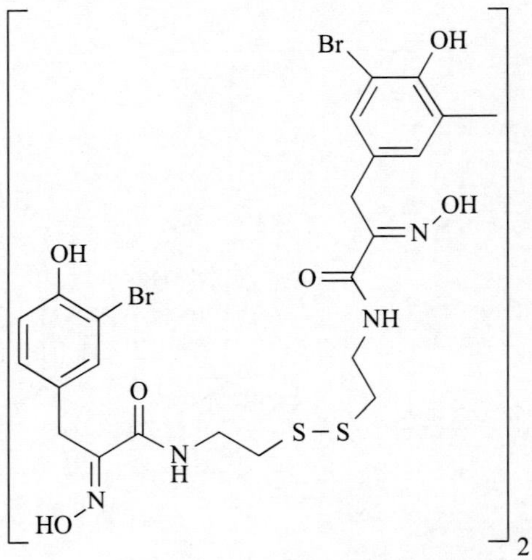

Fig. 5.87 Biprasin

Diterpenoid bromosphaerone

Diterpenoid bromosphaerone, obtained from the red alga *Sphaerococcus coronopifolius* and some other marine metabolites, are highly active against *Staphylococcus aureus*. They are fascalkaloid fascaplysin, macrolide forboxazole, etc., are characterized by strong antifungal action, have appeared too toxic for use in clinical testing.

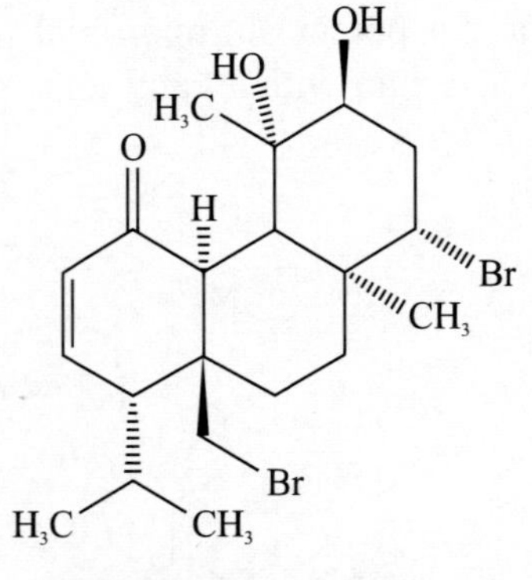

Fig. 5.88 Bromosphaeron

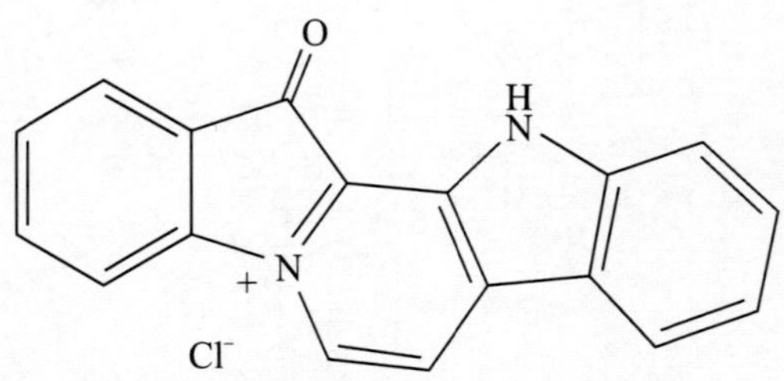

Fig. 5.89 Fascaplysin

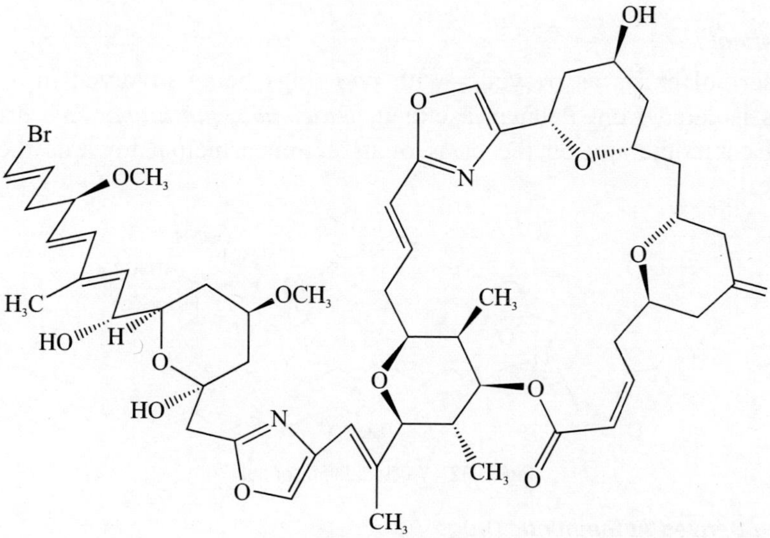

Fig. 5.90 Forboxazole A

Agelasines and Agelasimines

They are purine derivatives isolated from marine sponges of the genus agelas and show antimicrobial effect against various bacteria. More than ten agelasines are currently known, of which agelasine A-F have the highest antibacterial activity.

Agelasimines are also purine derivatives carrying a diterpenoid side chain, but they are neutral 3,7-dialkylated purines. Agelasine F having a potent antimicrobial activity against mycobacterium tuberculosis and along with Agelasine E possessed modest antimycobacterial activity.

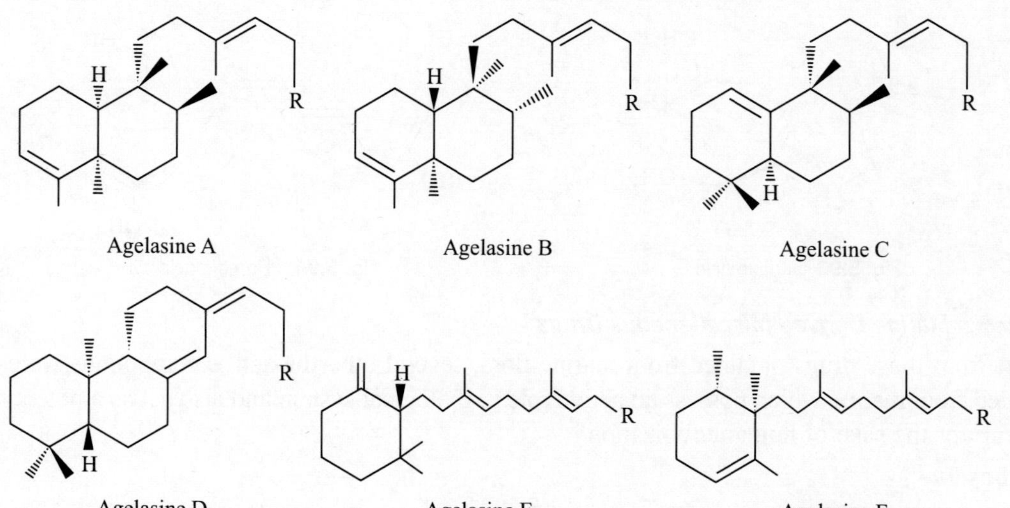

Fig. 5.91 Agelasine (A-F)

Cyclodidemniserinol

Cyclodidemniserinol exists as tricyclic, with two rings being involved in a bicyclic ketal ring system, is isolated from Palauan ascidian, *Didemnum guttatum*. This drug is used for anti- retroviral chemotherapy on the basis of its action principal towards the inhibition of HIV-1 integrase.

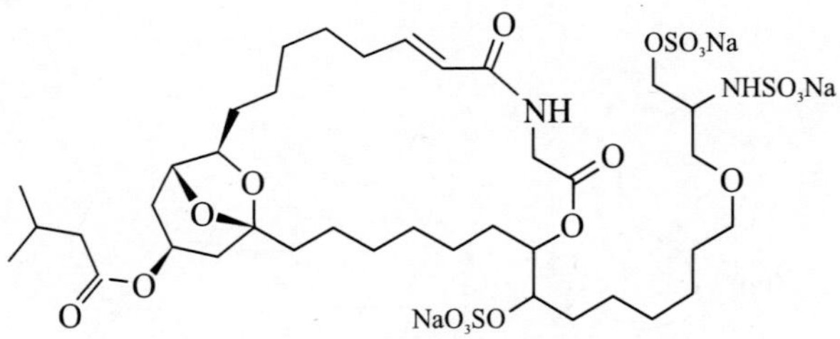

Fig. 5.92 Cyclodidemniserinol

5.4.6.4 Marine Derived Anthelmintic Drugs

Kainic and Domoic acid

Kainic acid (KA) is a marine acid obtained from seaweed. It is a specific agonist for the kainate receptor and is used as an ionotropic glutamate receptor which mimics the effect of glutamate. Kainic acid produces stimulating effect on CNS, and also acts as a neuroexcitotoxic and epileptogenic, acting through specific kainate receptors. This drug has been used for the treatment of different type of worm infections like round worm, tape worms and also ascariasis infection.

Domoic acid (DA), is a kainic acid analog. This drug is a neurotoxin that causes amnesic shellfish poisoning (ASP), obtained from the red algae *Chondria armata*. It is used in the treatment of ascariasis and pinworm infection.

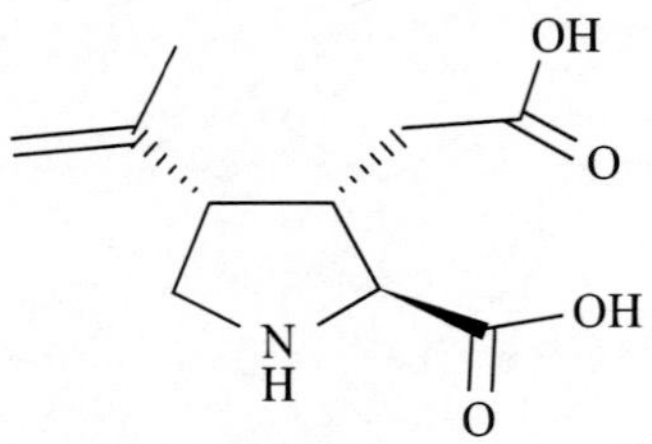

Fig. 5.93 Kainic acid

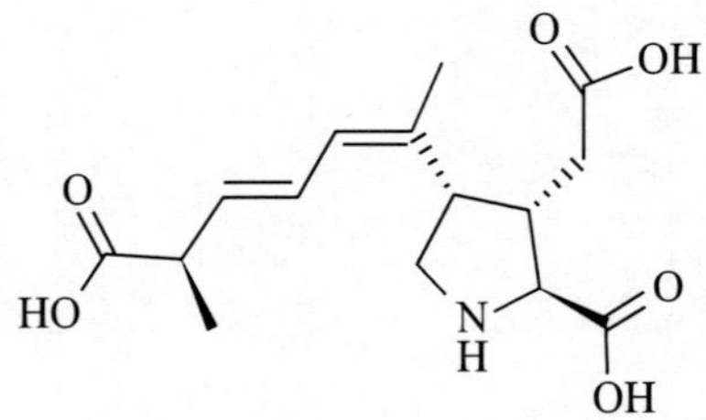

Fig. 5.94 Domoic acid

5.4.6.5 Marine Derived Miscellaneous Drugs

Apart from those drugs obtained from marine flora, several other bioactive compounds were also isolated from marine which possess an active role in biological system and also act as a potent hope of drug for the sake of human civilization.

Anabasein

Anabasein is a marine toxin was extracted from the sea worm hoplonemertea. The numerous anabasein analogues have several highly active compounds, including the pharmaceutical lead GTS-21, which has displayed cytoprotector properties and improved memory in test animals. Competing with the natural ligands, GTS-21 binds to α4β and the α7-subtypes of nicotinic receptors; the latter is considered to be important in control of β-amyloid neurotoxicity.Currently, substances of this series are being studied as potential drugs for the treatment of Alzheimer's disease.

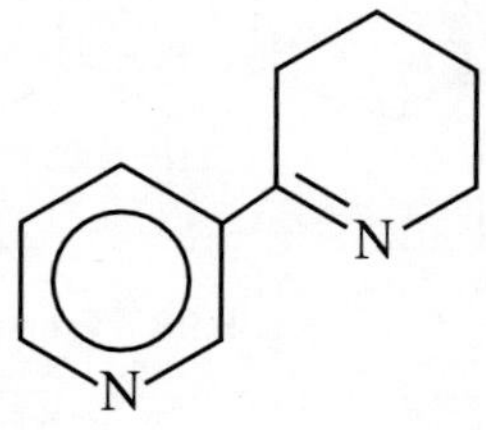

Fig. 5.95 Anabaseine

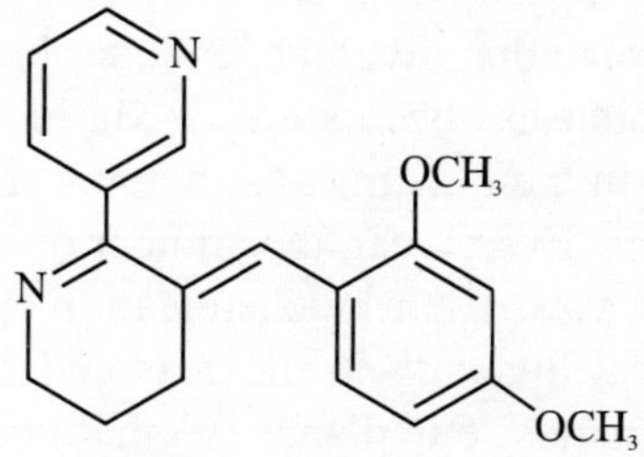

Fig. 5.96 33 GTS-21

Cumaside

The medical lead, so-called cumaside, is a monosulfated triterpene glycoside obtained from the sea cucumber *Cucumaria japonica*. Cumaside is a new immunomodulatory and cholesterol possesses significantly less cytotoxic activity against sea urchin embryos and Ehrlich carcinoma cells than the corresponding glycosides.

Echinochrome

The well-known pigment echinochrome is the major constituent of histochrome for ophthalmology and histochrome for cardiology drugs. It is an easily accessible natural source of echinochrome obtained from the sand dollar *Scaphechinus mirabilis*.

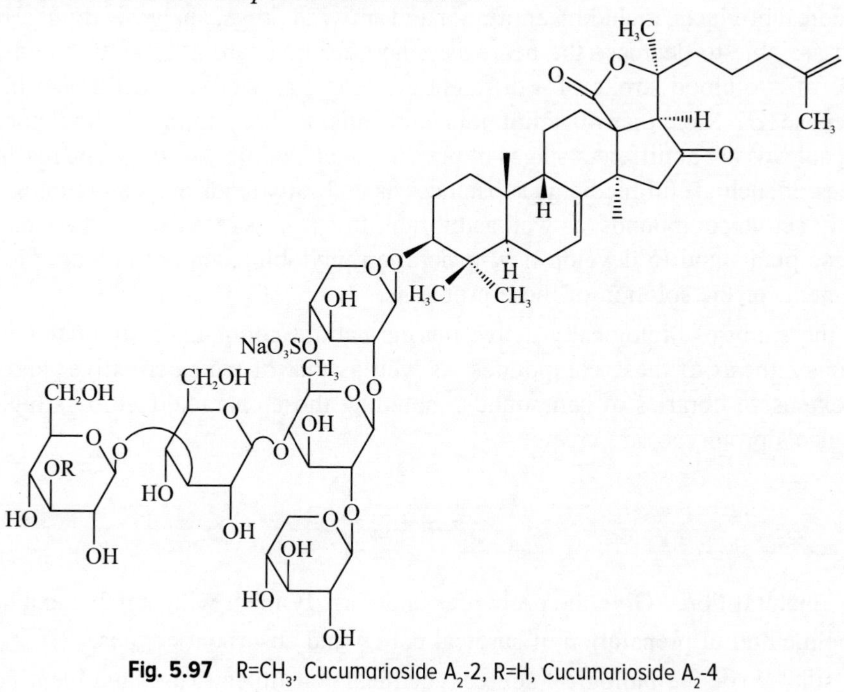

Fig. 5.97 R=CH_3, Cucumarioside A_2-2, R=H, Cucumarioside A_2-4

'Marine metagenomics', the study of marine natural products, has appeared very recently which leads to the direction of new search in marine natural products. Within the framework of this direction, not individual genomes, but a group of genomes from any habitat has been studied. Marine natural products are quite diverse in their chemical structures and also their different clinical actions. Every year, the number of known marine natural products increases. Their biochemical diversity is a result of the high biological diversity in the seas and oceans. According to different estimates, our planet is inhabited by several million species of marine microorganisms, as well as about a million of yet undescribed species of marine invertebrates and other marine organisms.

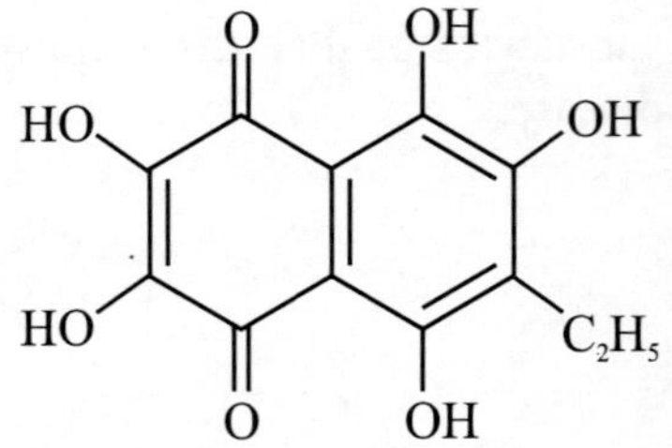

Fig. 5.98 Echinochrime A

Many marine secondary metabolites extracted from sponges, ascidians, and other marine invertebrates are biosynthesized by symbiont microorganisms. The frequently and most problematic side for the extraction of those metabolites is to only grow the microorganisms in an artificial environment and may be cultivated. An example is the extraction of the bacterium *Micromonospora* sp. from the deep-water sponge by American scientists. It produces manzamine and 8-hydroxymanzamine.These substances show very promising anti-parasitogenic and antituberculous activity, but they cannot be obtained in a large amount from the sponges. It is of interest that the biosynthesis of physiologically active alkaloids in this bacterium is possible only in a special environment, while the standard cultivation is not appropriate for their formation.

The investigation of marine natural products has led to the creation of a series of highly efficiency medical products, including antitumor and antiviral drugs, analgesic drugs, Histochrome series, which are able to decrease the necrosis zone after myocardial infarction and to treat the consequences of eye blood stroke of a different ethiology, as well as the Russian burn-treating drug, Collagenase KK. More than 40 antitumour, anti-inflammatory, immunostimulatory, and other pharmaceutical leads are at different stages of preclinical and clinical testing. The marine products are the sources of such useful medicine substances as ω-3 fatty acids and carotenoids, but, likely, of other highly active compounds, as well as biofuel. It is necessary to select the most promising strains of these plants and to develop new-generation phytobioreactors to obtain biomass in an amount sufficient for the solution of these problems.

Finally, the study of biologically active marine natural compounds stimulates work aimed at the organic synthesis of these compounds, as well as that of their derivatives and analogues. As a result, extensive libraries of compounds, including those characterized by a higher activity than a substance's prototype, are created.

EXERCISE

1. What is a natural fibre? Give the properties and classify them with suitable examples.
2. Write the method of preparation of surgical cotton and absorbent cottons.
3. What is silk? Write the biological source, chemical constituents, use, and identification tests for silk fibres.

4. What is natural hallucinogen? Write the mechanism of hallucinogens and classify them with examples.
5. What is teratogenicity? Classify teratogens with examples.
6. What is natural allergen? Describe the properties and mechanism of action of natural allergens.
7. Explain the various types of allergens with examples.
8. Write briefly about primary metabolites and their role in plant metabolism.
9. Explain the collection and preparation of agar.
10. What are proteins? Describe the structural chemistry and functions of proteins.
11. Define enzymes, their classification with examples, and their therapeutic.
12. Write a note on streptokinase and bromelin.
13. Explain the chemistry, classification, and identification tests of lipids.
14. Describe the analytical parameters of fats and oils.
15. Write a brief note on marine pharmaceuticals with their source and therapeutic actions.

Index